Psychiatrist in the Chair

Brendan Kelly is Professor of Psychiatry at Trinity College Dublin, Editor-in-Chief of the *International Journal of Law and Psychiatry* and author of *Hearing Voices: The History of Psychiatry in Ireland* (Irish Academic Press, 2016), among other papers and books. In addition to his medical degree (MB BCh BAO), he holds masters degrees in epidemiology (MSc), healthcare management (MA) and Buddhist studies (MA), and an MA (*jure officii*) from Trinity College Dublin; and doctorates in medicine (MD), history (PhD), governance (DGov) and law (PhD).

Muiris Houston is a medical writer and health strategist, a specialist in occupational medicine, Adjunct Professor of Narrative Medicine at Trinity College Dublin, and writer-in-residence at Evidence Synthesis Ireland, at the National University of Ireland, Galway. He is a columnist with the *Medical Independent* and *The Irish Times*. Muiris is a graduate of Trinity College Dublin and the University of Sydney. He is an honorary fellow of the faculty of pathology of the Royal College of Physicians in Ireland.

Psychiatrist
in the Chair

The Official Biography of
Anthony Clare

**BRENDAN KELLY &
MUIRIS HOUSTON**

MERRION
PRESS

First published in 2020 by
Merrion Press
10 George's Street
Newbridge
Co. Kildare
Ireland
www.merrionpress.ie

9781785373299 (Cloth)
9781785373305 (Kindle)
9781785373312 (Epub)

A CIP catalogue record for this book is
available from the British Library.

Typeset in Sabon LT Std 11/15 pt

Front cover image: Dr Anthony Clare, Professor of Psychiatry at Trinity
College, Dublin, *c.*1985. (Image © Morris/Hulton Archive/Getty Images)

Back cover image: Portrait of Anthony Clare, July 1989.
(Image © Richard Farley/Radio Times/Getty Images)

Contents

• •

'There's a divinity that shapes our ends,
Rough-hew them how we will.'

Hamlet, Act V, scene ii
William Shakespeare

Introduction:
Who Was Anthony Clare?

●●●●●●●●●●●●●●●●●●●●●●●●●●●●●●●●●●●●●●

In August 1996, BBC Radio 4 broadcast an interview with Uri Geller, the Israeli magician, psychic and spoon-bending illusionist. Geller had done thousands of interviews prior to this one and would go on to do thousands more. But this interview was different. This time, Geller was interviewed by Irish psychiatrist Anthony Clare (1942–2007), a generous, perceptive interlocuter with an extraordinary gift for communication, exceptionally well versed in human psychology and the wiles of human behaviour. This was no ordinary encounter.

The interview was lively and fantastical as Geller recounted tales of his extraordinary childhood and dramatic life as a spy, along with his abilities to stop clocks, bend spoons and read other people's minds. When the interview was later published, Clare reflected that he did not know what to believe, as the encounter was filled with so many colourful stories and fantastic descriptions of dramatic events that they made Geller's ability to bend spoons fade to the relative insignificance of a party trick.[1]

On the air, Geller used his apparently psychic powers to bend the car key of the programme's producer, Michael Ember, who had to take the train home. Clare was curious and perplexed in equal measure. Geller was just as mystified as Clare:

CLARE: And what is your explanation? Do you know how it's done? If it's not magic, how is it done?
GELLER: I have no explanation.[2]

This was gripping radio: elegant, erudite, entertaining. It helped that Clare was clearly impressed by Geller and that Geller could bend keys with his mind. But the real magic came from Clare's openness to Geller's performance and persona, Clare's willingness to express his bafflement at what he saw, and Clare's endless curiosity about people – not only about people who could bend spoons with their minds, but about everyone whom Clare encountered in his media and medical careers.

In 2018, more than two decades after the Geller interview, and a decade after Clare's untimely death, it is Geller who is lost in admiration, still deeply moved by his 'subliminal connection' with Clare: 'Clare was a great guy, a very elegant interviewer … It was one of the best interviews I've ever had, no doubt. Clare's questions penetrated my life, my psyche, and my psychological make-up. He was bang-on.'[3] Magic indeed.

In truth, Clare's remarkable connections with his radio guests were rooted in humanity and genuine engagement rather than magic, mysticism or psychic communication. Between 1982 and 2001, Clare interviewed hundreds of well-known figures for *In the Psychiatrist's Chair*, ranging from Stephen Fry to Spike Milligan, Maya Angelou to Anthony Hopkins, Barbara Cartland to Arthur Ashe.[4] Clare's gentle, robust, probing style changed the nature of broadcast interviews forever.

In the Psychiatrist's Chair was both critically acclaimed and popular with the radio-listening public, which helped attract more guests. The British Conservative politician Nigel Lawson agreed to an interview with Clare in 1988 solely 'because I had enjoyed his previous programmes', even though Lawson considers himself 'a very private person'.[5] Somehow, Clare created a space where even the introverted were willing to speak about their personal lives to an audience of millions on national radio. How he did so is one of the questions at the heart of this book.

Always the psychiatrist, Clare left indelible impressions on those he met. He interviewed businesswoman Nicola Horlick for the programme in 1998 when her daughter, Georgie, was critically ill with leukaemia. Horlick found the experience 'incredibly beneficial':

It wasn't just a radio programme, it became an actual therapy session. The interview was meant to take around an hour, but we actually spoke for over two hours … Anthony could feel the pain that I was suffering and was extremely kind to me. After Georgie died, he wrote me a lovely letter saying that he felt he knew her, even though he had never met her, and how tragic her death at the age of 12 was.

I thought he was a wonderful man. The two hours that I spent with him helped me to cope with the immense difficulties that I was facing at that time in my life and I was very grateful. It wasn't just that he was a psychiatrist, he was also a father and he felt a deep empathy for me as I watched my darling daughter battling for life.[6]

Clare's psychological astuteness and deft verbal skills allowed him to ask questions that few others dared to ask. Interviewing Conservative politician Ann Widdecombe in 1997, Clare established a rapport so effective that it seemed entirely natural for him to ask if Widdecombe believed she was ugly (Widdecombe: 'Whether I believe it or not I'd say, so what, so what?'),[7] if Widdecombe felt she would have made a 'good mother' ('What a very good question, I don't know the answer to it'),[8] and what, precisely, was the balance of logic and faith that underpinned her well-known religious beliefs? Widdecombe responded with characteristic assurance and even sought to turn the tables on Clare: 'Is your life sort of completely anchorless?', she asked him.[9] 'No, no. Don't do that to me!', Clare responded, with impeccable *faux* alarm. It was wonderful radio.

In addition to interviewing and commenting in the media, Clare was a qualified doctor, the best-known psychiatrist of his generation, an accomplished researcher in psychological medicine, a son, a brother, a husband, a father and a public intellectual who combined knowledge and experience in a way that was humble and assertive, expert and inquisitive, and – above all else – imbued with deep compassion, a genuine interest in others, and – when needed – a dispassionate sense of enquiry.

Born in Dublin in 1942, Clare studied medicine at University College Dublin (UCD) and won the highly prestigious *Observer* Mace

Trophy for debating in 1964, along with Patrick Cosgrave (future adviser to Margaret Thatcher). Clare graduated as a medical doctor in 1966 and trained in psychiatry at St Patrick's Hospital, Dublin for over two years, followed by five years further training at the famous Maudsley and Bethlem Royal Hospital in London. His first scientific publication appeared in the *British Medical Journal* in 1971[10] and many more were to follow, accompanied by multiple books, hundreds of broadcasts and (literally) countless newspaper articles.

In 1976, just ten years after graduating, Clare published an extraordinary, career-making book titled *Psychiatry in Dissent: Controversial Issues in Thought and Practice*.[11] Originally conceived as part of a textbook, Clare's lucid, incisive and endlessly compassionate text become an instant classic of twentieth-century psychiatry.[12] In it, Clare explored the concept of psychiatric diagnosis with unprecedented clear-sightedness, provided insightful discussions on schizophrenia, electroconvulsive therapy (ECT) and psychosurgery, and argued that it was unhelpful to conceptualise normality and madness as dichotomous, and better to see them as points on a continuum. More than four decades later, in a notoriously fickle field, all of these ideas have stood the test of time.

Most of all, Clare's 1976 book provided psychiatry with a clear, logical and persuasive response to its critics who were so vocal and ubiquitous during the 1960s and 1970s. Several decades later, *Psychiatry in Dissent* is still routinely cited as one of the most influential texts in twentieth-century psychiatry and beyond. Clare legitimised psychiatry not only in the eyes of the public but in the eyes of psychiatrists too.

In 1983, Clare was appointed Professor and Head of Psychological Medicine at St Bartholomew's Hospital, London (Bart's) where he continued to write, co-write and edit publications on psychiatric themes. His engagement with popular media deepened and he became a regular contributor to BBC Radio 4's *Stop the Week* programme. This led in turn to his best-known media work, *In the Psychiatrist's Chair*. But Clare was also involved in a range of other radio and television programmes, writing for a wide variety of publications, and speaking at countless meetings and events. A witty, generous and engaging orator, there were infinite demands on his time.

In 1989, Clare returned to Dublin to become Medical Director of St Patrick's Hospital and Clinical Professor at the Department of Psychiatry in Trinity College, Dublin. His many charitable activities included serving as chairperson of the Prince of Wales's Advisory Group on Disability from 1991 to 1997. In his personal life, Clare was a family man and enjoyed tennis, opera and cinema. Clare was due to retire in December 2007 but died suddenly in Paris that October, leaving both an unfillable gap and an extraordinary legacy in his wake.

This book, the first biography of this much-loved figure, examines the man behind these achievements: the debater and the doctor, the writer and the broadcaster, the public figure and the family man. The story starts with Clare's background and education in Dublin (1942–66; Chapter 1), his training as a psychiatrist (1966–76; Chapter 2) and the writing of his iconic book, *Psychiatry in Dissent* (1976; Chapter 3). Chapter 4 looks at Clare's career in London as a doctor, psychiatrist and scientist (1976–89) and Chapter 5 explores Clare the broadcaster, with particular focus on *In the Psychiatrist's Chair* (1982–2001), his most iconic co-creation. Chapters 6 and 7 examine Clare's return to Ireland in 1989 and the years leading up to his death in 2007, and Chapter 8 explores Clare's legacy.

While it is still too soon to engage in a truly critical examination of Clare's contributions to his chosen fields, this book describes Clare's professional life and his many achievements, places these in the contexts of his personal life and, especially, his broader professional worlds, and provides a portrait of the career of this remarkable man who was commonly hailed as the most multi-talented, brilliant psychiatrist of his generation.[13]

A Note on Language

Throughout this book, original language and terminology from the past and from various archives and reports have been maintained, except where explicitly indicated otherwise. This reflects an attempt to optimise fidelity to historical sources and does not reflect an endorsement of the broader use of such terminology in contemporary settings.

I

Background and Education
(1942–66)

· ·

'My earliest memory of Tony Clare is of a 6-year-old boy in an orange overcoat and wellingtons sitting on the floor of a Number 13 bus, laughing his head off. There was rainwater on the floor and his older sister Jeanne was telling him to get up and stop being a baby.'[1] Ross Geoghegan's first memory of his friend Anthony ('Tony') Clare is vivid, warm and memorable. It evokes a happy, energetic childhood in post-war Dublin, an upbringing that provided Clare with the right balance of core values, personal discipline and human curiosity to ensure an interesting life ahead.

The year was 1949 and Clare and Jeanne were on their way to school in the Loretto Convent on St Stephen's Green in Dublin's city centre, which chiefly enrolled girls but also educated boys to the age of 8. Just two years later, Clare and Geoghegan would be inseparable classmates in Gonzaga College, a new Society of Jesus (Jesuit) school for boys in Ranelagh, south Dublin. The school was located close to both their homes (in Clare's case, just over the back wall) and its extensive grounds offered plenty of space for the new friends to get to know each other over the following summer.

Little did either boy know at the time what their futures would hold: one, Clare, was destined for a career in medicine and broadcasting in the UK and Ireland, and the other, Geoghegan, for a future as a mathematics professor in New York. For then, both boys just enjoyed the summer.

Family Background

Anthony Ward Clare was born on 24 December 1942 in Hatch Street Nursing Home ('The Hatch') at 15 Hatch Street Lower in Dublin's city centre, just around the corner from the original UCD campus in Earlsfort Terrace, where Clare would later study medicine.[2] Clare was the youngest of three children; Jeanne was almost 2 when Clare was born and Wyn was 6.

Clare's father, Ben, was a mild-mannered, popular solicitor, the youngest of a family of seven children, with three sisters and three brothers. He was educated in Belvedere College, another Jesuit school in Dublin. Three of Ben's brothers fought in the British Army and one died in service: Leo and Freddy survived the First World War; Alfred died in the Second World War.[3] Alfred helped to set up an Irish battalion in South Africa[4] and stories of his uncles' wartime exploits had a big impact on Clare as he grew up. Geoghegan remembers a 10-year-old Clare with strong pro-British views. In their games, Clare would be a high-ranking British general in battles against the 'Mau Mau' in Kenya:

> This whole thing was a secret. We were Irish boys and other boys would have ridiculed us. Indeed, I was uncomfortable with so much pro-British stuff, but I was impressed by what Tony seemed to know about places and details. I vaguely knew that Kenya was in Africa – a place for which regular collections were made outside our church, collections to help the 'black babies' and the 'foreign missions'.[5]

Clare's mother, Agnes (Aggie) Dunne was a formidable presence and an especially 'emotionally formative' influence on Clare, according to his future wife, Jane.[6] Clare recalled being 'pushed' as a child, especially by his mother,[7] who had left school aged 14 years.[8] Clare felt that his mother found it difficult to let him grow up, possibly because he was the youngest child and only son.[9] Aggie, in turn, felt that Clare married too young (at the age of 23 in 1966) but, as Clare later commented, he never knew if anything he ever did was good enough for Aggie.[10] Ruth Dudley Edwards, historian, writer and friend of Clare, recalls that 'Tony was full of doubts. He said once that if he became Pope his mother would think he hadn't gone far enough in the Church.'[11]

At the time of Clare's birth, the family lived in Tudor Road, owning a small, semi-detached house on a short, narrow road in the leafy Dublin suburb of Ranelagh. The Tudor Road house was not especially Tudor but it had a solid, reliable aspect, tucked away in one of the more desirable areas of the city. It was very close to the future Gonzaga College, which Clare attended when it opened in 1950.

Shortly after Clare's birth in Hatch Street Nursing Home, a nurse allegedly dropped him to the floor, leaving him with a scar on his left shoulder for the rest of his life. A court case followed and the nurse was disciplined. Clare was made a ward of court and stayed in the nursing home for a further six months. Clare stated that Aggie later wondered if this affected his bonding with her. It certainly heralded the start of a somewhat fraught relationship that was never entirely resolved. Jane notes that Clare 'didn't cry when his mother died and he felt bad about that'.[12]

Many years later, one of Clare's sons, Peter, recalls visiting his grandparents when he was a child:

> I remember Dad wanting us children to visit his parents with him and there being no takers. They were my grandparents and we got on well, but while Mum's parents, Sheila and Sarsfield Hogan, were close and warming, there was a sense of distance and a coldness to my Dad's parents. I would accompany Dad to his parents' house. He'd always say, 'We won't be long', to reassure me or perhaps himself.[13]

Childhood and Education

Despite the difficulties in his relationship with his mother,[14] falling into a paddling pool as a toddler (and getting fished out),[15] and being bullied on his way to piano lessons,[16] Clare's childhood in post-war

Dublin was a happy one. His daughter Rachel recalls that 'Dad grew up listening to the BBC.'[17] Little did the young Clare know that he would go on to co-create and present one of the BBC's most celebrated programmes, *In the Psychiatrist's Chair*, on BBC Radio 4 (1982–2001; Chapter 5). Rachel adds that, 'for him, it was an honour to work in the BBC and he was truly engaged in what he was doing there. He really enjoyed the communication, the engagement.' And Clare's love of radio can be traced to his earliest childhood, watching his father listen to opera on Saturday afternoons and hearing dramatic news reports from all over the world, even as a child.

Throughout these years, Clare enjoyed an especially close friendship with Ross Geoghegan – a friendship that continued through university and all of his adult life. Crucially, both boys attended Gonzaga College, founded in 1950 as a day school for boys under the direction of the Jesuits. Clare greatly enjoyed his time at Gonzaga and his school reports show a reasonable, if not spectacular, level of application to schoolwork. There was a constant refrain that he would do better if he did not talk so much and did not distract his fellow classmates – a clear indicator of the oratory and rhetoric that would come to define so much of Clare's later life. Once Clare started talking, he never stopped.

Clare excelled in English and arithmetic, but not algebra or geometry. Languages were not a strong suit either. He enjoyed sport, especially tennis which he played for most of his life,[18] and he won prizes for running. Gonzaga had not yet built up a reputation for success in rugby and, being of slight build, Clare did not enjoy the game very much.

Throughout his school years, Clare remained close to his older sister Jeanne: 'He was always there for me,' she recalls.[19] As children, Clare and Jeanne played together and cricket was a big interest for both; Jeanne remembers accompanying Clare to Gonzaga where she was included in the games. She also remembers her brother reading newspapers forensically from the age of 10, especially the rather highbrow *Observer*.

Clare and Geoghegan cemented their friendship with endless after-school discussions on the relative merits of Ireland and England, and whether the British influence in Ireland had been good or bad. 'The one good outcome of all our silly debates, spread over several years, was that we both learned to put together an articulate argument for our age level and to think fast on our feet,' Geoghegan recalls.

Clare and Geoghegan were allowed to join the Gonzaga debating society, 'An Comhdháil', when they were aged 14.[20] Clare's maiden speech concerned the Suez Crisis of 1956, when Britain tried and failed to roll back the seizure of the Suez Canal by Egypt's radical President Nasser. An otherwise dull debate was enlivened by Clare's opening sentence, as he pounded his fist on the table and declared: 'Nasser is without doubt an out-and-out scoundrel.' Clare had an intuitive awareness that catchy sound bites have the greatest impact and tend to be remembered. Discursive and argumentative by nature, he took to the recently formed debating society at once and the school quickly became known for its clutch of very able speakers, with Clare and Geoghegan to the fore.

This was all highly consistent with Gonzaga's general ethos during those early years, which had a major impact on Clare. One of the key personalities in Gonzaga at that time and one of Clare's most lasting influences was Fr Joseph (Joe) Veale, a Jesuit priest who taught English and religion to Clare and Geoghegan from 1954.

To understand Clare, it is necessary to understand Veale. He was, as Jane notes, 'a very formative influence'.[21] The son of a civil servant, Veale attended school at Synge Street in Dublin and entered the Jesuits at the age of 17.[22] He studied English at UCD alongside writer and broadcaster Benedict Kiely (1919–2007), before becoming a teacher at Belvedere and then Gonzaga.

In 1957, Veale posed a number of rhetorical questions about Gonzaga in an effort to centre the fledgling school's philosophy on a series of key goals: What kind of boy do I wish to form by the time he is 18?[23] How shall we educate him so that he may be able to continue to educate himself, so that he is prepared and equipped to take his place in modern Ireland, to be a responsible citizen, to earn his living, and to use his life for personal fulfilment and for the benefit of others? And, Veale wondered, how could the school enable the boys to live effectively by a teaching that says blessed are the poor, blessed are they that mourn, blessed are they that hunger and thirst after justice?

The importance of these questions, and their answers, shaped Veale's teaching in the 1950s and had a decisive influence on Clare not just as a child but throughout his entire life – a life characterised by intense engagement with public debate, profound curiosity about human nature, and an endless desire to understand and help others. Clare also echoed Veale's intellectual hunger and ability to move between different fields of endeavour: Veale's approach to religious studies at Gonzaga, for example, included generous doses of sociology and philosophy, while Clare's professional work spanned medicine, management, oratory, journalism and broadcasting. For Clare, as for Veale, there was no question that could not be addressed through careful thought, rigorous argument and rational application.

Both Clare and Geoghegan remained close to Veale after they left Gonzaga. On the fiftieth anniversary of the school in 2000, Clare wrote movingly about Veale in the *Sunday Independent*, pointing to his teacher's firmly held principles of communal responsibility, collaborative action and moral responsibility – principles that Clare still held dear almost five decades later.[24]

But perhaps the greatest gift that Veale gave to Clare during the Gonzaga years was a love of words, both spoken and written. In a 1957 article titled 'Men speechless', published in the Jesuit journal *Studies: An Irish Quarterly Review*, Veale quoted the ancient Greek rhetorician, Isocrates, who held that 'the right word is a sure sign of good thinking'.[25] This position was reflected not only in the Gonzaga debating society, which Veale founded and both Clare and Geoghegan enjoyed greatly, but also in Clare and Geoghegan's early brush with journalism, when they decided, in the early 1950s, to produce a newspaper for the play-town ('Luxembourg') that they created in Geoghegan's home.

The first issue of the *Luxembourg Weekly* was handwritten and contained short articles about the population of Luxembourg. All two copies were brought to school by its two authors and offered to their classmates to rent at 2d ('tuppence' or two pennies) for one hour of possession. Some students duly paid this not inconsiderable sum and read the offering. The second issue was typed on Geoghegan's father's ancient typewriter and ran to four copies. Clare was editor; Geoghegan was typist. Clare wrote about the lives of saints and current news, while Geoghegan wrote a series on cars, among other contributions – some under his *nom de plume*, 'Edward Maguire'.

By the time the fourth issue appeared (10 February 1954), the *Luxembourg Weekly* had grown to three pages, acquired a slogan – 'For good reading, read the *Luxembourg Weekly*' – and the leading article announced, with no small drama, that there were 'general elections in sight' in 'Luxembourg':

> The Prime Minister, A. Clare, told the house of parlment [*sic*] that the elections were less than three weeks away. The main fight is between the Conservative party (A. Clare) and the Labour party (Gen. Ross Geoghegan). The present situation in seats is: Conservetives [*sic*]: 58 seats and Labour: 42 seats. It is expected to be a very fierce fight. A. Clare is to meet General Ross Geoghegan and other leaders … During the week there will be different talks by members of parlment [*sic*] on Radio Luxembourg.

Issue 4 also had advertisements for the Labour party ('If you want the prices low, then vote for Labour') and the Conservatives ('Keep the straight road with Conservatives'; 'Vote No. 1 Clare'), a 'Lost and Found' section (if you spotted a terrier lost from 'Clare Road' you were to contact PO Box '264 5/8'), and a twenty-question prize quiz that relied heavily on the honesty of readers: 'We trust that the entrants for this competition will not use the aid of books when answering the questions.' Clare also revealed the solution to 'the crime at the village' (spoiler: 'Derek Sandler must have done it') and, in 'Late News', the newspaper announced that 'a meeting has been called by the editor, printer and other members of the staff of this paper. The reason is still a secret' (and remains a secret to this day).

Building on this clear potential and the enthusiasm of its authors, the *Luxembourg Weekly* was duly followed by the *Gonzaga Observer*, a weekly publication about Gonzaga that appeared on Fridays. With a production run of thirty copies, the publication's business model evolved from rental to sales, still at two pence per copy. Producing the paper was complex, so Clare's sister Jeanne assisted with the messy duplication task on a school duplicator which they used (with permission) after they had typed up the content. The newspaper's occasionally outspoken content triggered the ire of the school authorities, but despite these challenges – or, possibly, *because* of them – Clare was well and truly smitten: his long career in journalism had commenced.

Clare also developed a penchant for dramatic public performance at Gonzaga. Most memorably, he played the part of Felix in *The Comedian* by Henri Ghéon (1875–1944), the celebrated French playwright and author.[26] Performed on 4 February 1960, during Clare's final year at Gonzaga, this was the first play produced on the school's original stage and it gave Clare another early taste of the joys of performing in front of an appreciative audience.

Clare had a serious accident during this period, in his early teens, when he ran with outstretched hand into a glass door at Geoghegan's house.[27] This event and Clare's subsequent treatment left him with fears of both pain and medical interventions of any kind. Although the surgical repair of his wound was a success, Clare's period of rehabilitation was more difficult, and he bore a heavy scar on his left wrist for the rest of his life. It was – paradoxically – during this time that Clare became interested in medicine and began seriously to contemplate a career as a doctor.[28]

By their final year in secondary school, however, both Clare and Geoghegan had other things on their minds: they were preoccupied with girls and they supported each other as they navigated this complex new world. Attending a boys' school meant that there were very few girls in their daily lives, apart from sisters. The strictness of Catholic teaching meant that sex was a minefield and the boys' parents monitored them closely. Clare, in particular, was under constant pressure from his mother to have nothing to do with girls as they would interfere with his studies. But, as Geoghegan recalls, 'the loves of a teenage boy are intense infatuations with a short half-life. The relief of having a friend in whom one could confide was not forgotten. The memory of this lasted through our college years and into adulthood. Tony and I grew up together. It was at the root of our lasting friendship.'

All told, Clare's childhood was a happy one, shaped not only by his family and friends, but also – to an unusual degree – by his time at Gonzaga, even if Clare's religious faith was to waver over the course of his life. Professor Sir Robin Murray, who worked with Clare in London in the 1970s and 1980s (and later become Professor of Psychiatric Research at the Institute of Psychiatry there) duly recalls that Clare 'spoke warmly about the Jesuits'.[29]

Looking back on his childhood in 1995, Clare described the Dublin of his youth as a grey and rainy place.[30] He said that, in one sense, nothing changed between 1942, when he was born, and 1959: the same dreary streets, the same local church, the same, unchanging Roman Catholic rituals. The two chinks of light that Clare recalled were his education at Gonzaga and his occasional trips to Northern Ireland where he acquired a taste for Bounty bars, among other delights.

But things were changing both in Dublin and for Clare towards the end of the 1950s, as he completed his schooling at Gonzaga. Clare was maturing rapidly and his horizons broadened: he increasingly enjoyed American and British cinema, and listened to Elvis Presley, Buddy Holly and Cliff Richard on (the real) Radio Luxembourg. And, when the time came, the former altar boy was more than ready to move on to the next phase in his education and personal development: studying medicine at UCD.

University College Dublin

The Catholic University of Ireland was founded in 1854 with John Henry Newman (later Cardinal Newman and now canonised) as its first rector, and UCD was chartered as a university in its own right in 1908. In Clare's time, the 1960s, the faculty of medicine was located in

Earlsfort Terrace in the centre of Dublin in a building that now houses Ireland's National Concert Hall.

Clare's decision to study medicine was an interesting one. His father, Ben, was a state solicitor in the Land Registry and it was generally expected that Clare would follow his father and grandfather into law. Clare, however, spent time doing work experience with O'Connor solicitors in Clare Street and did not enjoy it. And so, in the usual way of ambitious parents, if it was not to be law, it had to be medicine. This fitted with Clare's own interests since the time of his accident and thus, in 1960, at the age of 17, Clare started his 'pre-medical year', the first of six years of medical school in Dublin.

Once he arrived at UCD, Clare immediately gravitated to the Literary and Historical Society (L&H), UCD's legendary debating society which was founded in 1854 by Newman, based on the idea that there was a lot more to university than just studying for your degree. Clare would later say that he possibly should have done journalism or a degree in English, as these were his natural interests and more consistent with debating, rather than science or medicine. His closest friends during his university years were mostly from the arts and, although the L&H had a number of talented medical student speakers, by far the larger proportion of L&H participants came from arts and law.

Debating was Clare's great passion. His inaugural address at the L&H was on the suppression of critical opinion within the Catholic Church, entitled 'The Heresy of Secrecy and Fear'. Building on his experience in the Gonzaga debating society, Clare excelled in the L&H, mixing brilliant argumentation with humour, passion and a verbal virtuosity that left opponents reeling.[31] He duly won the silver medal for debating in the society's 1961/2 session, while his friends Charles Lysaght[32] and Liam Hourican[33] took the gold medal and medal for first year speakers respectively.[34]

Clare's colourful debating exploits were frequently reported in the media. As early as 1960, *The Irish Times* recounted that the 17-year-old Clare, just months out of secondary school, described Ireland's secondary school system as 'farcical' at the Dublin Institute of Catholic Sociology Debating Society.[35] Two years later, at the same venue, Clare, now representing the L&H, argued that, because of late marriages, many Irish parents had little contact with their children.[36] Despite his involvement with these debates and various other Catholic events, however, Clare resisted overtures to join the priesthood, lured away, in no small part, by the excitement of life at UCD and especially the L&H.

In February 1963, Clare and his long-term L&H debating colleague, Patrick Cosgrave, won *The Irish Times* trophy for student debate when they spoke against the motion 'That the lights are going out in Europe' at University College Galway.[37] A team from Queen's University, Belfast, came second and another UCD team, including Geoghegan, came third. The trophy presented to Clare and Cosgrave was a bronze figure by artist Oisín Kelly[38] and, most excitingly, the pair were put forward to the semi-finals of the prestigious *Observer* Mace debating tournament. Winning the *Observer* Mace was every debater's dream – without doubt the most prestigious debating prize in Ireland and Great Britain.

In March 1963, the first of the three semi-finals of the *Observer* Mace was duly held at the L&H in UCD, and Clare and Cosgrave roundly defeated teams from University College London and University College Cardiff to qualify for the final in Bristol in May.[39] The other semi-finals were held in Bangor and Leicester later that week. In May, the three teams in the final, drawn from an original entry of 111, battled it out in Bristol, debating the motion, 'That this house believes the world owes its progress to unreasonable men.'[40]

Crushingly, Cosgrave and Clare lost out to a team from the University of Glasgow, comprising Malcolm MacKenzie and Donald Dewar; the latter went on to become Scotland's first First Minister in 1999.[41] Dewar had the advantage of experience, having lost in the Scottish round of the *Observer* Mace in 1960, when he debated alongside John Smith, who was on the winning team in 1962 and later led the British Labour Party from 1992 to 1994. In 1995, the *Observer* Mace was renamed the John Smith Memorial Mace in memory of Smith, following his sudden death in May 1994.

But Clare and Cosgrave could profit from experience too, and in May 1963 they won *The Irish Times* debating trophy in the Scottish–Irish debating tournament in Glasgow, opposing the motion that 'This house regrets that the sun has set on the British Empire.'[42] The dynamic duo scored especially highly for teamwork, refutation and eloquence. In January 1964, they won the semi-final of the Union of Students in Ireland (USI)–*Irish Times* Debating Tournament at Trinity College Dublin, proposing the motion 'That marching to disarm is marching towards disaster.'[43] Clare argued that progress towards disarmament would have to be tedious and slow: 'Whenever you march,' he intoned, 'you march to disaster.' Mr Donald Smyllie of *The Irish Times*, announcing the results, said that the standard of speaking was the highest that the judges had ever heard at a semi-final.

Clare and Cosgrave duly won the USI–*Irish Times* final at UCD in March 1964 and qualified again for the semi-finals of the elusive *Observer* Mace.[44] The following month in Dundee, they defeated teams from University College London, University College Swansea and Jordanhill College of Education Glasgow, proposing the motion 'That this house believes that the British scientist should stay at home.'[45] And then – epically – on 26 June 1964, at the 11th Annual Student Debating Tournament at Nottingham University, Clare and Cosgrave won the *Observer* Mace, debating the motion that 'This house believes that general elections in Great Britain should be held at regular intervals on fixed dates, as in the United States of America.'[46]

Clare, who was elected unopposed as auditor (chairperson) of the L&H for its 1963/4 session,[47] and Cosgrave, who had previously won an outstanding speaker award at the tournament, were now *bona fide* heroes. Bringing the *Observer* Mace home to the cheering L&H was like Caesar's army returning in triumph to Rome. There would be few events in Clare's later life that could match the unadulterated joy and sheer exuberance of that evening. It was, without doubt, one of his happiest moments.

Clare's and Cosgrave's friends also exulted in their triumphs. Ruth Dudley Edwards 'met Tony through the L&H because I was Patrick Cosgrave's girlfriend':

I was in the same year as Jane. Tony and Patrick were an extraordinary combination. Patrick was one of the few working-class people at UCD. He was brought up in a depressing council estate in Finglas and went to the Christian Brothers. His mother was a devout Catholic and uncritical nationalist. As a child, Patrick was in bed for a year with rheumatic fever and he read every book in the local library, which helped him change his religious and political views and loyalties, becoming an English romantic Tory and anti-Irish Catholicism. As a result, he arrived at UCD as a fully formed intellectual. Tony was completely accepting of Patrick's attitudes. He and Tony made fun of each other a lot and just clicked completely as partners in the L&H. Patrick would do the reasoned demolition and Tony would do the peroration, full of throbbing emotion.[48]

Colm de Barra, a friend of Clare and fellow L&H devotee, recalls that 'Tony was a great respecter of tradition in the L&H but he coupled this with a sense of humour and drama':

One of the big nights of the year was the inter-varsity debate when speakers from the major UK universities were invited. On the day of the debate, one speaker cancelled by telegram. Tony approached me asking if I would adopt a disguise and replace that speaker. Tony was delighted that I got away with the subterfuge, even to the extent of enjoying the pre-meeting dinner!

On another occasion, when the candidates for election as his successor had been nominated at the normal meeting, Tony accepted a procedural motion 'That the race now be run.' At this, the candidates (Paddy Cosgrave and Tony Cahill) along with their supporters left the meeting and ran a symbolic race around the outside of St Stephen's green. This 'race' became a tradition for many years after.[49]

But despite his high good humour and fondness for pranks, there was also a seriousness of purpose to Clare, even at the L&H. De Barra recalls that, in early 1965, 'when Winston Churchill was dying, there was huge media coverage during the final few weeks':

> Some of the old extreme nationalist feelings were stirred up as Churchill was not popular in Ireland. Tony had been auditor for the previous session of the L&H and he broke with tradition and returned to the society after Churchill's death to propose that the meeting adjourn out of respect to Churchill's heroic stance in the face of Nazism. All the prominent members spoke against the motion but it was carried due to Tony's passionate delivery and flourishing rhetoric.

Looking back, Clare's future colleague Robin Murray got 'the impression he enjoyed undergraduate life'.[50] In fact, Clare *loved* every single minute of undergraduate life: debating constantly, meeting new people, attending lectures and participating fully in virtually every aspect of the university scene. Clare also started to write more during this period, defending Ireland's military neutrality in *The Irish Times* in 1962,[51] discussing contraception in UCD magazine *St Stephen's* in 1963,[52] and writing about 'students and intellectual freedom' in *Hibernia* ('The Nation's Review') in 1964:

> It would appear from conversations and discussions in which I have taken part that many people number among their impressions of University College Dublin, the picture of a totalitarian institution, the atmosphere of which is cramped by clerical bigotry, stifled by narrow minded pressure groups and pervaded by the odour of a stern autocratic censorship.[53]

Cosgrave, also wrote voluminously about a broad range of topics during this period, pre-figuring his extraordinary future as writer, editor and political adviser in the UK – as well as many busy, exciting years as Clare's debating partner.[54]

The other aspect of UCD that appealed to Clare was the social one. Jane Hogan, his future wife, came to UCD in 1961 to study arts. Prior to Clare and Jane becoming a couple in early 1962, Jane remembers encountering Clare just once or twice – notably in the middle of an argument with a group of arts students in the 'Annexe', the steamy, damp basement café in Earlsfort Terrace.[55] 'There were a few medics who percolated into the ranks of the arts and law students, not many though,' she recalls. Clare was definitely one.

On another occasion, Jane remembers Clare entering into the fray of a political controversy concerning the co-option of students on to the Student Representative Council in midterm, but without due process. Unfortunately, Jane was one of those about to be co-opted, so Clare's diatribe inadvertently involved his future wife: 'This was upsetting and I thought the usual fire and brimstone that was Tony's style was unnecessarily righteous.' None of this stopped Clare tentatively approaching Jane in the Main Hall to ask if she would go to a dress dance with him: the Goldburn Beagles on 6 March 1962. The pair 'hit it off' at the dance and 'by the end of the year, or towards the beginning of the next, we were an item', Jane recalls.

Many years later, Clare commented that the 1960s were a wonderful time to be a university student in Dublin and that the inauguration of John F. Kennedy as United States president on 20 January 1961 marked the emergence of a new kind of national consciousness that he relished at UCD.[56] Clare saw Kennedy as an American Irishman who exulted in being an American, bringing a sense of hope even to the streets of Dublin. Kennedy's assassination on 22 November 1963 brought, for Clare, a stark realisation that a harsh, unforgiving world could, in a moment, crush such promise. Eimer Philbin Bowman, a friend of Clare and future psychiatrist, has 'a lovely memory of standing on the corner of Leeson Street and Stephen's Green the day Kennedy died, and watching Tony cycle with Jane on the crossbar down to University church. I envied them their closeness on that sad day.'[57]

Before she met Clare at UCD, Jane had never been to an L&H meeting, which meant that she 'was not open to being impressed by his performance. This was a fact that continued to be a feature – in many ways a distinctive paradigm – of my relationship to this person, who was at this stage a pretty immature boy. In fact, most middle-

class university students in Dublin were pretty immature boys and girls
during this period – still children to their parents, still living at home
and still getting pocket money when they needed it for the odd coffee,
film or bus fare.' As one might expect following his Jesuit education,
Clare was also still a practising Catholic when he started at UCD.
Initially, he held a conservative position about contraception too, but
this – and much else – changed as his religious observance slipped
away over the following years.

At UCD, Clare applied himself to his medical studies with diligence
and spent the long summer holidays either working (at Aer Lingus, for
example, where his sister was employed) or doing medical electives (in
Glen Cove, Long Island, for example, in 1965). But it was the L&H
rather than the school of medicine that got the best of Clare during his
university years.[58]

Clare loved attention. He said that the 'greatest satisfaction' he got
was from holding an audience captive and conducting their emotional
response as a conductor controls the musical response of an orchestra.
'He often said to me he would have liked to be a conductor.'[59] And in
future years, long after he left UCD, Clare would occasionally return
to student debating[60] and to the L&H,[61] including one memorable
occasion in 2000 when he convened a group of former L&H auditors
and committee members to consider the centenary re-enactment of
James Joyce's 'Drama and Life' paper, which Joyce read to the L&H
on 20 January 1900, in the old physics theatre in Newman House.[62]
Jane provided the material to Gerry Stembridge who scripted the one-
act re-enactment, with Peter Clare playing James Joyce and Clare
playing Joyce's father. It took place – fittingly – in the old physics
theatre in Newman House. Clare also later funded the refurbishment
of the L&H 'auditor's chair' which had been rediscovered in 1985.[63]

But notwithstanding his enduring love of the L&H, Clare was still
a medical student and he always accepted that he had to do consistent
study in order to pass his exams. Despite all his other activities, he
could be a model of self-discipline when he put his mind to it. He did
not drink alcohol and only smoked because it was the 'cool' thing to
do. He did not socialise with 'mates' in the way that some boys did,

and nor did he play sports for the college, unlike several of his medical cohort who were or became Irish rugby internationals. Clare played tennis well and regularly later in his life, but not as a team player in UCD.

In the midst of all of this activity, change and excitement, Clare and Jane were soon committed to a relationship that both expected to last. From the time they started going out in earnest, they saw each other most days. Jane remembers Clare's lectures ending at 'around 5 or 5.30 p.m., and we walked or cycled, me on the cross-bar, home to our respective parents for dinner or tea'. Jane occasionally 'persuaded him to ditch a lecture and we would go for coffee and cakes in Merrion Row, usually the DBC or Kilimanjaro – the former was the regular venue for teasing out the approach of the team to the given proposition at an upcoming debate. Paddy Cosgrave and Ruth Edwards were a couple and the four of us met to concoct the best argument to be made and how it was to be developed by each in turn.'

Jane remembers her future husband as essentially a one-man band. In later life, 'he had no time for committees unless he was chairing them, or conferences – he only went to those if he was a speaker – and was at his best in intense but relatively short-lived collaborations, except for his long-lived collaboration with Michael Ember':

What marked him out for me from the other boys was that he was complicated and interesting, and funny, and could talk the talk and engage with me at an intellectual level. He was an angry young man who could be explosive, but was also kind, and, when he felt he could trust in my positive regard, could allow a measure of vulnerability to surface.

Jane remembers Clare as somewhat detached from his family, in the manner of a cuckoo in the nest, apart from his sister Jeanne. He remained close to Jeanne all his life. Jane feels that his mother regarded her as a distraction from her son's career, and that Clare's mother was central to the drive that propelled his somewhat frenzied trajectory through life:

She wound him up, in every sense of the word, and set him off to prove his worth to her and thus to himself. She so injected the instability and conditionality of her approval into his core that he was condemned to a life of performance-generated self-esteem. He essentially did not think much of himself, although he could parade his entitlement at the same time, and his occasional knee-jerk criticism of others who were competitors was often the result of envy or a lurking fear regarding his own worth in relation to them.

The influence of Clare's upbringing 'was a topic of conversation in the last phase of his life, when he likened his self-punishing regime at the height of his hyper-productive fame to an addiction – a fix, with its risk/reward, pain/pleasure kick. He identified fear as being an unacknowledged presence in most of his life.'

Back in his student days at UCD, Clare progressed through medical school with no clear sense of what specialty within medicine he wished to pursue. Surgery was not an option, owing to his hand injury, and while he enjoyed obstetrics as a student, it was ultimately psychiatry, arguably the most verbal of medical specialties, that eventually won him over.

And, despite his intense engagement with debating, Clare remained deeply committed to medicine. Indeed, when Jane first met him, he expressed the view that medicine was a truly noble profession – healing the sick – and he was disparaging about literary criticism, which Jane was engaged in:

I tended to agree and was glad to be associated with medicine at one remove, as I had intended to do medicine myself. In fact, we did not know each other long when he took me, at my request, to the anatomy room to see the 'stiffs' [cadavers or dead bodies for dissection by medical students] – me donned in a borrowed white coat. There were over forty students in his year, most of whom I knew slightly, so they were amused. But the lecturer hadn't a clue that I was not one of his students – how would he? I dutifully took up my post at one poor 'stiff' and looked the part.[64]

The medical student with whom Clare was closest at UCD was Brendan Canning, a brilliant scholar. He and Clare engaged in highly regarded student research together and Canning was groomsman at Clare and Jane's wedding, as well as record secretary to the L&H when Clare was auditor. After UCD, Canning, like Clare, moved rapidly through his postgraduate training, at St Vincent's Hospital in Dublin, the Mayo Clinic in Minnesota (where Canning was a fellow in internal medicine from 1970) and the University of California San Diego, when Canning decided to pursue neurology. Clare had moved to London by the time the Canning family returned to Ireland in 1976, and Canning died tragically at the age of 33. His death was an acute loss for Clare, who remained in contact with, and supportive towards, the Canning family over subsequent years. Canning's daughter, Sinéad, served as auditor of the L&H for its 1991/2 session and Clare was – of course – uniquely positioned to advise her about the role.

As medical school came to a close, Clare and Jane Hogan decided to get married after they graduated in 1966, Clare with a medical degree in June, and Jane with a Masters degree in September. At this point, Clare and Jane were both still living at home with their families. Jane's family lived in Clogheen on Shelbourne Road, near Lansdowne Road rugby stadium. Jane's father, Sarsfield Hogan, was a senior civil servant in the Department of Finance, later chairman of Irish Steel Holdings[65] and a senior figure in Irish rugby for several decades.[66] Clare was still living with his family too, now at Albany Road in Ranelagh, not far from their previous residence on Tudor Road. Like Tudor Road, the Albany Road house was semi-detached and solid rather than flamboyant, but it was larger than the previous residence and situated on a wider, more welcoming street.

In an interview with Sebastian Cody in May 1984, Clare reflected that his childhood was 'typical of the Irish middle-class life of the 1940s, 50s and 60s' and pointed in particular to the influence of Veale at Gonzaga:

My mother, a busy energetic doer, had time for me. My father is a lawyer, good with his hands, intuitive. I don't come from an introspective family. One of the things about my life that I think about a good deal includes the influence of a Jesuit at my school who taught English literature and RE [religious education]. He was going through his own personal crisis – he was in his early 30s – torn by uncertainty and doubt, and introduced those elements into what until then had hitherto been a settled Catholic upbringing. I have a Catholic sensibility – but my practise rather faded when I went to the States.[67]

In 2000, at the age of 57, on the occasion of the publication of *On Men: Masculinity in Crisis*,[68] Clare discussed his family relationships again with Kathryn Holmquist in *The Irish Times*, and re-emphasised the role of his parents' characters in shaping his childhood, education and young adult life:

When he met Jane, Clare had a precedent for loving women with fight. While his father, a state solicitor with the land registry, was 'gentle' and 'a romantic', his mother was a woman to be reckoned with and 'stronger' than his father. 'I was more afraid of my mother, who had a fairly explosive temper. She'd whack you, never in cold blood. She was a passionate woman – about everything,' he says.

Clare says that 'physically I am like my father, but I have a lot of my mother's passion. She was very argumentative. I am very argumentative behind the urbane face.' Clare's early life was also dominated by two older sisters – Wyn, a draftswoman with RTÉ [Raidió Teilifís Éireann, Ireland's national broadcaster] and Cablelink [a cable television relay company], and Jeanne [Clare's other sister].[69]

Jeanne worked in Aer Lingus and later married and moved to England.[70] Clare remained close to both his sisters over subsequent years. Back in Ireland in 1966, however, Clare was finally about to leave both UCD and his family home, and take decisive steps towards an independent life with his new medical career and his fiancée, Jane. Next stop: New York.

2

The Making of a Psychiatrist
(1966–76)

●●●●●●●●●●●●●●●●●●●●●●●●●●●●●●●●●●

Following graduation from UCD in June 1966, Clare completed a rotating internship in family practice at St Joseph's Hospital on Prospect Hill in Syracuse, New York.[1] During this mandatory 'internship' year, the new medical graduate is a physician in training who has a medical degree but does not yet have a licence to practise medicine unsupervised. It is often a gruelling year.

After internship, virtually all doctors do further training in a medical specialty. This involves supervised practice for many more years as the doctor proceeds through a succession of 'senior house officer' and registrar posts (known in the United States as 'resident' posts). Following this period of supervised training, and after completing further examinations, the doctor finally, around ten years after graduating from university, becomes a specialist who can practise independently and supervise trainees.

The intern year is, then, the first step in this lengthy postgraduate training process. St Joseph's, Syracuse was established in 1869, when Mother Marianne Cope and four other Sisters of St Francis, transformed a New York dance hall and bar into a small fifteen-bed hospital. Continually sponsored by the Sisters of St Francis, the establishment grew and St Joseph's Hospital Health Center eventually comprised a 451-bed comprehensive medical care institution, dedicated to providing quality healthcare to the residents of sixteen counties in Central New

York. The complex now also includes a college of nursing, psychiatric emergency programme and physicians' office building.

When Clare did his internship there between July 1966 and June 1967, he was shocked by his experiences in their emergency department[2] and later commented that he 'came as close as he ever has to a nervous breakdown' during this period.[3] But despite the stresses, this was also a happy time for Clare, as he returned to Dublin to get married to Jane on 4 October 1966. They were both 23. The wedding, in St Mary's Church on Haddington Road, was concelebrated by Fr Joe Veale, Clare's beloved mentor at Gonzaga, and Fr Diffney. After the wedding, Clare and Jane spent six days on honeymoon in Bermuda *en route* to Syracuse where they stayed in hospital residences until Clare completed his internship in June 1967.

Clare returned to Ireland in July 1967 and commenced his postgraduate training in psychiatry in earnest at St Patrick's Hospital in Dublin. Many years later, Clare's eldest child, Rachel, suggests that 'one of the reasons that Dad was drawn to psychiatry I think is because it's the most "verbal" part of medicine, it involves personal narrative and, with Freud, storytelling. He had to choose a profession; that was non-negotiable given his parents' expectations.'[4]

The late 1960s was an exciting time to enter psychiatry. For over a century, mental healthcare in Ireland had been defined by large public asylums designed in the 1800s.[5] By the time Clare arrived back from sunny Syracuse, however, change was in the air. Four months earlier, the report of the governmental Commission of Inquiry on Mental Illness was published, urging 'radical and widespread changes' to Ireland's mental health system.[6] It suggested a shift away from inpatient care towards community care and treatment by general practitioners, as well as better services for people with alcohol problems, among other recommendations. Both these areas quickly became key interests for Clare.

St Patrick's Hospital, Dublin (1967–70)

The old building at St Patrick's Hospital, now St Patrick's Mental Health Services, is grey and imposing, but not austere. Its story started in 1731 when Jonathan Swift (1667–1745), author of *Gulliver's Travels* (1726), announced his intention to provide in his will for the establishment of a hospital for the mentally ill in Dublin. Clare, who would become medical director of the hospital in 1989, wrote about Swift's comments on madness in *A Tale of A Tub* (1704) and *Gulliver's Travels*.[7] *A Tale of A Tub*, Swift's first major work, saw Swift divide madness into three types: religious, philosophical and political. In *Gulliver's Travels*, Swift portrayed people trying to extract sunbeams from cucumbers and an architect who sought to build houses from the roof downwards. In *The Legion Club* (1736), Swift treated the Irish Houses of Parliament as an asylum, complete with madhouse keeper.

Following Swift's bequest and death in 1745, a royal charter was granted to St Patrick's by King George II on 8 August 1746 and the board of governors held its first meeting three weeks later.[8] The hospital expanded rapidly, especially when Dr Richard Leeper (1864–1942) became medical superintendent in 1899, and Clare later wrote about its illustrious history with clear pride.[9] Leeper opened a branch asylum in Lucan, called St Edmundsbury Hospital, where Clare would later work.

Leeper's enthusiastic reforms were continued by Dr (later Professor) J.N.P. Moore (1911–96) who served as junior assistant medical officer at St Patrick's from 1938 to 1941, and medical superintendent from 1946 to 1977.[10] Moore was a leading figure in Irish psychiatry for several decades and had a profound influence on Clare. Clare first met Moore on a television programme about medical education on RTÉ when Clare was a medical student in the 1960s. After the programme, Moore offered Clare a job at St Patrick's once he qualified and Clare duly arrived to take up the offer in July 1967.

At St Patrick's, Clare hit the ground running. In addition to his clinical duties as a trainee, he performed a study of alcohol dependence syndrome and road traffic accidents, for which he recruited 100 male patients admitted to St Patrick's with alcoholism.[11] Clare found that alcoholic drivers had significantly greater numbers of road traffic accidents and violations in their driving records when compared to a non-alcoholic comparison group selected from general practitioners' patient lists. Alcoholic drivers had approximately four times as many prosecutions and twice as many accidents as the non-alcoholic comparison group.

Alarmingly, of the seventy-two accidents in which alcohol was stated by the alcoholic to have played a major part, Clare found that only nineteen reached the court system, for various reasons. Clare urged that the diagnosis of alcohol dependence should not be missed and that better treatment and rehabilitation should be provided. The paper based on this work was published four years later, in 1973, in the *Journal of the Irish Medical Association*, with Dr J.G. Cooney, psychiatrist at St Patrick's, as co-author. Clare would return to the theme of alcohol dependence repeatedly in his later writings[12] and public education work.[13]

Clare's early years in St Patrick's were formative not only in terms of his clinical practice and research career, but also in terms of his vision of the role of the psychiatrist. Much of this was linked to his mentorship by Moore, of whom Clare was very fond. Clare always had good relationships with father figures throughout his career, arguably better than the relationship he had with his own father.[14] In 1996, Clare wrote an especially warm obituary of Moore, emphasising the older man's therapeutic enthusiasm, reformist zeal and general optimism.[15] Under Moore, patient turnover at St Patrick's rose, length of stay declined, and the hospital underwent an extensive programme of redevelopment. In his early training years, Clare was a clear beneficiary of Moore's new dispensation at the old establishment.

Ivor Browne, chief psychiatrist of the Eastern Health Board (1965–94) and Professor of Psychiatry at University College Dublin (1967–94), however, injects a note of caution. He recalls Clare as 'a very good person who had a big impact', but also points to the lingering effects of Clare's training with Moore:

Tony was a mixture because his psychiatric training was in St Patrick's Hospital and he picked up Dr Norman Moore's drug orientation. Moore was an amazing man – the son of a clergyman. And he had a wonderful skill for communicating. Moore arrived to psychiatry a few years before me and became very infatuated with the arrival of the new medications. He did not see the side effects and the negative aspects until later.

I was working in St John of God Hospital [in Stillorgan, County Dublin] in 1957, but, luckily, I stayed on there a second year. I had the same reaction as Moore: early psychiatric medications such as phenothiazines would remove the symptoms, but when I stayed for the second year, the patients returned, relapsed. Moore, however, was more committed to the medications because he came in earlier and saw psychiatry before the drugs.

As a result, Tony was caught a bit by his basic training in St Patrick's and although he emerged from that to an extent with his public exposure, he was never fully free of it. He became a sort of psychiatric philosopher with *In the Psychiatrist's Chair* [Chapter 5] but at the same time he had his background training in St Patrick's.

Tony didn't develop expertise in psychotherapy. I remember him giving a talk and he said that psychoanalysis was the deepest form of psychotherapy and that it was not very effective. And, therefore, he concluded, all forms of psychotherapy were ineffective. That was mistaken: psychoanalysis is not the deepest form and much psychotherapy is effective.[16]

Back at St Patrick's in the late 1960s, during Clare's time there, Moore pioneered patient lectures to increase patients' understanding of mental illness and its treatment, supported voluntary organisations in their work, and facilitated the first branch of Alcoholics Anonymous in Ireland, which had held its inaugural Irish meeting in November 1946. In addition, Moore was a member of the Commission of Inquiry on Mental Illness whose '1966 Report' urged the modernisation of psychiatric services and training – precisely what Moore himself was trying to achieve at St Patrick's through his lengthy involvement with postgraduate training and his decisive influence on an entire generation of trainee psychiatrists, including Clare.

But Moore's greatest impact on Clare related not so much to Moore's specific accomplishments in particular areas of psychiatric practice, but rather to the way that Moore conducted himself and epitomised a new kind of psychiatrist that interested Clare greatly: energetic, progressive, outward-looking and willing to engage with society at large. Footage from an RTÉ News report on 26 July 1968, in which Clare discusses the arrival of the Church of Scientology in Ireland, shows the young Clare to be articulate, clear and confident even as he appears on national television again just two years after graduating as a doctor.[17] Moore's approach to training was clearly paying dividends.

It was, then, Moore who organised Clare's first period at St Patrick's from July 1967 to January 1970, and whose values and priorities shaped much of Clare's training, career and professional life. Like Moore, Clare followed his early period at St Patrick's with time abroad, before returning to Dublin to become medical director of the hospital at which both trained. But whereas Moore spent his later training years in Dumfries in Scotland in the 1940s, Clare went to London, to the Maudsley Hospital and Institute of Psychiatry (1970–83) and, later, St Bartholomew's Hospital or 'Bart's' (1983–9). These were, perhaps, Clare's most formative years, during which the indefatigable, charismatic psychiatrist who was to change the public face of psychiatry forever came firmly into focus.

The Maudsley Hospital, London (1970–6)

Clare's training at St Patrick's was followed by five years as a junior doctor in psychiatry (postgraduate psychiatric trainee) at the prestigious Maudsley Hospital in London, from 1970 onward. When Clare first travelled to London for his interview in 1970, he stayed with Jane's cousins, Dorothy and Oonagh Boland, in their rented flat in Redfield Lane in Earls Court. The Clares' first own home in London was a rented house in Sevenoaks from which Clare commuted to work by train, until they moved to Monks Orchard Road in West Wickham in 1971. This house, one of a series of abodes rented out to employees by the Bethlem Royal Hospital, which stood directly opposite, was the Clares' home for almost a decade while Clare worked at the Maudsley.[18]

The Maudsley was and still is one of the world's leading psychiatric facilities, renowned for clinical care, research, education and training. The hospital was named after Henry Maudsley (1835–1918), a pioneering British psychiatrist who, like Clare, combined clinical and research work with a distinguished writing career.[19] The hospital building was completed in 1915 and initially requisitioned by the War Office as a 'shell shock' hospital with the result that it did not open to civilians until February 1923.[20] Edward Mapother (1881–1940), a Dublin-born doctor, was the first medical superintendent of the Maudsley and creator of the Institute of Psychiatry.[21] Professor Aubrey Lewis (1900–75) was the first director of the Institute,[22] a post he held until his retirement in 1966, the year Clare graduated from UCD.

By that time, the Maudsley had a strong reputation as a centre for postgraduate training so it is not surprising that Clare gravitated there after his time at St Patrick's in Dublin. And while Clare arrived in London in 1970, four years after Lewis retired as director, Lewis still cast a long and not unwelcome shadow over the hospital and institute, and Clare referred to him frequently.[23]

Anthony Mann, a colleague of Clare at that time (and later head of the section of Epidemiology and General Practice and, for a time, Old Age Psychiatry, at the Institute of Psychiatry) recalls Clare during this period:

I joined the Maudsley Rotation six months before Tony did [in 1970]. We were long-term colleagues. We had a shared training experience with Frederick Kräupl Taylor.[24] He inherited the same patients after I had completed my six months. Kräupl Taylor's approach was Prokaletic or 'challenge therapy' – to counter a patient's damaging or self-destructive behaviours.[25] In the context of three-times-a-week, one-hour sessions with very difficult patients, most of whom would earn the term 'borderline' nowadays, the challenges were offered.

They only had a chance of success if the patient had attached to the registrar/therapist. Kräupl Taylor judged that before any challenges were given. They were of two broad types – predictions of therapist failure or implosion, always preceded by 'I am afraid that your case is too difficult for me' or 'Dr Kräupl Taylor is very dissatisfied with my lack of progress with you.' The alternative was to challenge an unwanted behaviour, usually self-cutting, by making an unpalatable sexual Freudian theory derived association with it. Years after this experience, Tony and I greatly enjoyed reminiscing about patients and Kräupl Taylor himself.[26]

Robin Murray, another contemporary of Clare at the Maudsley during these years and later Professor of Psychiatric Research at the Institute of Psychiatry, remembers Clare as a dominant figure in the 1970s, an impressive speaker, dressed in a velvet suit.[27] Murray's first encounter with Clare was several years earlier as a medical student at the University Union debating chamber in Glasgow:

Glasgow was a powerhouse of student debating with people like John Smith, Donald Dewer and Menzies Campbell debating there. We got used to Oxbridge people being slaughtered at debates in Glasgow University Union. Visitors were heckled in a rowdy atmosphere. Tony [Clare] and Patrick Cosgrave (who became Margaret Thatcher's biographer) started in the face of hostility but were just so funny and such good debaters that they beat the locals. This was quite an upset.[28]

Murray did not see Clare again until they met in the Maudsley in 1972:

By the time I arrived in London, he was a senior registrar. We had a two-day introduction which was all a bit tedious. Tony came to tell us about the on-call duties which for some reason he was organising. He was dressed in a velvet suit and was just so lively and interesting. He gave us an accurate view of what it was like being a junior doctor at the Maudsley which had a bit to do with psychiatry and had a lot to do with fighting with the Royal College of Psychiatrists and the GMC [General Medical Council].

During this period, Clare fought strongly for better conditions for doctors training in psychiatry, with considerable success.[29] As it happens, Clare had arrived in the Maudsley at a critical time in the development of his chosen profession. While an association of asylum doctors and, later, psychiatrists had existed in various forms since 1841, it was only in 1971, the year after Clare's arrival in London, that a Supplemental Charter accorded the association the status of 'Royal College of Psychiatrists'.[30] On foot of this development, an examination for membership of the College (MRCPsych) was being introduced in the early 1970s and this stimulated heated discussions about the objectives and nature of postgraduate training in this field. Inevitably, Clare was in the thick of it.

On 22 August 1971, a meeting of doctors training in psychiatry was held in Birmingham, with trainees from Birmingham, Edinburgh, Glasgow, London, Manchester and Sheffield in attendance.[31] Together, they developed the idea of founding an 'Association of Psychiatrists in Training' (APIT), with Clare as convenor, owing to concerns about the new membership examination and various other aspects of the nascent college, including the composition of the college council.

To further these concerns, Clare and over 300 other trainees wrote a letter to the editor of the *Lancet* on 11 September 1971, posing searching questions about the new examination: in an era of continuous assessment, why had the College introduced a highly formalised, expensive examination?[32] Was this to be a competitive examination with a predetermined pass-rate? Why was it introduced in such haste, apparently without appropriate consultation? Clare and colleagues asked all junior psychiatrists who were considering entering for the examination to reconsider their position until there was clarity about the examination's format, purpose and future. They also announced the formation of APIT.

The 1971 *Lancet* letter was a clear declaration of intent and an accompanying editorial strongly endorsed the trainees' concerns, noting that the new college had no president and no council, and that there were key unanswered questions about the examination.[33] The trainees found a strong voice in Clare: a further meeting of APIT, convened by

Clare, was agreed for Manchester on 31 October 1971. The matter was duly taken up by the GMC who accepted the concerns of APIT, according to Clare.[34] The following year, Clare elegantly distilled the key issues in this rather protracted debate in a *Lancet* paper based on his address to the Society of Clinical Psychiatrists in Sheffield on 3 October 1972.[35] Clearly, Clare was not for turning.

In his 1972 *Lancet* paper, Clare reflected on the similarity between the terms 'training' (as it was then being used) and 'indoctrination', both of which he juxtaposed negatively with 'education', the latter being concerned with formation of the mind rather than necessarily shaping behaviour to fit a predetermined paradigm. Clare felt that the examination framework proposed by the Royal College of Psychiatrists was a charade owing in significant part to the lack of training facilities and teaching staff in many parts of the United Kingdom. Other unresolved problems included the determination of appropriate education methods to be used, the position of research within the new framework, and confusion about what was considered basic as opposed to specialist training.

To bolster its arguments, APIT, of which Clare was now chairman, studied membership examination candidates and found that 70 per cent of candidates in Edinburgh had no clinical experience whatsoever in child psychiatry, forensic psychiatry or the psychiatry of intellectual disability. Clare finished his *Lancet* paper with a warning about the perils of bureaucracy and even quoted T.S. Eliot on this point, adding a dash of rhetorical colour that would become a regular feature of Clare's writing even on topics as apparently technical as this one.

Clare was to write much more for the *Lancet* over subsequent years, but in 1972 it was remarkable that someone at such an early stage of training (just six years after graduating) was being published in such a prestigious journal. The fact that Clare was sole author of the 1972 *Lancet* paper confirmed the emergence of a new, confident and articulate voice in psychiatry.

Clare returned to the *Lancet* the following year with another letter about training, this time co-authored with Paul Bowden, also from the Bethlem Royal and Maudsley Hospitals.[36] On this occasion, Bowden and Clare were concerned about the redeployment of registrar and senior-registrar trainee posts from certain hospitals to others, ostensibly in order to achieve more equitable distribution of trainees across the United Kingdom. While this policy itself was understandable at one level, Bowden and Clare were concerned that staffing problems in provincial hospitals were being solved at the expense of academic centres, which were effectively being told to dismember themselves. In addition, they added, redistributing posts would not necessarily equate with redistributing manpower and there might be effects on the recruitment of doctors into the specialties, with potentially serious consequences for services.

Murray points out that Clare's activism in relation to training had a considerable impact:

> The College had set up the MRCPsych and wanted to give it to anyone who was a consultant. So, the trainees had to pay a lot of money to sit the exam while all sorts of dunderheads were being given the MRCPsych just for being consultants. Tony led the revolt against this and refused to sit the exam. My recollection is that I arrived [at the Maudsley Hospital] and we had the Junior Common Room where all the junior doctors met. The first meeting I went to, Tony and various others said what we were going to do was resign from the GMC. Everyone else was doing it so we all resigned from the GMC. The House Governor of the Maudsley Hospital, Nicky Paine (Tony played tennis with him for several decades),[37] found a clause in the hospital by-laws which said he could employ doctors for a month even if they were not registered with the GMC. Eventually the College of Psychiatrists back-tracked quite a lot, saying they would never make a profit from the exam and trainees would be on all appropriate committees. Tony did that.[38]

Murray 'later became chairman of APIT and was on the Council of the Royal College of Psychiatrists':

Professor Kenneth Rawnsley, Dean [of the Royal College of Psychiatrists, 1972–7],[39] was very sympathetic to the trainees and democratised the college. In these days junior doctors had a lot of influence. This fuss got trainees onto all sorts of committees ... As a result, I was on the Maudsley Hospital board in succession to Tony.

Clare's activism on the issue of training tapped into his skills for framing an argument, debating it fiercely, engaging in discussion and distilling his thoughts in elegant speech and prose. As Murray points out, Clare liked to question norms:

He liked challenging authority. He just thought he could do it better and was totally fearless. Many would have said 'What about my career?', but Tony just decided what he thought was right. He was a very clever politician. He managed to have disagreements with people in relatively good humour. He wasn't somebody who would go to a journal club and tear somebody to shreds. He might demolish their arguments but not abuse the person.

At the Maudsley, Clare used his rhetorical skills not only to champion the cause of psychiatric trainees, but also to address leading critics of psychiatry including such counter-cultural heroes as R.D. Laing (1927–89), author of *The Divided Self* (1960),[40] and Thomas Szasz (1920–2012), author of *The Myth of Mental Illness: Foundations of a Theory of Personal Conduct*.[41] Murray recalls both critical psychiatrists visiting the Institute of Psychiatry during Clare's time there:

It was the back-end of Ronnie Laing and Thomas Szasz. Szasz came and gave a lecture at the Institute of Psychiatry and wiped the floor with the professors who argued with him. Tony was much better arguing with him. At that time, anti-psychiatry was a big force. Ronnie Laing also came, but was too nervous to come in at first, pacing up and down outside. He wore a pin-striped suit and spoke about the army – a great disappointment.

Clare would later interview Laing on *In the Psychiatrist's Chair* in 1985[42] and comprehensively demolish Szasz's arguments both in person[43] and in his 1976 book *Psychiatry in Dissent* (Chapter 3).[44] Professor James Lucey, later a colleague of Clare and one of his successors as medical director of St Patrick's, comments that Clare 'was passionately critical of psychoanalysis':

> Tony's resolution of the R.D. Laing view versus the Royal College of Psychiatrists' view of mental health was head and shoulders above everyone else. He never lost that; the debates just took another form. For example, there is no single cause of schizophrenia. Tony knew that. He was an intellectual. He struggled with people who either identified with a single idea or persisted with a single idea because it suited their purpose.[45]

This passion for engagement, discussion and debate, evident from Clare's student days at UCD, continued unabated throughout his time at the Maudsley and beyond, marking Clare out as an exceptionally articulate young voice in psychiatry in the 1970s, ready and willing to contribute to the development and understanding of his chosen field.

Addiction, Migration and the London Irish

Clare's busy years at the Maudsley were filled not only with clinical work as a psychiatry registrar (1970–2) and senior registrar (1973–5), campaigns for trainees' rights and debates with critics of psychiatry, but also with his early forays into the peer-reviewed scientific, medical and psychiatric literature. He had an auspicious start with a case report in the *British Medical Journal* in November 1971 on the theme of diazepam, alcohol and barbiturate abuse.[46] Diazepam is a benzodiazepine medication used to treat anxiety, seizures (fits) and alcohol withdrawal states, among other conditions. Launched in 1963, it was widely used until the addictive potential of the entire benzodiazepine class of medications became all too apparent. In 1975 the US Food and Drug Administration (FDA) introduced additional regulations governing dispensing and reporting.[47]

Four years earlier, in his *British Medical Journal* paper, Clare described the case of a 39-year-old woman admitted to the Bethlem Royal Alcoholism Unit in 1970 for treatment of dependence on alcohol and barbiturates (medications used for anxiety, seizures and sleep problems). Following four months of treatment, the woman was discharged on a greatly reduced dose of barbiturate and on diazepam at a dose of 20 milligrams three times per day (quite a high dose).

After she left hospital, the woman's dependence on diazepam grew to a point where she was taking 500 milligrams of diazepam per day (a potentially fatal dose) and substituting it with sherry when she ran out of tablets. She was readmitted in an undernourished, underweight, bruised and broken state. She was restless, anxious and demanding. After what must have been a difficult first week of treatment, however, she had withdrawn from all drugs and alcohol, and was discharged two months later on no tablets. After five months, Clare's patient was symptom-free, living in the community, sleeping well, and working in a full-time job.

Discussing this case in his paper, Clare noted the speed with which the woman had developed dependence on diazepam and warned that the sanguine view of many doctors towards such minor tranquillisers inured the public to their very significant risks. Four years later, the FDA strongly endorsed Clare's concerns.

Clare's brief 1971 paper is notable in the context of his development as a psychiatrist and writer for two key reasons. First, it is highly unusual for someone's first clinical scientific paper to appear in a journal as prestigious as the *British Medical Journal*. This early publishing success, along with his 1972 *Lancet* paper,[48] was a clear indication of the long and accomplished career in writing, researching and publishing that lay ahead of Clare. His 1971 case report was also notably clear and concise, and its timing impeccable, just as the tide was about to turn against the benzodiazepines.

Second, it is unusual for a trainee to publish such an early paper without listing a senior figure as a co-author (e.g. a consultant or professor). At the end of his 1971 *British Medical Journal* paper, Clare acknowledged the permission and advice of Dr Griffith Edwards (1928–2012; psychiatrist and director of the Medical Research Council-funded Addiction Research Unit from 1968), but the case report itself had just a single author: Clare. For most people at that early stage of training, a senior author provides guidance and support and, not unusually, re-writes the entire paper for the trainee. The fact that Clare was the sole author listed on his first paper in the peer-reviewed scientific literature was another early indicator of his ability to think, write and publish in his own distinctive voice from the earliest stages of his career.

The following year, 1972, saw this aspect of Clare's career formally develop further, with the emergence of his first major research theme as he was awarded a Masters degree in philosophy (MPhil; *Magister Philosophiae*) in psychiatry from the University of London for a dissertation concerning psychiatric illness in the Irish immigrant population in London.[49] Clare's choice of theme was, perhaps, unsurprising: Clare himself was a migrant to London and, as Murray notes, 'when you migrate you're interested in the mental health of your compatriots'.[50]

Clare's dissertation was centred on a study of seventy-six patients from Ireland who made their first contact with the psychiatric services of the Camberwell area of London in 1970.[51] In a characteristic flourish, Clare started his thesis by quoting author George Bernard Shaw, another famous emigrant from Ireland, to the effect that the ambitions of all Irish people turn on their opportunities for leaving their native land. Clare went on to note that despite the fact that there were then almost one million Irish immigrants in Great Britain, there had been little study of their psychiatric status to date. Clare aimed to change this.

Clare started his 1972 thesis by providing a brisk, efficient run-through of the distribution of the Irish population in the United Kingdom, an analysis of stresses specific to migrants, and a summary of relevant research findings to date (limited as they were). He noted that migrants faced many different stressors related to, *inter alia*, loss of external supports, changes to routines, greater self-reliance, social isolation, prejudice and a possible excess of paranoid illnesses. He also identified stressors more specific to Irish immigrants, including racial stereotyping of the Irish as hard-drinking, delinquent, violent and unreliable.

Noting reports of high rates of hospitalisation with mental illness among the Irish in Ireland, Clare also noted apparently increased rates of psychosis (serious mental illness involving a break with reality) among Irish migrants in New York compared to other migrant groups there. Clare's own study in London, performed while he occupied a full-time clinical job, centred on the Camberwell Case Register, a record of all contacts with psychiatric facilities in a defined geographical area of London, in order to compare rates of mental illness among Irish migrants in London with rates in Ireland and New York.

Clare looked at referral data concerning seventy-six Irish migrants and seventy-six natives of England, Scotland and Wales living in Camberwell, with an average age around 38 years. He used population data to calculate rates of illness per 1,000 population in the Camberwell area.

Clare found that psychiatric referral rates were higher in the Irish migrants compared to the indigenous population, but that the rate of schizophrenia was not higher among the Irish migrants, despite the reportedly higher rates in Ireland and New York. Clare also found that Irish migrants presenting to the Camberwell psychiatric services were no more socially isolated than their UK counterparts and did not seem to be at greater risk of mental illness as measured by previous psychiatric history, family history of psychiatric illness, early age of onset of symptoms or disturbed early life.

The Irish migrants had, however, higher rates of alcohol problems and mood disorders compared to UK natives, and were more likely to use psychiatric services (as opposed to general practitioner services) and to do so at an earlier stage in their illness compared to the indigenous UK population. There was no difference between the Irish migrants and the UK natives in terms of likelihood of admission to inpatient psychiatric care, involuntary treatment under mental health legislation ('sectioning'), duration of inpatient treatment, or outcome.

Overall, Clare concluded that, contrary to the expectations of many, there was little evidence to support the idea that immigration *per se* was a specific factor in precipitating serious mental illness such as schizophrenia among the Irish in London.

Clare's findings of higher rates of referral, alcohol problems and mood disorders among Irish migrants in London were, of course, interesting, but it is the unremarkable rate of schizophrenia among the Irish migrants that is, in retrospect, the standout finding in this work, along with the increased likelihood of the Irish to seek psychiatric care rather than care from general practitioners for their early symptoms.

The idea that the Irish have an increased rate of serious mental illness was a long-standing one and, as Clare noted in his thesis, the idea was still prevalent in 1970s Ireland. It was to take several more decades of research and discussion to dismantle this idea of the 'mad Irish' and to prove definitively that the Irish do not have, and never had, a higher rate of mental illness than any other people.[52]

Clare's 1972 thesis actually contained a clue as to one of the real factors perpetuating the myth of the 'mad Irish': that the Irish became engaged in psychiatric care (as opposed to general practice care) at an earlier stage in their illness compared to other people, leading to an apparently higher rate of serious mental illness among the Irish. This was just one factor among many contributing to the idea of the 'mad Irish', but it was a significant one that has been relatively neglected in the relevant literature. If greater attention had been paid to Clare's 1972 study, much of the anguished hand-wringing and baroque theorising of the intervening decades might well have been avoided.

Clare's finding of high rates of alcohol problems among Irish migrants was significant if not surprising. In 1974, he published a paper on alcoholism and schizophrenia in Irishmen in London in the *British Journal of Addiction to Alcohol and Other Drugs*, exploring this theme further.[53] In that paper, he presented more data from his MPhil thesis and concluded that his findings did not support the idea that alcoholism in the Irish masks schizophrenia. On the contrary, the diagnosis of alcoholism was often missed and it was likely that the prevalence of alcoholism was under-reported in this population. In this way, Clare helped shed light on this hidden suffering among the Irish in London, many of whom clearly had serious problems with alcohol (among other challenges). Clare later became a founding patron of the charity Immigrant Counselling and Psychotherapy which worked chiefly among the Irish community in the United Kingdom,[54] only retiring from this position in mid-2007, shortly before his death.[55]

Clare's concern about the adverse effects of alcohol among Irish migrants in London in the 1970s was consistent with his 1969 study in St Patrick's in Dublin, linking alcohol with road traffic accidents, published in the *Journal of the Irish Medical Association* in 1973.[56] The following year, 1974, saw the same journal publish more of Clare's MPhil findings, emphasising again the high rates of mood disorders and unremarkable rate of schizophrenia among the Irish in London.[57] Interestingly, both papers that stemmed directly from Clare's MPhil were, again, published without a senior author, emphasising the self-directed nature of Clare's early work and the confidence of his early scientific voice.

Clare was to return to these themes, alcohol and migration, many times throughout his career. He spoke and wrote particularly extensively about alcohol misuse,[58] its causes,[59] its links with mood disorders,[60] approaches to treatment,[61] and attitudes within the medical profession.[62] He also returned to the theme of migration and mental health in the *Irish Journal of Psychological Medicine* in 2002, some three decades after his original studies in 1970s London.[63] Ironically, Clare's 2002 paper centred on the mental health of migrants arriving *into* Ireland, rather than those who left Ireland and settled in London or elsewhere. The decades since his MPhil research had seen a startling reversal of migration patterns, as the net outward migration of some 2 per cent of Ireland's entire population in 1988/1989 reversed, with the number of immigrants *into* Ireland between 1995 and 2000 amounting to an extraordinary 7 per cent of the entire population.[64]

Clare's 2002 paper on this theme acknowledged the challenges presented by mental illness among migrants into Ireland but also made the valuable point that immigration itself is not always associated with proneness to disease. He noted that migrants coming to live among fellow immigrants are able to continue to contribute to their own culture as well as that of their host country. What is challenging, he argued, is the abrupt exposure to different social demands and social expectations that are unfamiliar and intimidating. The critical issues were, he wrote, broader than treatment of mental illness and centred on Ireland's overall social response to the increased inward migration of recent years.

As with much of Clare's work, his 2002 paper on immigration contained clear echoes of Aubrey Lewis's analysis of health as a social concept, deeply embedded in prevailing social, economic and political conditions.[65] In his 2002 paper, Clare combined this keen social awareness from his years at the Maudsley with an acute psychological sensibility that was highly appropriate to his consideration of the mental health of migrants both into London in the 1970s and into Ireland in the 2000s.

As early as 1976, Clare demonstrated his considered awareness of these complexities when he elaborated on his work with Irish migrants in an interview with journalist and novelist Maeve Binchy in *The Irish Times*.[66] In this discussion, Clare spoke about the high rate of alcohol misuse among the Irish migrants in London and possible reasons for the disparity in treatment rates between the Irish in London and the Irish in Ireland. In reflective, speculative mood, he suggested that there was, in Ireland, a desire for urgent treatment, to be cured *immediately*, meaning that people were anxious to go to hospitals for treatment they think will provide rapid cures, rather than availing of outpatient treatment with general practitioners or others. A more considered, dispassionate and analytical approach would, he felt, be helpful.

Clare himself would soon play a key role in fostering such a thoughtful approach both within the profession of psychiatry and in the public eye. Much of this was attributable to his groundbreaking, career-making 1976 book, *Psychiatry in Dissent: Controversial Issues in Thought and Practice* (Chapter 3).

Life in London in the 1970s

Clare's crowning achievement in psychiatry, *Psychiatry in Dissent*, emerged not only from Clare's evolving academic work and research, but also from his clinical activity and personal life in 1970s London. Jane recalls that the family 'lived at Monks Orchard Road, opposite Bethlem Hospital' alongside many colleagues.[67] 'There was blurring of lines between work and home life. We knew each other very well, like an extended family, especially at the Maudsley.'[68]

Clare's eldest child, Rachel, agrees that 'Dad enjoyed the easy sociability of Monks Orchard Road. There were parties in people's gardens during the hot summers, with us kids running off to play in the woods at the back. As psychiatrists' kids, we all went swimming in the hospital pool at the weekend.'[69] Clare 'was not an absentee Dad. He was very good at having debates with us children about the issues of the day. When I was age 14 or 15, he would give me things he had written to read, and I loved that.'

At home, Clare was prone to letting the family cats fall asleep on him. Pushkin, their first cat, surprised them all by having kittens. Later, Clare's daughter Eleanor got a black cat whom they named after Mimi in Puccini's *La Bohème*. Peter, too, recalls the pets:

> We also had rabbits and Eleanor had a gerbil who trapped his tail in a drawer at one point. When we returned to Dublin, Mimi came with us and we got dogs: Mossie, a sheepdog whom we looked after and who then became our own, and Bonzo who showed up one day, chose to stay and became a welcome additional member of the family. Sebastian had goldfish that used to die and be replaced; this went on for some time before he found out.[70]

Rachel points out that Clare, like his father, relaxed by listening to music:

> He listened to popular opera (Puccini, Verdi, Tchaikovsky, Wagner) and the Beatles, Queen, and later Oasis. We would always listen to the top 40 on Sunday and he would often watch *Top of the Pops* with us. Dad's passions crossed disciplines and maybe that's what

made him able to move easily between the academic and the media worlds. Dad just loved going to the theatre or opera in London. I remember as a real treat my parents took me out of school to see Placido Domingo in *Cavalleria Rusticana* and *Pagliacci* at the Royal Opera House, Covent Garden [February 1976].

Dad loved actors. I grew up thinking that everyone believed acting was an incredibly noble profession, that being Laurence Olivier was the highest possible achievement. I was with him at an event once where he sat and talked with Jeremy Irons forever.

Dad absolutely loved Billy Wilder, he loved sharing *Some Like It Hot* with us, introducing us to the movies that he loved. He enjoyed going to the cinema throughout his life. I remember him being fascinated by Meryl Streep in *Kramer vs. Kramer* [1979] and then having quite long chats about *The Queen* [2006] with him.[71]

This was also a very busy time for Clare. His friend Ruth Dudley Edwards recalls that 'Tony was always the star of things, but he did live very much on his nerves':

He was a prodigious worker, and needed all the income he could get as the children were being educated privately. We would arrive over for the evening and we would hear Tony's typewriter from another room, writing a column for the *Spectator*, perhaps. He would appear later on and would often do the cooking.[72]

Dudley Edwards recalls that 'Tony was the great provider.' All told, Clare and Jane had seven children. Robin Murray describes a period of happy busyness in a well-established community of people working in psychiatry and living close together during this period:

We lived in the same road ... We were very, very friendly. We were very different. Tony was flamboyant and could dominate any argument. It was a principle of mine never to argue with Tony Clare in public. He was brilliant as an intellectual jouster or provocateur. Because we lived in the same street, if we were coming home at midnight or 1a.m., we'd drive past Tony and Jane's house, and the light would be on as Tony was at his desk trying to complete some article to a deadline.

Tony seemed to do a lot of the housework and regular visits to the supermarket. He was a very good, hard-working clinician. He was writing all his articles and academic work. And he was going off to the supermarket. Tony was always late because he was doing so many things. He was always rushing around from one thing to another.[73]

While Clare's involvement in the media deepened rapidly as the 1970s progressed, he always 'admired Robin Murray's devotion to psychiatry'.[74] Murray, who later became Professor of Psychiatric Research at the Institute of Psychiatry, recalls that, even before *Psychiatry in Dissent* appeared in 1976, 'Tony had started writing regularly for *World Medicine*, which came out once a month. It reviewed advances in specific areas of medicine and Tony wrote a monthly piece for that':

He was also beginning to write odd pieces for the major newspapers which did not make him popular among many senior staff at the Maudsley. They thought who was this jumped-up little Irish bugger who had not just plagued the Royal College of Psychiatrists, but now also appeared on radio and television pontificating about psychiatry, when it should have been them?

You knew that if you were having a discussion with Tony over lunch there was a chance the comments would appear in a newspaper or magazine in the next few days. Or he was trying out something. You would go into the Maudsley canteen and there would be fifteen people grouped around one of the tables, and a huge argument going on as Tony provoked a discussion about classification of psychosis, or the treatment of dissidents in Russia in the early 80s,[75] or something else.[76]

Clare's burgeoning career in journalism dated from his time in secondary school working on the school newspaper, his years in UCD writing for *St Stephen's*,[77] and his postgraduate training in psychiatry in Dublin. When he was a psychiatry registrar in St Patrick's in 1968, he wrote courageously in *The Irish Times* about the dilemma that *Humanae Vitae*, a 1968 papal encyclical, presented to doctors who prescribed oral contraceptives.[78] Two years later, he again took to the pages of *The Irish Times*, this time from London, to bemoan the polarisation of the debate about abortion law in the United Kingdom[79] and to comment again – not without controversy – on the thorny issue of contraception in Ireland.[80]

In a more scholarly vein, Clare wrote a measured and insightful essay in *Studies: An Irish Quarterly Review* (published by the Jesuits) in 1969 before leaving Dublin, looking at the work of Konrad Lorenz (1903–89), the Austrian zoologist, ethologist and Nobel prize-winner (1973) who wrote about aggression in his 1966 book, *On Aggression*.[81] In his notably eloquent 1969 essay in *Studies*, Clare asked a simple question that cut to the core of Lorenz's argument: 'Is aggression instinctive?'

> The disenchantment with the structures of Western industrial democracy, often incompetently formulated and incoherently expressed, has spawned a philosophy and a theology of violence which portrays force – *la violence, die Gewalt* – as a necessary, creative drive, the final assertion of life in the face of a sterile, oppressive, bureaucratic totalitarianism. This cult of violence derives its philosophical basis from the writings of Sartre and Fanon, the studies of existential psychiatrists such as Laing, the revolutionary tactics of Debray and Guevara. Now it appears to have found in the work of the Austrian ethologist, Konrad Lorenz, scientific justification for its position. It is the purpose of this article to examine Lorenz's position on aggression and to discuss the implications of his claims with reference to the presentation of violence, education and discipline.[82]

Clare was fundamentally unimpressed with Lorenz's essential argument that animals, including humans, are biologically programmed to fight over resources. *On Aggression* left Clare with a 'feeling of profound disappointment' for its lack of 'cautious, critical, scientific detachment':

> Its major defect is that the opening assertion that aggression is an instinct is regarded by the end of the book as proven, the ultimate blind-alley result of the inductive method in science. In addition, the astounding ease with which Lorenz first compares and then identifies animal behaviour with that of man is capricious and misleading.[83]

Clare also honed his growing critical faculties with a series of book reviews in *The Irish Times* in the early 1970s, looking at topics such as the history of the unconscious,[84] western and eastern psychotherapies,[85] and, most of all, the state of psychoanalysis,[86] with Clare, controversial as ever,[87] fundamentally unconvinced by anything that the Freudians had to offer.[88] This position pre-figured Clare's later, more trenchant criticisms of the persistence of psychoanalytic thought throughout the twentieth century (although this did not deter him from making a pilgrimage to Freud's consulting rooms in Vienna in 1983).[89] Clare also wrote in *The Irish Times* about the parlous state of Irish medicine in the early 1970s[90] and the social and family dynamics of bigotry and fear in conflict-ridden Northern Ireland,[91] a well-received article that took him, ironically, back to the work of Lorenz.[92]

In 1972, Clare reviewed *The Manufacture of Madness*[93] by contrarian Thomas Szasz in *The Irish Times* and was generous enough to give a careful hearing to the controversial psychiatrist, whom Clare also encountered at the Institute of Psychiatry and elsewhere,[94] although Clare was ultimately withering in his critique of Szasz's core arguments.[95] Clare returned to Szasz's provocations again and again over the following years, most notably in *Psychiatry in Dissent* in 1976 (Chapter 3), but also in *The Spectator* in 1972 after attending the recording of a televised debate involving Szasz.[96] Clare simply could not resist a good argument.

A year earlier, in 1971, Clare's former UCD debating colleague, Patrick Cosgrave, had been appointed political and deputy editor of *The Spectator*, a weekly UK magazine, after working for some time at the central office of the Conservative Party (1969–71).[97] Clare contributed extensively to *The Spectator* over the following years, reviewing books on topics as diverse as educability and group differences,[98] and the psychology of military incompetence,[99] as well as a volume of letters by psychiatrist Carl Jung.[100] Clare liked the Jung letters very much, possibly because Jung, like Clare, did not deify Freud (to put it mildly).

Clare's other *Spectator* articles (and there were many) touched on themes such as psychological techniques for handling sieges,[101] the use of psychiatric medication in prisons,[102] and, in 1973, the 'return' of R.D. Laing, the anti-psychiatrist who had, paradoxically, significantly influenced Clare's initial path into psychiatry.[103] Clare's rather balanced critique of Laing triggered a horrified response from a sociologist in Keele University[104] to whom Clare duly responded in kind, with a robust defence of his views.[105] Clare visibly relished these exchanges (and, again, there were many of these too).

Even greater controversy followed Clare's 1973 *Spectator* article about psychologist Hans Eysenck (1916–97) in which Clare questioned whether the celebrated Eysenck was really a scientist at all.[106] He also disputed Eysenck's view that the Irish scored poorly on IQ tests, a claim that Clare had already mercilessly demolished in *The Irish Times* some two years earlier, fundamentally questioning Eysenck's interpretation of the research on which he based his view.[107] Eysenck's response to Clare's essay in the *Spectator* was rapid and colourful,[108] as was Clare's inevitable riposte to Eysenck,[109] as each man described the other as a controversialist and argued their respective points to the bitter end. In truth, of course, there was no end: these debates just went on and on.[110]

Clare loved it all and the *Spectator* was the perfect venue for such exchanges in the early 1970s. Cosgrave remained in his editorial position with the magazine for four years from 1971 and this was, according to the *Guardian*, 'the bright time of [Cosgrave's] life':

If [Cosgrave] had been another sort of journalist – cooler, less rash, also physically healthier – he ought to have advanced to national editorship or a ministerial career. But not only did Patrick never calculate, he had a drink problem, which itself derived from his health problem. Stricken by rheumatic fever as a boy, he suffered from a permanently weakened heart. The drinking was steady and spectacular, and it became clear to both the Tory command and editors that Patrick, though brilliant, learned and profoundly loveable, was 'impossible'.[111]

And Cosgrave really was brilliant: a superb debater,[112] a gifted writer, biographer[113] and journalist (even as a student),[114] and a commanding mind.[115] In this sense, Cosgrave and Clare were natural allies, but Cosgrave's politics were to the right of centre; as the *Guardian* noted, he worked at the highest level of the Conservative party and was a special adviser to Margaret Thatcher.[116] In this respect, as Murray points out, Clare's 'choice of debating partner was interesting. Patrick Cosgrave was politically to the right of Margaret Thatcher. Tony debated not only with those he was familiar with.'[117] Nevertheless, Clare and Cosgrave had a strong bond and, many years later, in September 2001, Clare would deliver a moving, if bleak, tribute at Cosgrave's funeral service in Clapham Common.

As the 1970s progressed, Clare contributed less and less to *The Irish Times*[118] and more to *The Spectator* and various other UK publications including *New Society*, *The Times* and the *Guardian*. He would go on to contribute to many more, including the *New Statesman* and various others, over the following decades.[119] Clare was also commonly quoted in the media during the 1970s, be it concerning training in psychiatry[120] or the need to increase the number of psychiatrists in the National Health Service (NHS) by some 50 per cent (he claimed).[121] As a 1976 *Irish Times* article about Clare noted, 'people listen to him and discuss with him',[122] and it was this ability to command an audience that increasingly shaped Clare's work in print and broadcast media during the 1970s.

But Clare kept a firm foot in the medical and scientific literature too, and focused most of his popular media writing on various aspects of psychology, psychiatry and the mind, and how they related to the broader world. In 1976, he wrote in the *Nursing Mirror and Midwives Journal* about the psychology of kidnapping[123] and the evolving role of nurses in psychiatry, to take just two examples.[124] And in the *Lancet*, he wrote bluntly and movingly about the coruscating film *One Flew Over the Cuckoo's Nest*, readily acknowledging its perceptiveness, persuasiveness and implicit criticisms of psychiatric power.[125]

These were tempestuous times in England, during the 1970s, with all kinds of established power structures being questioned. Rachel recalls that 'the political climate was such that there were strikes, three-day weeks and bread shortages; the unions were very active; Britain went to the International Monetary Fund [in 1976]; and there was the Winter of Discontent' [1978–9].[126] Even so, and despite his growing medical, academic and media commitments, 'Dad was very home-centred':

When there is a big family, the home is the heart of it – you don't just have your brothers and sisters, you have all the friends coming over as well. My Mum was very welcoming, she loved having lots of people coming over. Dad would come home and say 'It's like a railway station in here.' He needed a lot of recharging downtime. He loved watching TV with the family. We would sit and watch *Dallas*, talking and commenting through it. But his study was a retreat. He liked the bustle *and* he liked to escape it.

A key thing about Dad was that, given how famous he was, he was in no way interested in being part of the London dinner party set. He would have been more than welcome but he was genuinely not interested in that sort of thing.

Editors of newspapers were often on the phone asking for 1,000 words or 500 words on the theme of the day, and he'd get very irritated after putting the phone down: 'Don't they realise this is not my day job?' It would be usual to open the Sunday papers and there would be a piece by Dad. He had an opinion on anything and everything. He was interested in everything around him: history, cities, cultures, what makes people tick.

David Knowles was a colleague, friend and next-door neighbour of Clare during this period, from 1971 to 1976, and then a friend for the rest of Clare's life. He notes that 'Tony was pre-eminently someone who connected with people through his verbal skills and his sheer charm, which was very different to some of his peers.'[127] Clare 'had the gift of the gab', called himself 'the eclectic psychiatrist', and was 'competitive to the nth degree'.

In his clinical work at the Maudsley, Clare was engaging, bright and witty, always ready to spend extra time with patients to relieve their anxieties.[128] He was, according to colleagues, a breath of fresh air. That breath of fresh air would soon turn to a bracing blast with the publication of Clare's magnum opus, *Psychiatry in Dissent*, in 1976.

3

Writer: *Psychiatry in Dissent* (1976)

●●●●●●●●●●●●●●●●●●●●●●●●●●●●●●●●●●●●

When Clare graduated as a doctor from UCD in 1966, psychiatry, the field to which he would devote his career, was – as usual – experiencing an existential crisis. The psychoanalytic revolution that started with Freud in the late nineteenth century and informed much of psychiatry in the early twentieth century was in clear decline. The emergence of new forms of psychological therapy (such as behaviourism) and the failure of several biological therapies (such as insulin coma and lobotomy) saw psychiatry come under attack from all sides and from within. The onslaught crystallised in 1961 when three key texts were published, each presenting fundamental challenges to the very existence of the profession of psychiatry and each shaping Clare's thinking in subtly different ways.

In the United States, sociologist Erving Goffman published *Asylums: Essays on the Social Situation of Mental Patients and Other Inmates* based on his personal observations within a American psychiatric institution.[1] Goffman, with a keen eye for oppression and an ear for the absurd, reported that mental hospitals functioned as 'total institutions' in which adjusting patients to institutional roles was accorded greater priority than treating them. For Goffman, mental hospitals were places of custody, not cure.

Goffman's critique resonated strongly with that of French philosopher Michel Foucault in *Folie et Déraison: Histoire de la Folie à l'Âge Classique*, later published in English as *History of Madness*.[2] Foucault wrote that 'madness' in the modern world was associated primarily with exclusion and repression, and had little connection with 'mental illness' (however defined). Foucault's arguments were baroque in the extreme and rooted in an idiosyncratic version of history, but they complemented perfectly the grounded, anthropological observations of Goffman: for both Goffman and Foucault, the mentally ill were repressed and excluded by a society that did not care about their real needs and sought only to control them through coercive rituals such as labelling and disempowering, distancing and oppressing. Psychiatry was the chief vehicle for achieving these nefarious aims on behalf of society.

The third key text to appear in 1961 came from within psychiatry itself, when US psychiatrist Thomas Szasz published *The Myth of Mental Illness: Foundations of a Theory of Personal Conduct.*[3] A gifted polemicist, Szasz argued that by diagnosing unwanted behaviour as mental illness, psychiatrists inappropriately absolved individuals of personal responsibility. He argued that 'mental illness' was non-existent and that psychiatrists dealt with personal, social and ethical problems in living, rather than 'mental illnesses'. In a virtuoso whoosh of rhetorical frenzy, Szasz issued a bracing warning against psychiatric overreach, denounced Freudian psychology as a pseudoscience, and outlined his alternative 'theory of personal conduct' which, he said, better articulated the *moral* dimensions of human behaviour in the psychiatric context.

Psychiatry in the 1960s

To the visible disappointment of these critics of psychiatry, many psychiatrists responded to their loudly proclaimed arguments by agreeing with them to greater or lesser degrees. There could be little doubt that mental hospitals were routinely used for social warehousing and that a diagnosis of mental illness was sometimes used to evade personal responsibility. The complicity or otherwise of psychiatrists in these processes was, perhaps, a matter for greater debate. All told, the popular impact of the three 1961 texts was soon dwarfed by a single novel published the following year: Ken Kesey's iconic *One Flew Over the Cuckoo's Nest.*[4]

Kesey's novel presented a no-holds-barred picture of life in a US mental hospital: wrongful incarceration, casual cruelty by staff, punitive ECT and brutal lobotomy. Placing the novel's shock tactics to one side, there was also great subtlety in Kesey's portrayal of many of the characters and an especially keen sense of the negative effects of institutions not only on patients but also on staff. In 1975, the book was made into a celebrated film by Miloš Forman, and went onto win all five major Academy Awards: best picture, actor in lead role, actress in lead role, director and screenplay.

Clare, reviewing the film for *The Lancet*, drew attention to one key, neglected aspect of the story, which reached to the heart of both Kesey's original novel and Clare's worries about psychiatry more broadly.[5] With elegant insight, Clare highlighted that it was not the misuse of specific treatments such as ECT and psychosurgery that posed the greatest danger in the film, but the absolute belief of some practitioners of psychiatry that their own authority and power were incorruptible. This underlying assumption, Clare argued, presented the gravest threat.

Ten years prior to the appearance of the film, back in the early 1960s when Goffman, Foucault and Szasz added pre-emptive academic weight to Kesey's concerns, the new era of critical psychiatry had been carefully noted by Clare, who understood better than most that this was a defining period for his chosen branch of medicine. The emergent critiques presented an opportunity and, arguably, created a necessity for someone to step forward with a response, to articulate clearly the merits (if any) of contemporary psychiatry and to offer a reasoned path forward. After all, despite their philosophical flourishes and verbal virtuosity, the critics offered virtually no suggestions about how better to assist people in severe psychological distress. Perhaps psychiatry still had something to offer?

As a medical student and keen reader, Clare was also aware of the work of another critic from within psychiatry, Ronald Laing, whom Clare would later interview for *In The Psychiatrist's Chair* in 1985. Laing published his best-known book, *The Divided Self*, in 1960, in which he argued that ontological insecurity (being insecure about one's existence) prompts a defensive reaction whereby the self splits into various different components, and that this process generates the psychotic symptoms commonly seen in schizophrenia (loss of contact with reality in certain respects).[6] Laing, who truly blossomed in the media spotlight, went on to articulate many of the key tenets of what became known as the 'anti-psychiatry' movement, based on the idea that psychiatric treatments do more harm than good. This movement gained momentum during the 1960s, just as Clare graduated as a doctor in 1966. As Robin Murray notes, 'because of the anti-psychiatrists and people like Ronnie Laing, all of this stuff was quite familiar to the media. At that time, any half-decent psychology student had a paperback of Ronnie Laing in their back pocket.'[7]

Faced with this onslaught of criticism from both without and within, orthodox psychiatry clearly needed a defender – if, in fact, there was anything still worth defending. In 1951, Dr David Stafford-Clark, an English psychiatrist, had written an influential account of contemporary psychiatry titled *Psychiatry Today* (1952), largely defending conventional practice.[8] Stafford-Clark was a popular broadcaster and media psychiatrist in his day, but his credibility diminished sharply over the years as he slipped into media overexposure and lost the peculiar combination of intimacy, focus and academic gravitas required to sustain such a complex public role.[9] By the late 1960s and early 1970s, it was clear that a new voice was needed.

A New Voice

Following his graduation in 1966, as he trained in New York, Dublin and London, Clare became increasingly aware that an updated defence of psychiatry was now an urgent necessity. Such a defence needed to not only address psychiatry's critics but also articulate all that was positive about psychiatry, acknowledge the weaknesses of the discipline (although not at the expense of its strengths) and note both the imperfections and the promise of what was still a relatively new branch of medicine.

In this way, the idea underpinning Clare's single greatest contribution to psychiatry was born and, in 1976, a mere ten years after he graduated, Clare's defining book was published, *Psychiatry in Dissent: Controversial Issues in Thought and Practice.*[10] The book arrived with a foreword by Professor Michael Shepherd, professor of epidemiological psychiatry at the Institute of Psychiatry in the University of London, with whom Clare worked. Anthony Mann, a colleague of Clare, emphasises that Shepherd was 'a very positive influence on Tony' during this period:

> [Shepherd] knew just how far to go with his sarcasm to challenge you how to do better. *Psychiatry in Dissent* was Tony's big step forward although Shepherd, as per usual, having provided study leave for him to do it, still referred to it as 'Dr Clare's little book'. *Psychiatry in Dissent* was great, perfect for teaching anyone who needed the contradictions in psychiatry to be explained.[11]

At the time of publication, Clare was a research worker with Shepherd at the Institute of Psychiatry in London, honorary senior registrar at the Bethlem and Maudsley Hospitals, and just 33 years of age.

Originally conceived as part of a textbook, Clare's lucid, incisive and endlessly compassionate text became an immediate classic.[12] In it, Clare explored the concept of psychiatric diagnosis in considerable depth and pointed out, among other things, the importance of diagnostic classification systems in protecting people from being labelled as mentally ill for purposes of societal or political convenience. He provided clear-headed, pragmatic discussions on schizophrenia, ECT and psychosurgery, as well as a fascinating chapter on responsibility and involuntary psychiatric admission.[13] These were all controversial topics, carefully and systematically examined in nuanced, measured tones by Clare.

Clare argued that it was unhelpful to conceptualise normality and madness as dichotomous, and better to see them as points on a continuum. He cautioned against too crisp a divison between 'organic' (biological) and 'functional' (mental) disorders, a warning that remains as relevant in the twenty-first century as it was in 1976.[14] Most of all, *Psychiatry in Dissent* provided psychiatry with a clear, logical and persuasive response to its critics from the 1960s and 1970s. Over four decades later, it still merits and rewards close reading.

Clare's daughter Rachel recalls that Clare 'sacrificed quite a lot to do that book':

> We remember falling asleep to the sound of the typewriter. In later years, when he was writing in his study, I remember Simon and I saying we would never live like that – as children, you can't see the enjoyment, the internal reward that comes from that kind of work. Dad would eat, go back to the typewriter, watch television with us, and then go back to typewriter again. I think in another life he might have liked to be a journalist.[15]

Following Clare's death in 2007, Professor Peter Tyrer, editor of the *British Journal of Psychiatry*, recalled not only Clare's intellect, logic and charm, but also the period when Clare was working on *Psychiatry in Dissent*.[16] Tyrer was completing his MD (*Medicinae Doctor* or Doctor of Medicine) thesis at that time and both Tyrer and Clare had the same secretary working for them on their projects, out of hours. Tyrer later told Clare that he was not using his academic abilities sufficiently, given Clare's myriad different interests, but also acknowledged that Clare was such an excellent communicator that it was the right thing for him and for psychiatry to allow his talent for communication to flourish.

And, if *Psychiatry in Dissent* proved anything, it was that communication in psychiatry was more than *just* communication: good communication could redefine and revitalise an entire field. This was much needed in the 1970s because psychiatry was then – and arguably still is – the medical discipline that generates the highest level of dissent, both from inside and outside the profession: no other medical discipline, for example, has some of its own members consistently argue that its very foundations are rooted in a series of harmful myths and that the illnesses it treats do not exist – as Szasz had argued over a decade before *Psychiatry in Dissent* appeared and continued to argue for many decades to follow, despite the increasing untenability of his position.[17]

The best responses to the types of criticism levelled by Szasz and his companions identify the core concerns of the critics, dissect their most relevant arguments dispassionately, and develop ways to integrate useful suggestions with existing knowledge so as to advance the field in a pragmatic, sensible, democratic and still evidence-based fashion. Such constructive responses to controversy are very rare but *Psychiatry in Dissent* is one of them and it deserves close attention as a result.[18]

Controversy, Commentary, Reason

Clare started *Psychiatry in Dissent* by focusing on the concept of mental illness and addressing the criticisms of psychiatric diagnosis and classification presented by Szasz, Laing and Foucault, among others. Clare acknowledged the problems presented by psychiatric classification and explored several diagnostic dilemmas that illustrated the limitations of existing systems, including the case of a 16-year-old boy who was described as aggressive, disruptive and remorseless, but did not show signs of affective or psychotic disturbance. Clare noted that in this case most psychiatrists would consider a diagnosis of personality disorder, but there would be significant disagreement over whether or not the person is actually ill. He might be disturbed or unhappy, but is he *ill*?[19]

In the early twenty-first century, some four decades after *Psychiatry in Dissent* appeared, the values of specific psychiatric classifications continue to be debated within the profession, often centred on cases such as the one Clare outlined in 1976. Indeed, many of the issues highlighted by him have, arguably, become more acute in recent years following the emergence of such novel diagnostic categories as 'dangerous severe personality disorder', the societal and legal convenience of which appear to substantially exceed their clinical provenance.[20] We still need, perhaps, more of the dissent advocated by Clare.

Clare's explicit defence of psychiatric classification in *Psychiatry in Dissent* was a clear reflection of the turbulent times in which the book first appeared, when psychiatry was facing radical criticism in relation to such fundamental issues as the validity of the concept of mental illness and the usefulness of classification. These debates, once a dominant feature of psychiatric discourse, have, over the intervening decades, become more measured but at the same time more peripheral. This is attributable to a number of factors, including the evolution of classification systems that are designed as diagnostic and research tools rather than absolute systems.[21] While there is still much research to be done, classification systems at least help to ensure that we all know what we are talking to each other about, if only in general terms.

Another defence of diagnosis and classification offered in *Psychiatry in Dissent* was that, contrary to the claims of the anti-psychiatry movement, clinically based classification systems *protect* the individual from being labelled mentally ill for purposes of societal or political convenience.[22] Someone can be diagnosed with mental illness only if they have certain symptoms or signs, and this protects the dissident and the outsider from being inappropriately labelled as ill, Clare argued.

In the decades since *Psychiatry in Dissent* first appeared, the importance of Clare's defence of clinical classification has been demonstrated again and again, particularly in the context of the alleged labelling of political dissidents as mentally ill in the former Soviet Union in the 1970s and 1980s[23] and more recently in the People's Republic of China.[24] Robust diagnostic and classification systems facilitate accountability and responsibility in diagnosis and treatment, not least in involuntary care.

At the same time, although generally defending the usefulness of the concept of disease entities, Clare warned that it was an error to see normality and mental illness as dichotomous, and it was better to see them as opposite ends on a continuum, with most of us located in the large grey area in the middle.[25] When these words were written, the idea of a continuum of illness had a long history in relation to mood disorders (e.g. depression, bipolar disorder), but the subsequent forty years have produced considerable evidence of another, less obvious, continuum in relation to the psychoses, based on increasing evidence of the surprisingly common occurrence of psychotic and quasi-psychotic phenomena (such as hearing voices) in the general population who do not meet the formal criteria for psychotic illness such as schizophrenia.[26] In other words, many people hear voices, but not all are ill: there is a continuum of experience in this and many other regards, just as Clare argued in 1976.

Focusing further on the ways in which clinicians conceptualise psychological disorders, Clare argued that it was no longer possible to identify any disease or state as being *either* psychological *or* physical. A condition such as anxiety could equally be described in psychological terms such as terror and fear, or in physiological terms like nervous system function or hormonal systems. Required, for practical reasons, to use one set of terms or the other, psychiatrists inadvertently created the impression that there were two distinct kinds of disease: psychological or functional and physical or organic.[27] This simply was not the case.

Even today, more than four decades after Clare made this point, the misleading distinction between 'psychological' and 'physical' phenomena remains as unhelpful as it was in 1976, and it still supports a false dichotomy between mind and brain that distorts perceptions of mental illness.[28] We are embodied human beings; our brains are parts of our bodies and we cannot separate the two.

Conflict, Discussion, Dissent

Throughout *Psychiatry in Dissent*, Clare did not shy away from contrary arguments or awkward positions, and did not hesitate to acknowledge the relative merits of conflicting approaches to different issues. Today there may be less fundamental dissent about issues such as the validity of the concept of mental illness or the overall usefulness of psychiatric classification, but there remains an active critical psychiatry movement based on ideas that continue to challenge and illuminate many controversial areas within psychiatry.[29] As Clare understood, dissent remains a key path to progress.

There is, in addition, also increased concern today about various other specific issues, such as the effects of the pharmaceutical industry on psychiatric practice[30] and the merits or operational validity of particular diagnostic categories in clinical care.[31] Clearly, the reasoned, logical and balanced approach to conflict and dissent, reflected in Clare's 1976 text, is still as necessary and relevant as ever.

Moreover, even though some of the themes of conflict have changed over the past forty years, many of the specific topics explored in *Psychiatry in Dissent* remain very relevant in the early twenty-first century, albeit in different ways. For example, Clare's discussion of psychosurgery in children as young as 5 years now serves as a strong defence of contemporary models of evidence-based medicine, even though Clare was writing some twenty years before the recurring concept of evidence-based medicine enjoyed its most recent renaissance.[32] Clare's comments on schizophrenia also serve as a poignant reminder of how little has changed in certain areas, as it broadly remains the case that, despite certain advances in understanding, the origins of this condition remain largely mysterious and the suffering it causes is often very great.[33] While treatments have improved, a cure is still sought.

Finally, in an era when much psychiatric debate is still characterised by confrontation rather than engagement,[34] and psychiatric training is increasingly based on characterless, vapid multi-author texts, *Psychiatry in Dissent* serves as an affirmation of the ability of the thoughtful individual psychiatrist to make sense of the controversies that rage within the field. It is also a testament to the importance of applying recent advances in thought and practice to the development of models of patient care that are equitable, acceptable, evidence-based and, most of all, effective. Clare's calm, logical approach to controversy and care is his book's most lasting legacy.

The value of *Psychiatry in Dissent* was recognised immediately following publication. In May 1976, just prior to the book's appearance, Angela Neustatter wrote in the *Guardian* that Clare's upcoming book was 'likely to take psychiatry by storm', and that

Clare felt contemporary psychiatry was a 'shambles', a 'mess' and 'at a very primitive level':

> [Clare is] volatile and angry at the state of chaos which he blames on an unwillingness within the profession to meet and discuss ideas, an omission very disturbing for the public and destructive to the profession. He talks quickly, the words hopscotching over each other to complete sentences; arms flail the air like windmill blades in a force nine gale.
>
> He does not expect to receive bouquets from his colleagues for this effort; rather he is waiting, like a medieval villain in the stocks for an onslaught of abuse.[35]

Clare had, however, underestimated the appetite for change among his colleagues: the 'onslaught of abuse' he expected never came. Fellow psychiatrist Professor Sir William Trethowan in the *British Medical Journal* found much to think about in *Psychiatry in Dissent* and noted with approval that Clare dealt thoroughly with Szasz, presented reasoned discussions of ECT and psychosurgery, and covered important topics with a clear grasp and a gift for sharing his understandings with others.[36]

Clare's book was widely reviewed in the professional literature, generally, although not exclusively, positively; one reviewer felt that the book did not devote sufficient attention to clinical studies, biochemistry or psychoanalysis.[37] Clare's communication skills came in for widespread praise and most reviewers agreed with the *Canadian Journal of Psychiatry* that *Psychiatry in Dissent* addressed many of the most important controversial issues in contemporary psychiatry and that Clare's presentation style kept the reader interested for the most part.[38]

Peter Sedgwick in the *Guardian* described *Psychiatry in Dissent* as a 'liberal riposte to the last ten years' anti-psychiatric and radical campaigning against mental medicine'.[39] Sedgwick, a revolutionary socialist activist whom Clare discussed in *Psychiatry in Dissent*[40] and who later authored *PsychoPolitics*,[41] found much to praise in

Clare's book, including Clare's criticism of inadequate psychiatric facilities. Sedgwick felt that Clare underestimated the importance of lay alternatives such as the Samaritans, the National Schizophrenia Fellowship or the Mental Patients' Union, possibly owing to Clare's 'medical loyalties':

> However, an individualistic training like that in medicine or psychology is bound to leave some traces of non-dialectical thought in its wake. Clare's book is a courageous journey into dissent which one senses may be just beginning to define itself. Latent within it is a critique of a social order which continually summons us out to perform on the high wire of competitive striving, and then chops away at the last remaining safety net if we ever falter and crash.

In *The Irish Times*, journalist and novelist Maeve Binchy interviewed Clare about *Psychiatry in Dissent* in June 1976 and wrote that he 'wanted lay people to read it, since psychiatry has always had the reputation of attracting the eccentric, the charlatan and the faith healer. His intention was to make people less confused, to point out that no branch of psychiatry has yet unlocked the key to human behaviour, but that great advances are being made down a lot of different paths. It's because there are so many paths, that he called the book *Psychiatry in Dissent*.'[42]

Long-term Impact

In the months and years following its publication, *Psychiatry in Dissent* featured regularly in public and professional discussions about mental illness and its treatment.[43] Later in 1976, Clare wrote an article in the *Nursing Mirror and Midwives Journal* with the same title, 'Psychiatry in dissent', arguing that this was a period of crucial change in psychiatric nursing.[44] The book's reputation also grew steadily within the psychiatric profession as a second edition appeared in 1980 and was reprinted repeatedly, festooned with praise from *The Sunday Times*, the *Times Higher Education Supplement*, and the *Journal of*

Analytical Psychology.[45] The *Journal of the Royal College of General Practitioners* said it was a joy to read.[46]

Over the following decades, *Psychiatry in Dissent* was routinely discussed by psychiatrists in the popular 'ten books' series in the *British Journal of Psychiatry*, praised as generally excellent,[47] good-humoured and eloquent,[48] and exerting a powerful impact on an entire generation of psychiatrists.[49] In 2016, forty years after the first edition appeared, Dr Trevor Turner paid fulsome, forthright tribute to a book that had clearly stood the test of time and, far from prompting a torrent of abuse, had boosted psychiatrists' morale at a time when morale had been affected by various historical issues, criticisms from sociology, and general disbelief in mental illness.[50] To counter this, Clare argued clearly in favour of psychiatry, saying that mental illnesses such as schizophrenia really did exist, and that diagnosis and hospitalisation were acceptable interventions for people who could not look after themselves.

For Professor Sir Simon Wessely, later President of the Royal College of Psychiatrists (2014–17), Regius Professor of Psychiatry at King's College London (2017) and President of the Royal Society of Medicine (2017–20), it was Clare who persuaded him that psychiatry was worthwhile after all.[51] Four decades after *Psychiatry in Dissent*, Wessely is still clear why the book had such an impact: 'It was the *ideas*. The book showed that psychiatry was a place where things happened and I never changed my mind on that.'[52] And Clare made it all seem so logical: 'normal intelligent people without any technical knowledge could take part in these debates in psychiatry', unlike in neurosurgery, for example, which was too technical a topic for most people.

Wessely emphasises Clare's gift as a communicator and recalls his after-dinner speech at the 750th anniversary of Bethlem Royal Hospital in 1997: Clare's delivery was a model of 'humour, timing and irony', with at least one prominent psychiatrist falling from his chair with uncontrolled laughter. Clare 'was a kind man, a superb teacher, literary, well read, and with a sense of humour. He made you feel good about being a psychiatrist and was the kind of person you so look forward to meeting. It made your day.'

Professor Tom Fahy, Consultant Psychiatrist and Professor of Forensic Mental Health at King's College London, recalls the influence of Clare on an entire generation of psychiatrists:

> He was an inspiration to me and to many of my peers when we decided to train as psychiatrists. I spent my prize money from a medical school case presentation competition on a copy of *Psychiatry in Dissent*. This book created an atmosphere of excitement at entering a controversial, multifaceted profession. Most of the cohort of trainees who started psychiatry at the Maudsley in the late 1980s were similarly inspired.[53]

Clare himself later commented that the book was 'all about avoiding extending psychiatry, making it a mass business, making it say things about war, pollution, prostitution. It's a warning about what happens to psychiatrists – I read it every now and then!'[54]

'There is Still an Enormous Conceptual Problem'

For these and other reasons, *Psychiatry in Dissent* remained prominent in the psychiatric literature for many decades following its publication in 1976[55] and featured strongly in Clare's citation when he finally, reluctantly accepted honorary fellowship of the Royal College of Psychiatrists in 2007.[56] Four years later, Professor David Cunningham Owens pointed out that, despite the book's undoubted strengths, some of the arguments in *Psychiatry in Dissent* might benefit from reworking,[57] a point anticipated by Clare in 2005, when he wrote (in a letter to one of the authors of this book) that 'some of the debates of the 1960s [discussed in *Psychiatry in Dissent*] do indeed take on a different perspective' today (in 2005):

> When I was defending the emphasis on classification, for example, I never anticipated a situation whereby a preoccupation with classification bordering on the obssessional would develop and that arguments of a religious intensity would surround such

dubious concepts as borderline personality or that concepts such as rapid cycling [bipolar disorder] and ADHD [attention deficit hyperactivity disorder] would grow so elastically. Now I might be somewhat more sympathetic to Szasz's argument about the medicalisation of problems of living and the subjectivity of psychiatric descriptions.

I had forgotten that I had favoured the continuum notion of mental health/mental illness but [am] relieved that I did! As I get older, I worry increasingly at the implicit assumption that those of us helping are perfectly sound psychologically while those we help are ill and there is a gulf between us.

Now I feel there are new controversial issues that have taken over from such concerns as the existence of mental illness and the efficacy of ECT. I think of the remorseless psychiatrisation of so much of human experience – with the diagnostic looseness of notions such as depression, rapid mood cycling, post-traumatic stress and attention deficit disorder. I think of the laughable use of words such as caring and community in systems and programmes that relate to neither. I think of the pusillanimous stance of the psychiatric profession in the face of the persistent neglect of the mind in political planning and in particular education, health and social services – our too ready acceptance of, in Ireland for example, skeletal child psychiatric services, primitive long-term facilities for the elderly and lamentable numbers of skilled non-medical professional staff such as psychologists, behaviour therapists and psychotherapists.

I remain concerned about the seemingly irresistible tendency on the part of human beings to dichotomise – in psychiatry this leads to an incorrigible desire to assign primacy to this or that cause – biological over psychological – when the evidence such as it is suggests a more systems-appreciation might well be more defensible.

I am uneasy about the extent to which psychiatry – here [in Ireland], in the UK, the US and elsewhere – tacitly accepts widespread inequalities in service provision. I believe it is a right that a person has a degree of choice in the selection of a doctor.

Other issues remain – the dreadful role psychiatry has played in draining the Third World of valuable and expensively trained doctors, the quite pathetic way that we psychiatrists endorse each and every product from the pharmaceutical industry ... This is not to say that newer drugs are not to be welcomed – but could we not by now have developed a more sober process of welcome? There is the inexorable process of 'professionalisation' whereby a simple treatment, relatively easy to learn and efficient and effective in application, such as cognitive behaviour therapy, is remorselessly turned into an educational industry and becomes something that can only be practised after a lengthy, expensive and 'approved' training. The effect: very few practitioners on the ground and treatment for equally few.

The fact that the universities have utterly reneged on their original historical remit as temples of learning and now are just money raising training centres has not helped. Other issues of dissent? Many but I must stop or you will never get this letter!

In short, I believe there are still plenty of grounds for dissent within psychiatry but there seems less appetite within the profession (no shortage outside it) to engage in it. You and your colleagues live at a most interesting time [2005] and, if I live long enough, I will watch the outcome with interest![58]

Clare 'was often tempted to write a follow-up' to *Psychiatry in Dissent* but 'never got round to it':

Of the issues raised in the book some thirty years ago the one that perhaps worries me most now concerns the issue of 'dichotomies'. I know that theoretically there is so much emphasis on multi-axial approaches [to diagnosis] and you rightly draw attention to the evidence [in] support of a more dimensional way of thinking,[59] but I am afraid what I never foresaw back in the 1970s was the massive swing in the United States away from the dogma of psychoanalysis to the dogma of DSM [*Diagnostic and Statistical Manual of Mental Disorders*]![60] It may well be that in years to come people will look back at the age of the American empire and one of the manifestations of it will be the domination of international classification by American ways of thinking. I know ICD [*ICD-10 Classification of Mental and Behavioural Disorders*][61] makes a spirited WHO [World Health Organisation] defence but in fact DSM is at the moment all conquering. With the rise of the Chinese empire who knows what kind of psychiatric classification our successors and yours too will be working with in thirty or forty years time!

There is a book to be written about the current controversies in psychiatry ... There is still an enormous conceptual problem regarding psychiatric illness. For example, I no longer say to patients that psychiatric illness is 'the same' as any other illness. Of course it is not and it has been a cheap and shoddy lie to pretend that it is. It is like equating the brain with the heart or the liver or the lungs.

Psychiatric ill health strikes at the very heart of our humanity. It affects our reasoning, our perceptions, our thought processes, our very identity. Anyone, and that includes most of us, who have suffered from time to time the terrifying experience of being out of control, psychologically speaking, knows that it is in a completely different domain from physical ill health.

That is why the stigma concerning psychiatric illness exhibits such robustness. That is why there is such fear and denial and rejection. The medical profession unwittingly, it seems to me, actually ferments such a view by relentlessly insisting on the differences between the ill and the healthy, rather than the similarities. Perhaps I will write something on these issues but at the present time [2006] I have other things preoccupying me and this will have to wait.[62]

Psychiatry in Dissent was, in many ways, a perfect distillation of the strengths and character of its author: fluent, thoughtful, witty and provocative. It provided a robust riposte to Goffman, Foucault, Szasz and Laing, and it restored the credibility of psychiatry in the eyes of the public and, perhaps most of all, in the eyes of psychiatrists themselves.

This was and still is an important task that rarely receives the attention it merits. While Stafford-Clark's 1952 *Psychiatry Today*[63] was comprehensively eclipsed by Clare's *Psychiatry in Dissent* in 1976, it was not until 2013 that another substantive volume explored and explained psychiatry, warts and all, for public and professional audiences, in Professor Tom Burns's *Our Necessary Shadow: The Nature and Meaning of Psychiatry*,[64] which proved a worthy successor to Clare's work. Burns recalls Clare as 'a central figure in UK psychiatry when I was training':

> [Clare] projected a coherent and attractive image of psychiatry, one that was intellectually stimulating and humane but also clear headed and honest about what we did and did not know. It was enormously important that he was so high profile in the media. I guess now we would call him a celebrity but it meant that people took us seriously and that the psychiatric voice was heard where it matters. How we could do with that voice now. How would he comment on reports of 75 per cent of students having 'mental health issues' or the rate of methylphenidate prescribing going through the roof? Eloquent, witty, but undeniably authoritative and sensible, I'm sure his charm would puncture the hubris of so many current commentators and anchor discussions in clinical reality.
>
> I invited him to come and talk about 'Psychiatry and the Media' in one of our monthly academic meetings at St George's [Hospital Medical School, London] in the 1980s. In my letter I commented that he was probably fed up with endless such requests and might want to choose another topic. He replied that he had never been asked to talk at a psychiatric meeting on the topic, would be delighted to, and gave a bravura performance. He didn't say, but I'm sure he knew that it was envy that got in the way.[65]

While demystifying psychiatry in the media and even within the profession itself can seem like a Sisyphean task, *Psychiatry in Dissent* not only demonstrated the value of such an undertaking, but also legitimised public engagement as an essential academic pursuit if psychiatry was to develop as a vital branch of medicine and a key element in the public health of nations.

For this, we have Clare to thank.

4

Psychiatrist, Scientist, Professor
(1976–89)

••••••••••••••••••••••••••••••••••••••

For most of the 1970s the Clare family lived contentedly on Monks Orchard Road opposite Bethlem Royal Hospital. They then moved to Whitmore Road, also in Beckenham, where they stayed until December 1984.[1] Clare particularly liked the new house. As Rachel recalls, he even turned his hand to DIY, helping to put cork tiles down, and renovating his study in the midst of his busy professional and family lives. Later:

> Dad commuted to work in the car and dropped us kids to school (at Alleyn's School on Townley Road). He'd come to plays, watch my brother's cricket matches, that kind of thing. Family holidays were very important, the focus of the year: everyone got into the car, and we headed off to Italy or France, with minimal preparation.
>
> Dad was very, very funny. He had a strong anti-authoritarian streak, so he loved *Private Eye*, and was always doing impressions of our headmasters, encouraging us not to take 'the establishment' seriously. We would all watch *Spitting Image*, *(Not) The Nine O'Clock News*, *Blackadder*. He made up some great stories on holiday, on long car journeys these would mutate into sketches that involved all of us as different characters, we would be crying with laughter.

Peter, too, recalls that 'we went on amazing holidays on the continent. What a life we were given – incredible! Sometimes, we'd stay in Clogheen on Shelbourne Road [in Dublin], with my mother's parents. I have great memories of that too.'[2]

These were good times in London: a happy, breezy family life, Indian takeaways in the evenings, and weekend trips to the cinema. Clare loved London and had a mug bearing the words of Samuel Johnson on the mantelpiece at Whitmore Road: 'When a man is tired of London, he is tired of life.' Rachel recalls:

Being in London was a kind of freedom, because he felt he was always an outsider. He could look at what was going on around him, evaluate the culture and current events, without being at stake himself. In the UK, he always felt that separation.

Dad loved London, Paris, Florence, Rome – all the great cities. He really enjoyed taking us to them, spending time wandering the streets, sitting at a café taking in the atmosphere. I think he was positive about human endeavour, not in a rose-tinted way, but he was an optimist. He liked change and the new.[3]

Clare's professional career was moving on rapidly too. In 1976, the year in which *Psychiatry in Dissent* made its dramatic appearance, he commenced a six-year period working and training at the General Practice Research Unit of the Institute of Psychiatry in London, working chiefly with Professor Michael Shepherd (1923–95), who wrote the foreword to *Psychiatry in Dissent*. Clare held positions as both researcher (1976–9) and senior lecturer (1980–2) in Shepherd's department. This period saw the emergence of two of Clare's key research interests (psychiatry in general practice and premenstrual tension) and a deepening of his involvement with popular media. But it was the figure of Shepherd that dominated Clare's professional development during this time, as the older man became yet another father figure with whom Clare developed a close, productive working relationship over many years.

Psychiatry and General Practice

Born in Cardiff, Michael Shepherd studied medicine at Oxford University Medical School and the Radcliffe Infirmary in Oxford.[4] He spent his entire career at the Maudsley in London, apart from a one-year attachment to the School of Public Health at Johns Hopkins University in Baltimore (1955–6). He was elected to a personal chair in epidemiological psychiatry at the Institute of Psychiatry in 1967, three years before Clare arrived there. Shepherd had a huge influence on the direction of Clare's research interests. As Murray notes, Clare 'worked for Michael Shepherd who did epidemiological research. So, Tony got into pre-menstrual tension and depression':

> Michael Shepherd was one of the major figures. The tradition of the Maudsley at that time was not to be very creative with new ideas but to puncture everyone else's ideas with data. Shepherd was someone who did surveys and David Goldberg, another protégé of Shepherd, produced the General Health Questionnaire [a method of psychiatric case identification].[5] Shepherd had a research unit funded by the Department of Health. He was also in charge of a clinical unit and appeared once a week, when the senior registrar would walk with him to the hospital – Shepherd in his white coat – which was unusual even in those days. There would be coffee and biscuits on the ward. Shepherd would meet a quivering member of the junior staff who knew he or she would be asked lots of questions about things he or she knew nothing about. Occasionally colleagues could be reduced near to tears by demands from Michael Shepherd. The function of the senior registrar was to protect the junior and mollify Shepherd.[6]

Anthony Mann, another colleague at the time, also recalls Clare's time with Shepherd:

> Tony and I were lecturers and then senior lecturers in Michael Shepherd's General Practice Research Unit. I joined in 1974,

two years before Tony. Shepherd was difficult with many of his consultant colleagues but captivating as a supervisor to Tony and me. He was caustic in his comments, but at the same time both very intelligent and shrewd.

I once gave a research paper to Shepherd for consideration for *Psychological Medicine* [a psychiatric journal with Shepherd as founding editor, from 1969 to 1993], and he stood in his doorway, saying 'How dare you submit something like this to me?' You either find that behaviour appalling or incredibly challenging. I found it the latter and was hooked. I had an indulgent family so I was attracted to a stringent father figure as supervisor.[7]

Clare fitted in well to Shepherd's unit, putting his full repertoire of clinical, academic and interpersonal skills to immediate and excellent use. He also maintained his personal links with the Dublin psychiatric community, presumably with an eye to returning there in the future.[8] But for now, Clare was utterly immersed in the London scene and, especially, the Institute of Psychiatry. As Murray notes:

Shepherd's unit had a rolling five-year grant. Tony would be exceptionally good at negotiating with the Department of Health for that grant [...] Shepherd liked being involved in controversy, but did not like to say things in public, so Tony would write them in articles. He was a front man for Shepherd and therefore had a much more equal relationship with Shepherd. Tony was very good at running the unit as Shepherd was a bit distant [...] The research focussed on the frequency of common disorders like anxiety and depression, aircraft noise and psychiatric disorder, PMS (Tony's area), and early intervention in psychosis (Ian Falloon[9] was just leaving at that time).[10]

Mann recalls Clare's ability to write 'beautifully' and the 'strange' atmosphere when working with Shepherd:

Shepherd was very hot on good English and Tony could write beautifully. Shepherd once said: 'It's funny having you and Dr

Clare on the unit: Dr Mann, you do good work but, reading your prose, no one would have a clue. On the other hand, there's Dr Clare ...' The atmosphere could be strange. We were situated along one corridor with Shepherd's office at the far end on the right. Shepherd went in in the morning, closed his door and never opened it till leaving for lunch and returning late afternoon.

To get to Shepherd you had to go through the office of his secretary, Michelle, whose affability meant that one chatted to her while waiting. She served as a conduit for gossip through to Shepherd who otherwise was completely out of the loop. There was also the office of Professor Denis Hill, the Head of Psychiatry, in the corridor.[11] Shepherd and he mutually disliked each other and avoided meeting. Tony and I, as Shepherd's senior lecturers, were dispatched to see him or the dean to deal with departmental business (grant signing, promotions, space, etc.) on Shepherd's behalf – being greeted not that jovially as the ambassadors.[12]

Consistent with Shepherd's research interests, which Clare increasingly shared, Clare published prodigiously on various aspects of psychiatry in general practice during his time at Shepherd's unit and afterwards. Clare's first paper on this theme appeared in 1978 in Shepherd's *Psychological Medicine* and concerned the 'design, development and use of a standardised interview to assess social maladjustment and dysfunction in community studies'.[13] Co-authored with Victoria E. Cairns, the paper presented a new interview to evaluate social maladjustment and dysfunction. The interview comprised items grouped under three headings: 'material conditions', 'social management' and 'satisfaction'. Interviewers made ratings on a four-point scale and the interview took approximately forty-five minutes to administer, covering housing, finance, occupation, social and leisure activities, and relationships with significant individuals in the patient's life. Clare and Cairns's paper examined the reliability of the interview, various methods of scoring, and its use in a number of studies in the setting of general practice. This rather technical paper was based on research initiated by Judith Sylph at the General Practice Research Unit directed by Shepherd. It clearly recognised the need for a reliable way to assess social functioning and adjustment in the relatively neglected fields of psychiatric care, social services, probation work and other areas.

Clare reprinted a version of the 1978 paper[14] in a 1979 book he co-edited with Paul Williams, lecturer at the Institute of Psychiatry, titled *Psychosocial Disorders in General Practice*.[15] For that volume, Williams and Clare wrote a preface in which they pointed out that twenty of the twenty-three papers in the book (including that by Clare and Cairns) had previously been published elsewhere, but they nonetheless felt that the recent explosion of interest in psychiatry in general practice justified collecting them into a single volume.[16] To reflect the balance between specialist psychiatry and general practice with immaculate even-handedness, the book had two forewords: one written by Shepherd, a psychiatrist at the Institute of Psychiatry,[17] and another by David Morrell, Professor of General Practice at St Thomas's Hospital Medical School in London.[18]

For their part, Williams and Clare introduced the book by noting the enormous burden psychiatric ill-health places on doctors working in general practice and social care services, and emphasising the centrality of the general practitioner in detecting psychiatric illness.[19] Later in the volume, Clare and Williams argued for a more systematic approach to research in this area focusing on two main themes: identifying psychosocial disorder (especially hidden psychiatric morbidity and people who do not consult general practitioners or who use non-medical coping strategies) and the management of psychosocial disorders with both medication and non-medication based approaches.[20]

Clare developed these themes at much greater length over subsequent years, writing in the *Journal of the Royal Society of Medicine* about 'community mental health centres' following a trip to the National Institute of Mental Health in Washington.[21] He argued with co-authors, including Paul Williams, that it was necessary to shift the focus of diagnosis of mental illness from hospitals into the community in order to address the very real problems faced by people with minor psychiatric disorder in their own communities.[22]

In 1981, the second edition of a book titled *Psychiatric Illness in General Practice* appeared, co-edited by Shepherd[23] and with a foreword by Aubrey Lewis,[24] who had a deep influence on both Shepherd[25] and Clare (Chapter 2).[26] The first edition had appeared in 1966[27] and, for the second edition, Shepherd and Clare added another rather technical update on recent developments in this field, focusing on questionnaires and standardised interviews for diagnosing mental illness in general practice and various issues relating to screening, sex differences (including premenstrual complaints), outcome studies, interventions and classification.[28]

The largest step forward in this field during that period, in which Clare played a pivotal role, occurred in September 1981 when the Mental Health Foundation held a conference in Oxford, and Clare co-edited the resultant book, which appeared in 1982, entitled *Psychiatry and General Practice*.[29] In the preface, Clare and his co-editor Malcolm Lader noted that the 1981 conference brought together people not only from psychiatry and general practice but also from the allied disciplines of social work, health visiting, community medicine, psychology, nursing and relevant divisions within the Department of Health and Social Security (which funded Shepherd's unit at the Institute of Psychiatry).[30] The conference dinner was addressed by Sir George Young, then Parliamentary Undersecretary of State for Health, who emphasised his department's commitment to community care and the need for government to be more sensitive to mental health issues.[31] This was also a recurring priority for Clare.

Clare's contribution to the 1981 conference and the 1982 book explored the problems of psychiatric classification in primary care, a theme that was, by now, a familiar one for him.[32] He also co-authored, with Karl Sabbagh, an account of an intriguing exercise that involved showing conference participants a video recording of a general practice consultation with a 44-year-old woman with symptoms of depression and various other problems.[33] One hundred and thirty six participants responded to three questions about the video, of whom fifty-nine were general practitioners, thirty-eight psychiatrists, and the remainder psychologists, social workers, sociologists, counsellors, community physicians, community psychiatric nurses, civil servants, medical journalists and lay people, as well as one probation officer and one 'health visitor'. Of general practitioners, 70 per cent made a tentative or definite diagnosis based on the video (mainly depression or anxiety), compared to 58 per cent of psychiatrists; 32 per cent of general practitioners recommended a 'reassurance, wait and see' approach with the patient, compared to 22 per cent of psychiatrists; and 15 per cent of general practitioners disapproved of the way the consultation was handled, compared to 32 per cent of psychiatrists.

The 1981 conference was a great success and the video exercise with the multi-disciplinary audience was heralded as groundbreaking in a 1984 review of the book in Shepherd's *Psychological Medicine*.[34] The review highlighted the overall importance of the conference and drew particular attention to the exemplary way that the conference material was treated and edited by Clare and Lader for the book.

Clare continued to work intensively in these thematic areas over the following years, co-writing a letter to the editor of the *British Medical Journal* in 1982 about the key role of 'health visitors' in identifying emotional problems and psychiatric ill-health in families,[35] and reporting, with colleagues, on a pilot study of a self-report questionnaire aimed at identifying social problems, difficulties and dissatisfactions in general practice.[36] In *The Practitioner* in 1983, he emphasised the value of the *consultation* in general practice, highlighting the importance of giving time to patients who are depressed or anxious, the use of various medications, and the role of other professionals in the primary care team.[37] He devoted particular attention to research about social adjustment and functioning,[38] and the importance of social workers providing emotional support and practical assistance to women with depression.[39]

All of these writings were suffused with Clare's deep awareness of the social context of psychological suffering and the need to move psychiatry away from hospitals and into people's lives in their communities. This was the first big theme of Clare's research career, as he studied, wrote and co-wrote voluminously about psychiatry in general practice[40] with a particular focus on depression and its treatment,[41] alongside other, more specific concerns in day-to-day care, such as the role of the general practitioner when people present with marital problems.[42] The overarching theme was Clare's emphasis on social as opposed to biological psychiatry, and the need to classify and understand mental disorders in a way that took account of people's lived experience of psychological suffering.

Murray notes that these themes in Clare's work were consistent with those of both Shepherd and Shepherd's own guiding light at the Institute of Psychiatry, Aubrey Lewis:

> Shepherd had been involved in the classificatory discussions with the ICD-9 [*International Statistical Classification of Diseases and Related Health Problems*],[43] so classification was very important at this time. We've become impatient with classification now. Tony did not live to see the re-engagement of biological psychiatry and social psychiatry. He was always on the social psychiatry front and was not wildly sympathetic to the latest advances in biological psychiatry. Biological psychiatry was not sufficiently sophisticated to engage him at that time. He was a classical social and epidemiological psychiatrist. He admired Aubrey Lewis.[44]

The next major research theme in Clare's career was, perhaps, less predictable but was nonetheless consistent with Lewis's general approach to psychiatry, Shepherd's emphasis on mental disorders outside of hospitals, and Clare's own concern with psychological suffering in the community, especially among women.

Premenstrual Syndrome

Between 1976 and 1980 Clare performed a detailed study of premenstrual syndrome that formed the basis of his thesis for the degree of Doctor of Medicine (MD) awarded to him by the National University of Ireland in 1980. When he graduated as a medical doctor at UCD in June 1966, Clare received the degrees of MB BCh BAO, the usual entry-level professional degrees for medical doctors in Ireland. MB BCh stands for *Baccalaureus in Medicina et in Chirurgia* (Bachelor of Medicine and Surgery) and BAO stands for *Baccalaureus in Arte Obstetricia* (Bachelor of Obstetrics). This is a basic medical degree in Ireland and it qualifies the bearer to practise as a medical doctor although further professional training usually follows.

In the United States, Canada and elsewhere, MD (*Medicinae Doctor* or Doctor of Medicine) is the equivalent of MB BCh BAO and is the basic entry-level first professional degree required to practise medicine in those jurisdictions. But the meaning of 'MD' varies internationally and in Ireland an MD is a postgraduate research degree in medicine, analogous to a PhD. (*Philosophiae Doctor* or Doctor of Philosophy). In Ireland, an MD is awarded upon submission of an original research thesis and, in some universities, a successful *viva* or oral examination. Clare received his MD from UCD in 1980 for his rather lengthy two-volume thesis titled 'Psychiatric and Social Aspects of Premenstrual Complaint'.[45]

Clare performed his research into premenstrual syndrome at the General Practice Research Unit of the Institute of Psychiatry under the guidance of Shepherd and with the assistance of Dr Clifford Kay, Chairman of the Research Committee of the Royal College of General Practitioners. Kay gave Clare access to the research register of the college and facilitated recruiting the twenty-five general practitioners involved in selecting the patient sample. Clare's sister, Wyn, helped with the preparation of figures, graphs and diagrams for Clare's thesis.

Clare started his MD thesis with a discussion and review of the literature regarding premenstrual syndrome, a condition with a long, complex and contested history. The first systematic medical description of premenstrual tension appeared in 1931[46] and one of the earliest uses of the term 'premenstrual syndrome' (as opposed to 'premenstrual tension') was in the *British Medical Journal* in 1953.[47] But Clare, of course, traced a much deeper history, drawing on epidemiology, medicine and science, as well as the work of writers such as August Strindberg, Anaïs Nin, Doris Lessing, William Faulkner, John Fowles and Fay Weldon. Clare would later (amicably) debate the merits of psychotherapy with Weldon at a public event in London in 1994,[48] but, back in 1980, his rather eclectic MD thesis was already classic Clare, taking a broad sweep across multiple disciplines before delving into the science.

The key purpose of Clare's research was to examine the relationship between premenstrual complaints and psychiatric morbidity. He hypothesised that women who complained of premenstrual symptoms would also have more psychiatric ill-health than those who did not complain of premenstrual symptoms. Clare included two groups of women in his work: 591 women attending general practitioners (of whom 521 were included in his final sample) and 170 women attending a special premenstrual tension clinic at St Thomas's Hospital, a teaching hospital in London. A range of interviews and assessments were performed and the following conclusions reached:

- There was a strong association between premenstrual complaints and psychiatric ill-health; i.e. women who complained of premenstrual symptoms also had more psychiatric ill-health than those who did not complain of premenstrual symptoms;
- Psychiatrically ill women with premenstrual symptoms reported more 'psychological' but not more 'physical' premenstrual symptoms than those who were not psychiatrically ill; more specifically, psychiatrically ill women with premenstrual symptoms experienced more depression, mood swings, tension, irritability, tiredness, confusion, crying spells, forgetfulness and taking naps, but did not experience more weight gain, headache, stomach pain, skin disorder, backache, feeling swollen or bloated, or painful or tender breasts, compared to women with premenstrual symptoms who were not also psychiatrically ill;
- In the general practice sample, fewer than 5 per cent of women reported absolutely no premenstrual symptoms, confirming that the vast majority of women experience at least some premenstrual symptoms;

- There was no overall association between premenstrual symptoms and social maladjustment, although there was an association between psychiatric ill-health and social maladjustment, chiefly relating to disturbances in social contacts and leisure activities;
- Premenstrual symptoms were associated with marital problems such as poor satisfaction with marital compatibility, poor marital harmony, and having few shared marital interests, activities, responsibilities or decisions; and
- There was no significant association between premenstrual complaints and lowered levels of progesterone in the premenstrual phase of the menstrual cycle or high levels of prolactin.

Discussing his findings, Clare argued that his work broke new ground by focusing on premenstrual complaints in general practice as opposed to hospital settings. In addition, Clare assessed psychiatric ill-health using the General Health Questionnaire[49] and premenstrual symptoms using the Modified Menstrual Distress Questionnaire,[50] two reliable, validated research tools, adding further to the strength of his work. In fact he designed and published a modified version of the latter tool in 1977 in the early phases of his research.[51]

Overall, Clare concluded that there was a significant association between psychological and behavioural premenstrual symptoms on the one hand, and psychiatric illness on the other, and a similar association between premenstrual symptoms and disturbances in marital function. He found no evidence that premenstrual symptoms were decreased by use of oral contraceptives. Most significantly, he reported that over 95 per cent of women attending general practitioners reported some level of premenstrual symptoms, although only 12 per cent reported levels like those seen in the specialist premenstrual tension clinic at St Thomas's Hospital.

Four decades after Clare was awarded the degree of MD, his thesis remains interesting for several reasons. From a scientific perspective, his work advanced the understanding of premenstrual symptoms significantly, highlighting their links with psychiatric illness and their ubiquity in women attending general practitioners. His detailed, almost obsessional methodology has also stood the test of time as he used various different interviews, multiple blood tests and detailed menstrual diaries, etc. From the outset, it was apparent that Clare took premenstrual syndrome seriously.

From a personal perspective, Clare's thesis demonstrated many of the features rapidly becoming characteristic of his work: elegant formulations of practical, unresolved issues in psychiatry, the use of literary references to set the scene more broadly and deepen understanding, and a focus on the lived experience of psychological problems and mental illness outside of specialist hospital settings. First and foremost, Clare was concerned with *people* – understanding the realities of their suffering and elucidating how such suffering impacted on their day-to-day lives.

Perhaps the most intriguing issue raised by Clare's MD, however, is why he chose to focus on premenstrual symptoms in the first place. In this context, it is important to note that most early-career researchers do not have full freedom to choose their research topics themselves and, because Clare worked in the General Practice Research Unit at the Institute of Psychiatry, his research was bound to focus on conditions that were common in the community. And, as Clare demonstrated in his MD, premenstrual symptoms were very common indeed, present in over 95 per cent of the women he studied.

In addition, Clare was always interested in human stories and his work on premenstrual syndrome allowed him to explore fully the stories of many of the participating women – not only their medical and psychiatric histories, but also their personal lives and social situations. In an appendix to his thesis, Clare duly presented detailed case histories of nine women with serious marital problems in order to illustrate the complex relationships between marital issues and the premenstrual symptoms they described.

One case concerned a 44-year-old woman, with a 13-year-old child, attending her general practitioner complaining of headaches during menstruation, along with tension, irritability and depression. Interviewed about possible social difficulties, the woman revealed significant marital problems with sexual compatibility and worries about the possibility of pregnancy. She was very defensive about these issues, but there was still plentiful evidence of considerable marital disharmony complicating her presentation to her general practitioner.

Another case concerned a 24-year-old mother of a 2-year-old boy attending her general practitioner with hay fever. On interview, this woman described premenstrual weight gain, cold sweats, feeling swollen, hot flushes and painful, tender breasts before her periods. Like the other patient, this woman described difficulties with sexual compatibility and family planning. She was not using any form of contraception and was worried about becoming pregnant. Her husband was anxious for a second child. In both of these cases, and many more, there appeared to be a link between marital problems and premenstrual disturbances, and Clare explored these issues fully both through these case histories and in the main body of his thesis.

Another reason why Clare chose to focus on premenstrual symptoms was likely his over-arching interest in relationships between women and men, and in the differences in gender-related hormones. This is evident not only in his MD thesis but also in many of his other research papers[52] and, most notably, his book *On Men: Masculinity in Crisis*, published in 2000.[53] Much of the public discussion of *On Men* centred on Clare's views about the relationships between women and men (Chapter 7) and this theme was also apparent in the emphasis on marital relationships in his MD thesis and his other publications concerning premenstrual syndrome in the late 1970s and 1980s.

Perhaps the final reason why Clare focused on premenstrual symptoms is a much simpler one: throughout his life, Clare was intrigued and, arguably, dominated by women. His wife, Jane, points out that Clare 'related better to women than to men'.[54] In a 2000 interview with Kathryn Holmquist in *The Irish Times* following the publication of *On Men*, Clare readily acknowledged that his life trajectory was shaped by strong, powerful women.[55] He had, according to Holmquist, 'a precedent for loving women with fight': Clare stated that his mother was 'argumentative' and 'stronger' than his father, with a 'fairly explosive temper' ('I was more afraid of my mother'); his childhood was dominated by his two older sisters (Wyn and Jeanne); and his wife, Jane, was 'the rock' upon whom he was 'utterly dependent'.

Holmquist reported that Clare 'says he gets on better with female patients than male ones'; 'female colleagues, too, have both engaged and informed him'; and 'a woman partly inspired the book [*On Men*]: Lesley Rees, to whom Clare refers often and generously', and whom he described as a 'very powerful' endocrinologist and former colleague at St Bartholomew's Hospital in London. Therefore, while the overall structure of Clare's professional life was dominated by a variably successful search for father figures (Moore at St Patrick's, Shepherd at the Maudsley), his day-to-day life was always dominated by the presence of women – and he liked it that way.

Back in the late 1970s, even as he prepared his MD thesis for submission in September 1980, Clare was – typically – already publishing scientific papers on themes relating to premenstrual symptoms.[56] In 1979, he published a paper in the *British Journal of Psychiatry* highlighting the current understanding of the condition and calling for better studies of symptom levels and treatment options.[57] He also explored specific aspects of premenstrual complaints in letters to the editors of the *British Medical Journal* in 1980[58] and *British Journal of Psychiatry* in 1981[59] (as letters to the editors of journals rapidly became one of Clare's favoured forms of publication: rapid, pithy, incisive).

More substantively, Clare published a lengthy paper on 'psychiatric and social aspects of premenstrual complaint' as a *Monograph Supplement* to Shepherd's *Psychological Medicine* in 1983.[60] The monograph was later reviewed in the same journal, noting that, notwithstanding Clare's contribution, there was still much more work to be done in this field.[61] Clare also published a paper on psychological aspects of premenstrual tension in a supplement to the *Irish Journal of Medical Science* in June 1983.[62] This paper stemmed from a symposium held by the Department of Obstetrics and Gynaecology at Trinity College Dublin on 19 June 1982 devoted to 'pelvic endometriosis and menstrual disorders', to which Clare contributed.

Clare wrote tirelessly on the subject over the following years, exploring 'the relationship between psychopathology and the menstrual cycle' in the journal *Women and Health* in 1983 (proposing a multifactorial model),[63] asking if there were 'single or multiple causes' for premenstrual symptoms in the *Canadian Journal of Psychiatry* in 1985 (he favoured multiple causes),[64] and reviewing the literature on hormones, behaviour and the menstrual cycle in the *Journal of Psychosomatic Research* in 1985, concluding that no specific hormonal abnormality had been consistently linked with premenstrual symptoms to date (consistent with his own MD work).[65] In 1984 Clare critically reviewed a book on behaviour and the menstrual cycle in the same journal[66] and in 1989 co-authored, with Roslyn H. Corney, a very useful overview of 'treatment of premenstrual syndrome' in *The Practitioner*, providing practical advice about managing the condition in general practice – always a key concern for Clare.[67]

Throughout all of these papers and reviews, Clare maintained a steady focus on understanding the complexity of premenstrual symptoms in women's lives and acknowledging the role of the personal and social circumstances in which such symptoms occurred. He was especially wary of explanations that attributed all premenstrual symptoms to detectable changes in hormones; the condition was, he felt, vastly more complex than that – a point he emphasised publicly in *The Times* in 1981.[68]

In 1985, Clare co-authored an especially outspoken leading article along these lines in the *British Medical Journal* with Rachel Jenkins, consultant in psychological medicine at Bart's.[69] Jenkins recalls her first meeting with Clare in the Junior Common Room at the Maudsley when she was elected secretary and her contemporary Marisa Silverman elected chairman.[70] Jenkins, then a registrar at the Maudsley, subsequently became Professor of Epidemiology and Mental Health Policy and Director of the WHO Collaborating Centre at the Institute of Psychiatry (1997–2012), having also worked as consultant and senior lecturer at Bart's (1985–7) and Principal Medical Officer at the Department of Health (1988–96). Clare 'came to vote for us'; he 'strode in to the meeting, simultaneously charming, captivating and elucidating the discussions on current Maudsley politics. My second early memory of [Clare] was in the Institute of Psychiatry small lecture theatre in fierce debate with Larry Gostin about what would become the Mental Health Act 1983, as ever, elucidating the issues with immense clarity and passion.'

Jenkins went on to work with Clare on a number of occasions over several years:

[Clare] was a brilliant and insightful colleague to have had the pleasure of working alongside ... both in the General Practice Research Unit, headed by Michael Shepherd, at the Institute of Psychiatry and later on at Bart's where he became Professor of Psychiatry for a number of years and I was senior lecturer for three of those years. On a personal level, conversations were always wide ranging, insightful and intellectually stimulating, and he had a very engaging and rather Celtic self-deprecating sense of humour. It was clear that his Jesuit education had been an enormous influence on his intellectual and personal development.

Like Michael Shepherd, he was very much a family man, devoted to his wife and children throughout his immensely busy working life. He was a multitasker par excellence, but with the inevitable consequence that he would frequently find himself double and triple booked, but was usually forgiven as his contributions when they came would be unfailingly helpful. One of the many practical things I learned from him was the therapeutic importance of clearing one's desk at the end of each week, however hectic and busy ... it cleared the head and saved one from totally drowning in the overload!

In their 1985 paper on 'women and mental illness' in the *British Medical Journal*, Jenkins and Clare argued that while sex differences in the rates of various illnesses (including psychological complaints) were traditionally linked to female biology, such a link was not supported by evidence and discussions of these topics needed to take greater account of differences between women and men in important social variables such as occupation, education and income.[71] They advised against attributing higher rates of depression in women to their reproductive biology or their constitution in general, and pointed instead to the importance of social and environmental factors.

This argument was highly consistent with Clare's MD work: not only did he report no consistent link between premenstrual complaints and specific hormones, but he found evidence to situate the syndrome firmly in the personal and social lives of women, demonstrating and articulating deep connections between premenstrual symptoms and the marital and social contexts in which women found themselves. In this way, Clare's early research work on premenstrual syndrome was not only academically and scientifically successful, yielding him an MD, multiple papers and professional recognition, but it also mapped onto one of the key themes that dominated so much of the rest of his career and personal life: understanding women.

Clare was especially outspoken about the position of women in society in a 1987 interview with Irish journalist and author Deirdre Purcell for the *Sunday Tribune*. Clare noted that 'society currently gives women a very difficult time, whether she is in a full-time career or not. For instance, society reinforces a man who devotes himself twenty-four hours a day to a job – indeed it's held up as a goal – whereas a woman who does that is regarded as quite seriously unbalanced':[72]

Professor Clare's considered view is that the women's movement, or the new consciousness, has had precious little actual effect beyond the boundaries of Fleet Street and the women's pages of the average Irish daily. 'There is very little evidence that women are beginning to penetrate real power, And there is no evidence that this new consciousness (where it is OK for a man to cry, for instance) has left any trace on personal behavior patterns.'

Clare did, however, see cause for hope in the next generation. At that point (in 1987), Clare and Jane had seven children, ranging in age from late teens to under two years: Rachel, Simon, Eleanor, Peter, Sophie, Justine and Sebastian. Clare was profoundly proud of all of them all his life, later remarking to Jane: 'You were right. My greatest achievement is our children.'[73] With Purcell in 1987, he said that the younger generation made him optimistic for the future:

> There is hope, however. 'I'm looking at my own kids (he has seven) – I think that's where there may be change. Our generation is the transition generation. We can't go on being like our parents. But the world has changed, even though we can't. Our children are picking up a new world – very complicated and disturbing, but new ...'

St Bartholomew's Hospital ('Bart's'), Smithfield (1983–9)

Following his years at the Maudsley (1970–6) and the Institute of Psychiatry (1976–82), Clare's next move was to St Bartholomew's Hospital ('Bart's') in Smithfield in central London. This is an especially historic part of the city and Clare fell in love with the district when he arrived there as Professor of Psychological Medicine in 1983.

At this point, Clare had spent six years at the General Practice Research Unit in the Institute of Psychiatry with Shepherd, from 1976 to 1982. He had applied unsuccessfully for a chair (professorship) of psychiatry in Bristol and had also applied for a chair in Trinity College, Dublin in 1977, but withdrew in favour of another candidate, Professor Marcus Webb. Rachel does not think that her 'father was especially concerned about academic progression. I know that as a younger man, he felt he was judged as lacking gravitas. There is a cultural assumption that to be professional, you need to be quite "dry" about your subject, quite detached. Dad was not dry, he was quite passionate, enthusiastic.'[74]

And, so, Clare remained in London where, in 1982, Robin Murray became Dean of the Institute of Psychiatry. Murray invited Clare to be Vice-Dean, based on Clare's persuasive skills and abilities, rather than his respect for bureaucracy:

> [Clare] was certainly hyperactive in the best sense. He would hope to convince people by the power of his argument, to sweep

them along. He wanted to get things done. He was hopeless with bureaucracy; he was not interested in the formal channels at all.[75]

Clare accepted Murray's offer, but ultimately it was time for Clare to move on from the Institute and so in 1983 he was appointed Professor and Head of Psychological Medicine at Bart's. Anthony Mann recalls that both he and Clare applied for the Chair at Bart's but Mann 'soon withdrew because they clearly wanted Tony', with his 'vivacity, enthusiasm and budding media career, to lead a department that was not inspiring at the time, certainly not for students. Tony was greatly liked by everyone in Bart's.'[76]

During these years, the Clares were particularly friendly with Professor (later Dame) Lesley Rees, professor of chemical endocrinology at Bart's and first woman dean of the medical school (1989–95), and her husband Mr Gareth Rees, a consultant cardiothoracic surgeon there. Clare was 'very fond of Lesley and Gareth', according to Rachel: 'He and Mum spent a lot of time with them. They had a lot of fun together. They came to the house a lot, and the family went for a few summer holidays to their place in Lucca' (a city in Tuscany, Italy).[77]

Bart's was a very venerable institution, founded in 1123 by the Anglo-Norman monk Rahere, a favoured courtier of King Henry I. Clare later wrote in some detail about the history of the hospital, noting that it found its roots in the visual hallucinations experienced by Rahere who fell ill on a journey to Rome to seek forgiveness for his sins, vowed to establish a hospital for the poor if he survived, and, on his return journey, had a vision of St Bartholomew.[78] Thus, Bart's.

Clare's medical predecessors at Bart's included such notable figures as William Harvey (1578–1657), an early advocate of the links between body and mind; Robert Gooch (1784–1830) who had a particular interest in insanity; George Burrows (1801–87) who linked mental illness with cardiac disease; James Paget (1814–99) who lectured in nervous diseases and said two of his brothers died of anxiety and overwork; Thomas Claye Shaw (1841–1927), the first formal lecturer in mental diseases at Bart's (1871–1909); and Erwin Strauss, who became lecturer in 1938, translated the work of Ernst Kretschmer (1888–1964) into English, and was an early advocate of ECT. All told, an illustrious group of people dedicated to advancing the treatment of mental illness.

In 1983, Clare was appointed as Professor ('Chair') and Head of Psychological Medicine at Bart's. As Murray notes, 'Bart's was one of the most desirable chairs to get at that time', and 'they wanted him at Bart's':

> For an academic career you need to be a good teacher and a standard bearer for psychiatry in your medical school and region. Tony was brilliant at that. He was very good as professor at Bart's. He got very good people at Bart's. Although he wasn't running an MRC [Medical Research Council] unit, he was good at spotting able young researchers. He was very good at Bart's in impressing the physicians and surgeons and getting them to take psychiatry seriously. He didn't have the interest in complex statistical analysis but was very good at stimulating other people to do research.[79]

Three years after Clare's appointment to Bart's, the 'major department research projects' of the Department of Psychological Medicine listed in the 1986 annual report clearly reflected Clare's interests: '1. Psychological aspects of physical disease. 2. Psychopharmacology. 3. Community psychiatry. 4. Psychiatric epidemiology. 5. Stress research.'[80] There was also a strong emphasis on teaching, although 'current manpower restrictions' hampered recruitment of lecturers in specific areas (e.g. drug dependence and psychogeriatrics).

Clare's public profile continued to grow during this period. *In the Psychiatrist's Chair* started in 1982, just before he went to Bart's, and grew steadily in popularity (Chapter 5), with the result that Clare was ever more present in the media. Dr (later professor) Ted Dinan worked with Clare as senior registrar and lecturer at Bart's in the 1980s and recalls that Clare's 'communication skills were second to none':

At the time, he was high profile, especially on TV. In all my time in psychiatry I have never met anyone who could interview a patient like Tony could. They would often provide information they would give to no one else. I also saw him handle hostile anti-psychiatry audiences and at the end of the session they would be completely won over by him. On one occasion I heard him speak on community psychiatry. The first two speakers were world authorities. I know for a fact Tony had nothing prepared. He listened carefully and when he spoke a neutral observer was definitely of the view that Tony was the world authority.[81]

Clare's authority only grew with time, as he was appointed to the general council of King Edward's Hospital Fund for London and, in 1987, identified by the *Sunday Times* as one of the 100 'powers that will be' in the 1990s.[82] Purcell's interview in the *Sunday Tribune* in 1987 described Clare as 'a compact, springy man in dark clothes with longish dark fine hair' and 'a huge briefcase to take home with him' from Bart's:

His office does have a couch – a bed really – but is dominated by a huge desk and decorated with family photographs. It is not a cosy place for a tête-à-tête. It is large and efficient, as befits a man who not only treats individuals but leads conferences, teaches his students, promotes research, writes papers and books – and who is also a media personality with his own series on the BBC [...] He is polite but patently bored with boring questions. He loves the variety of his work – as a university professor running a large department in a busy medical school, working with other physicians and surgeons, training junior psychiatrists, working on various committees ...[83]

Clare remained especially interested in psychiatric training throughout his career, even after his time with APIT (the Association of Psychiatrists in Training) ended.[84] In 1979 he co-authored, with Murray and others, a study of seventy-nine junior psychiatrists in the

Maudsley, noting a shift from a psychoanalytical to a biological model of psychiatry with increasing psychiatric experience.[85] The paper concluded that an interest in psychoanalysis appeared to be antipathetic to the development of scientific attitudes conducive to research. Clare was also highly regarded as a teacher at St Patrick's Hospital in Dublin after he returned as medical director in 1989 and is remembered as a hugely positive influence on trainees in psychiatry.[86]

Although not a psychoanalyst, Clare told Purcell in 1987 that he saw some value in the work of Sigmund Freud and drew a comparison between obsessive disorders and religious belief:

> In some respects, I think Freud was close to the truth. We have turned some religions into obsessional neuroses, where, if we don't obey certain things, terrible things will happen to us. If we don't put five coins of appropriate mintage into our right pockets, God will strike us ... if we don't obey the laws of God, He will visit AIDS on us ... There's a terrible lot of superstition involved which I see as a doctor.[87]

Working in Bart's from 1983 to 1989, Clare saw people from many different cultural and religious backgrounds, but was initially 'reluctant to discuss his own faith' with Purcell:

> But despite his reluctance, he does discuss it. 'I suppose I believe in a God in the sense that there *is* a point and a purpose to human existence.' However, he is 'much more shaky' on whether or not God intervened historically and inserted His Son at an historical moment. Neither does he believe that it is worth sacrificing major efforts to make this life better, in the fervent expectation of a better afterlife. 'I've seen people get to the end of their days and confront the possibility that maybe there isn't an afterlife ... and not drawing consolation – which I think is all that Christianity is about [...].

In Ireland we have got terribly hung up on the relationship between Christianity and morality. We have turned Christ's message into a series of prohibitions every bit as hard and fast as the fundamentalists in America. What Jesus had to say about abortion. What Jesus had to say about homosexuality. What Jesus had to say about women priests. What Jesus had to say about working women. All of this is appalling. Monstrous. Jesus had precious little to say about any of those things ...'

Clare told Purcell that Christianity was not about prohibitions, but about 'love and acceptance', and this was clearly expressed through – of all things – the NHS in the UK, where he now worked:

Christianity, *per se*, however, has made a 'noble contribution' to human existence, with its message of love and acceptance and loving one's neighbour, which was really a revolutionary idea. Take the National Health Service, for instance. Most people do not realise that this system is not a Lefty imposition but a Christian one. 'The British may not realise this – neither do the Irish – but the progenitors of the National Health Service were all stout Victorian Christians, who realised that we all had responsibility for our fellow man and the poor in particular. Some of that is lost, I notice, in current Irish discussion about the responsibility of the state – the state is nothing more in a sense than the personalised will of the community.'[88]

Rachel recalls her father's awareness of the social inequalities he witnessed in his clinical work:

Dad always made it very clear to us that we were very privileged. He was keen to emphasise the struggles faced by many of his patients in Hackney; that many of them were experiencing not mental illness, but a sane response to a difficult situation. He wanted us to be aware of how lucky we were, how random life

could be for people ... He was also very proud of working for the
NHS. With all its flaws, he felt it was a great social achievement
and something to be defended. He resisted private practice for
many years, he felt everyone was entitled to the same treatment
on the same basis.[89]

As is apparent from his *Sunday Tribune* interview with Purcell,
Bart's provided Clare with not only his first major academic position
as a head of department, but also a base from which to pursue his
myriad other interests ranging from writing to broadcasting, and from
researching to commentating in the media on matters as diverse as
mental health, religion, politics and the position of women in society.[90]
Within the hospital community, Clare was popular with medical and
surgical colleagues, joining with them to write to the *Lancet* in 1986
objecting to the proposed removal of preclinical medical education
from purpose-built facilities close to the clinical school at Bart's to a
location some four miles away.[91] He continued to stand by Bart's in
future years.[92] On this and more or less every other issue that raised
its head, Clare was tireless, opinionated and never afraid to express his
view.[93]

From a research perspective, in addition to his own work,
Clare became involved with field trials of new proposals for the WHO's
ICD-10 Classification of Mental and Behavioural Disorders which
appeared in 1992.[94] This is the WHO's international standard diagnostic
tool for epidemiology, health management and clinical purposes. Clare
assisted with initial drafts of the diagnostic classification system and
guidelines, which are still in use today. This work was highly consistent
with the importance that Clare placed on accurate, flexible diagnosis
in *Psychiatry in Dissent* in 1976,[95] and this remained a key research
interest throughout Clare's career, even after he left Bart's to return to
Dublin in 1989.[96] This also fitted with Clare's prolonged involvement
with the Health Education Council (later Authority) in the United
Kingdom.[97] Clearly, psychiatric diagnosis needed to be reliable,
systematic and compassionate – and Clare was determined to play his
part to make it so.

Writing, Writing, Writing

During the 1970s and 1980s at the Institute of Psychiatry and Bart's, Clare wrote rapidly, voluminously and insightfully on a broad range of topics in both popular and professional publications. His move to England in 1970 prompted him to reflect on the state of 'Britain's mental health' in *The Irish Times* in 1977, noting that 'one contemporary observer has advanced the considered opinion that the English suffer from an "obsessional hypochondria"':

And like the individual, self-obsessed patient, Britain cannot acknowledge that there is anyone sicker than herself. There are round-table TV discussions, chaired by Robin Day, who increasingly resembles some anguished elderly physician haunted by his ability to diagnose a plethora of fatal diseases while utterly incapable of arresting even one, in which unflattering comparisons are drawn between the feeble, geriatric British hulk, utterly dependent on regular transfusions of international money, dementedly indifferent to its shabby decline, contentedly besotted by a maudlin orgy of nostalgic reminiscence, and the stolid physical vigour of the Germans, the redblooded vitality of the French and the competitive bellicosity of the Japanese. God help us but even the Irish seem in better physical and mental shape.[98]

Even so, Clare concluded that while there were 'no grounds for complacency', there were 'no grounds either for presuming the British to be losing their nerves as they lose their Empire':

It was Alan Herbert [1890–1971; English writer and member of parliament] who claimed that the Common Law of England was laboriously built around a mythical figure – the figure of 'The Reasonable Man'. Yet the figure may not be all that mythical. Indeed, it may well be if the Englishman, bereft of his pride, his power and his self-esteem, does finally go mad, he will do it like he does everything else – he will go reasonably mad. That way he may not need us doctors.

Having lived and worked in England since 1970, Clare's view of the English was clearly informed by not only his own experiences living in London, but also his research in the area of community mental health. He noted in *The Irish Times* that 'approximately one in every seven patients attending their family doctor are suffering from psychological ill-health'. In addition, Clare had found more alcohol problems and mood disorders in Irish immigrants than in the native English (Chapter 2), although he emphasised in his 1987 *Sunday Tribune* interview with Purcell that the situation of the Irish in London, although difficult, was not remarkably different to that of other migrant groups:

> Contrary to some reports, Professor Clare believes that the Irish in Britain, even the new wave of young immigrants, are not suffering stress in any greater proportion than the stress prevalent in any immigrant group. In fact the contrary is the case. 'They are no worse than any immigrant group. They have not been remarked on by my British colleagues. In fact there is a perception that the Irish are the most successful immigrant group here – the group that has assimilated best.'[99]

Clare was one of those who assimilated especially well and he continued to write, co-write and edit publications on diverse themes including mental illness in general practice, social work, primary health care and various aspects of psychiatry.[100] He also wrote book reviews in *Nature*, arguably the world's leading scientific journal.[101] In the popular media, he wrote columns, articles and book reviews in multiple other publications including the *Times*,[102] *Daily Mail*,[103] *Sunday Times*,[104] *Sunday Telegraph*,[105] *Sunday Correspondent, Sunday Express*,[106] *New Society*[107] and the *Spectator*.[108] In *The Listener*, a weekly BBC magazine published from 1929 to 1991, he wrote about topics as diverse as the purpose of marriage,[109] psychotherapy[110] and primal therapy,[111] and reviewed books about autism,[112] neurosis,[113] Freud,[114] Jung,[115] cancer,[116] flagellation,[117] the disintegration of industrial society[118] and – most memorably – Susan Sontag's book

Illness as Metaphor which he admired, albeit with reservations.[119] In 1991, he wrote about Germaine Greer's views on the menopause in the *Daily Mail* and while he was a little unclear about Greer's ultimate message, he had to admit that she was a damn good read.[120]

Clare also wrote about politics[121] and politicians,[122] most notably Margaret Thatcher[123] and Garret FitzGerald.[124] In addition, he penned letters to the editor of the *Times* about matters as diverse as premenstrual problems[125] and the troubles in Northern Ireland,[126] and wrote and co-wrote letters to the *Guardian* on topics including ECT[127] and mental health legislation.[128] He even wrote a weekly column for *Riva*, an ill-fated women's magazine that lasted for just seven issues in the late 1980s.[129]

As a result of this somewhat frenzied activity, Clare was frequently invited to comment in the media on various topics,[130] launch books or videos,[131] and deliver lectures such as the 1983 Herben Lecture of the Royal Institute of Public Health and Hygiene (on the subject of 'sex and mood')[132] and a talk on 'power and the public man' in the 'What Do Men Want?' series at the Institute of Contemporary Arts in London in 1985.[133] Clare's wife Jane recalls the *Times* literary lunches where 'Tony would be at the top table' and Jane was seated on one occasion with novelist William Trevor and on another with biographer Michael Holroyd: 'The great and the good were there.'[134] In addition, Clare was friendly with such well-known figures as Malcolm Muggeridge (1903–90), the English journalist, satirist and anti-communist.[135] He was continually invited to attend dinners such as – to take random examples – those of the Association of Anaesthetists of Great Britain and Ireland at Plaisterers' Hall in London in 1986[136] and the Asthma Research Council in the Great Hall in Bart's in 1987, at which he commonly spoke.[137]

Clare attended thousands of similar meetings and events over the years and Robin Murray recalls that 'there would be few prominent people in the 1980s and 1990s that [Clare] had not had dinner with'.[138] Despite this – or possibly because of it – Clare expressed especially virulent disdain for 'dinner parties' in his 1987 *Sunday Tribune* interview with Purcell:

Professor Clare suffers interviews. He is genuinely very busy and an hour of his time could be spent doing better things. He also despises dinner parties and goes to as few parties of any sort as possible: 'They're a waste of time. It's one of the reasons I don't miss Ireland. An awful lot of time is wasted – an awful lot of people of great talent, particularly in Dublin, have let the talent dissipate. You can spend a lot of time doing nothing in Dublin [...] Dinner parties are the great curse of the Western world, save for those parties where the guests are people of very different backgrounds.' But of course that seldom happens. 'It's much more common to have a dinner party of doctors or lawyers or architects or – God help us all – politicians. Usually, spouses are bored silly ...'[139]

Not everyone was charmed by Clare's ubiquity in the media. Journalist Bernard Levin repeatedly expressed a sort of general, free-floating irritation with him in the *Times*,[140] and Clare himself 'was worried about over-exposure', according to Jane, although he generally managed to avoid it.[141] And Clare remained, at heart, an orator and debater, unable to resist an argument, an intellectual engagement or a robust discussion. In 1985, for example, he wrote two provocative articles in the *Times* expressing fundamental doubts about psychoanalysis[142] and these elicited strong responses from such figures as Dr Clifford Yorke, medical director of the Anna Freud Centre in London,[143] Dr Lawrence D. Phillips, director of the Decision Analysis Unit at the London School of Economics and Political Science,[144] and Dr Dennis Friedman of the Priory Hospital.[145] This was all just grist to the mill, of course: more discussion, more debate, more dissent. Clare loved every minute of it.

In addition to his popular media work, Clare continued to author and co-author papers in the peer-reviewed psychiatric and medical literature throughout the 1970s and 1980s. Increasingly, these publications concerned alcohol misuse, its causes,[146] its links with mood disorders,[147] treatment paradigms[148] and attitudes within the medical profession.[149] Other themes included an exploration of the diagnostic concept of 'cycloid psychosis' (a severe, atypical mental illness)[150] and the appropriate uses of psychiatric medications,[151] psychotherapy[152] and ECT.[153] Proper understanding and use of ECT was an especially long-standing concern of Clare's, which he explored in unprecedented depth in *Psychiatry in Dissent*.[154] And in 1980 Clare, with others, objected strenuously to the reported use of unmodified ECT (ECT without anaesthetic or muscle relaxation) at Broadmoor, in both the *Guardian*[155] and the *Lancet*.[156] This controversy raged for quite some time in the popular and professional media and, ultimately, at Westminster.[157]

Clare's concern about appropriate use of ECT was linked with his much broader interest in ethical psychiatric practice and professional standards, topics to which he repeatedly returned. In 1977 he wrote an especially penetrating working paper about clinical responsibility and psychiatry in the *British Medical Journal* based on a tape-recorded conference in which he participated in Pangbourne on 7 and 8 October of that year.[158] In the *Lancet*, he argued (yet again) against anti-psychiatrist Thomas Szasz[159] and in favour of compulsory psychiatric intervention when needed, based on papers Szasz and he delivered at a symposium entitled 'A Balance of Views Towards a Better Mental Health Act' held at the New London Centre on 8 December 1977.[160] This theme also featured heavily in *Psychiatry in Dissent*[161] and Clare consistently argued that the simplistic arguments presented by certain critics of psychiatry would inevitably be exposed over time.[162] He was right.

Clare was tireless in his exploration of these key controversial and ethical issues in psychiatry and broader medicine, and wrote again and again about consent to treatment,[163] compulsion, confidentiality, psychosurgery[164] and even doctors' involvement in the death penalty, which he opposed.[165] He also reflected on the 'clinical process in psychiatry'[166] and wrote a notably progressive paper about social methods of treatment for neurotic disorders and self-help approaches to mental illness, in the *Journal of the Irish Medical Association*, based on the proceedings of an 'International Symposium' on 'Alternatives to Drugs' held at the Killiney Court Hotel in Dublin on 16 February 1979.[167] Sponsored by the Irish Medical Association in conjunction with the Health Education Bureau of Ireland, the 1979 conference was also addressed by Mr C.J. Haughey (1925–2006), Minister for Health and Social Welfare (1977–9) and later Taoiseach (1979–81, 1982, 1987–92).[168] Haughey noted increased consumption of pharmaceuticals across Europe and questioned the necessity for so many vitamin preparations and tranquillisers. Clare, for his part, was positive about the potential of self-help groups and urged greater involvement of patients and families in psychiatric care.

Throughout this period, Clare not only spoke and wrote about these themes – ethical psychiatric practice, better mental health services, and enhanced patient and family involvement in care – but also became deeply involved with efforts to improve services on the ground. He did this not only through his own clinical practice, teaching and research, but also through his growing involvement with mental health charities and patient groups such as Mind.

The National Association for Mental Health was founded in 1946, was re-named 'MIND' in 1972, and became 'Mind' in the 1990s. Clare served as national medical adviser with MIND until 1982 when he took the view that the Mental Health (Amendment) Bill would make the management of severely mentally ill patients even more difficult, owing to excessive bureaucracy and legalism, as he outlined in the *Guardian*:

> I have consistently argued these points as MIND's medical adviser with that association, but without much success. Recently, the tendency to expand inexorably the boundaries of legal involvement [...] has again surfaced. MIND, not content with the process of a multi-disciplinary review being applied to ECT and psycho-surgery, is still pressing for virtually every psychiatric treatment to be controlled in this way.
>
> I do not believe that such a policy is in the best interests of the patients whom MIND seeks to represent and, as a consequence, with reluctance and sadness, I have resigned as MIND's national medical adviser.[169]

Even so, just three years later, in 1985, Clare co-wrote an outspoken report about conditions in the psychiatric wing of Holloway women's prison in London, commissioned by MIND and the National Council for Civil Liberties.[170] In 1991, he pointed out, at a meeting in Plymouth, that daily NHS spending on the mentally ill was just 29 pence per community patient per day – the price of a cup of tea.[171] Clare's gift for a sound bite never left him.

SANE, another mental health charity, was founded in 1986 by Marjorie Wallace whom Clare interviewed on *In The Psychiatrist's Chair* in 1997. Clare also found much common ground with SANE, calling for accurate public education about mental illness and its treatment, and greater research into its causes.[172]

Throughout this period, it was Clare's communication skills and the sheer joy he took in writing, speaking and broadcasting that defined much of his activity, as it did so much of his life. As Murray notes, 'communication is what he was good at':

Tony was fantastic at communication and he knew he was good at that. He got more and more invitations to do things in that area and therefore he followed that line [...] He sometimes did voiceovers and suddenly, as you were watching TV, you'd be hearing Tony.

Tony's success in the media meant he was a celebrity. We teach young psychiatrists how to do a psychiatric interview. Just listen to Tony interviewing people on the BBC recordings. He was a brilliant interviewer. He had the ability to get people to say things they had no intention of saying, by being so obviously interested in them. If someone was to write a history of politics and influential people in the 1980s and 1990s, you could publish these interviews, one after the other.[173]

5

Broadcaster: *In the Psychiatrist's Chair* (1982–2001)

●●●●●●●●●●●●●●●●●●●●●●●●●●●●●●●●●●●●●

During the 1980s, Clare's engagement with popular media deepened. He was a regular contributor to BBC Radio 4's *Stop the Week* programme and this in turn led to his best-known media work, *In the Psychiatrist's Chair*. This series ran from 1982 to 2001 and saw Clare interview a broad range of guests in unprecedented depth. His engaged, inquisitive charm elicited fascinating insights from Bob Monkhouse, Anthony Hopkins, Eartha Kitt, Arthur Ashe, P.D. James, Derek Jarman and R.D. Laing, among hundreds of others.

Before exploring *In the Psychiatrist's Chair*, it is worth noting that Clare worked on many radio programmes during this period and into the 1990s, including *Let's Talk About Me* (a six-part 1979 BBC Radio 4 series and book about novel psychotherapies),[1] *Thicker than Water* (a three-part 1981 BBC Radio 4 series about the influence of blood relationships), *Everyman*, *Father Figures* and *All in the Mind*, which he presented from 1989 to 1998, also on BBC Radio 4.[2]

Television and film work included *Motives* (BBC 2, 1982), a series of interviews with subjects including Petula Clark, George Best and Richard Ingrams[3] (to which critical reaction was distinctly mixed, as was Clare's),[4] *Beyond Belief* (a 1986 Channel 4 series exploring how beliefs shape actions), *Lovelaw* (a 1986 BBC 2 series and book about love, sex and marriage around the world),[5] *After Dark* (a television discussion programme, from 1987 to 1991),[6] *Seven Ages of Man* (a 1996 BBC 2 series in which Clare talked to public figures about ageing)[7] and *QED* (various documentaries between 1982 and 1991).[8]

Clare also participated in *Nationwide* on BBC 1 (with Frank Bough), *Friday Night, Saturday Morning* (1980), *Everyman* (1991), *Evolving Soul* (1992), *The Enemy Within* (1995),[9] *The Burgess Variations* (1999), *Saints and Sinners: The History of the Popes* (2005) and *The Unseen Spike Milligan* (2005), as well as dong voiceovers and guesting on countless other television and radio shows.[10]

But it was *In the Psychiatrist's Chair* on BBC Radio 4 that was to prove Clare's most enduring contribution to media, with the programmes regularly repeated for decades after they were first broadcast and many still available on the BBC Radio 4 Extra website.[11] Four volumes of the interviews were published (in 1984, 1992, 1995 and 1998);[12] a cassette set was produced by BBC Worldwide in 1996; and twelve interviews were released on CD by BBC Worldwide in 2016, in an extraordinary tribute to the enduring value and appeal of Clare's skills as a psychiatrist, interviewer and radio broadcaster.

Origins

In the Psychiatrist's Chair was produced by Michael Ember (1932–2017) who came from Hungary to the United Kingdom in 1956 and made multiple talk-radio programmes for the BBC.[13] In the early 1970s, Ember devised *Stop the Week*, a light-hearted programme that Clare appeared on and that ran for eighteen years, until 1992. Ember also revived *Start the Week*,[14] devised *Midweek* and, with Clare, co-created *In the Psychiatrist's Chair*, which was probably Ember's most iconic work.

In the Psychiatrist's Chair was originally to be titled *What Makes You Tick?* and its aim was to reveal the real person behind the façade of celebrity. Ember had studied psychology and criminology at the University of London and shared with Clare a deep curiosity about human motivation and behaviour. Ember retired from the BBC in

1992 but he and his wife Liz established an independent company to continue producing *In the Psychiatrist's Chair* beyond that point.

Clare described the idea for the series as a joint one that grew out of discussions between Clare and Michael Ember over several years.[15] In addition, Judith Jackson, who worked in the biochemistry department at the Maudsley, expressed an interest in knowing about the inner lives of well-known people: did these apparently successful and celebrated people suffer like ordinary mortals? Ember had noted articles and book reviews that Clare wrote for the *Spectator* and *New Society*, and was, of course, familiar with Clare's involvement in *Stop the Week*, *Thicker than Water* and *Let's Talk About Me*, the latter being a fascinating exploration of the burgeoning boom in self-exploration and experiential psychotherapy in California, and a joint enterprise with BBC producer Sally Thompson.[16]

The format of *In the Psychiatrist's Chair* was that Clare would interview guests in considerable depth and without haste, in an effort to explore their childhoods, self-image and current motivations. The format was not entirely new: Clare was keenly aware of *Face to Face*, a series of television interviews by John Freeman that ran on the BBC from 1959 to 1962 and enjoyed considerable success.[17] Clare was also aware that reactions to such in-depth and sometimes emotional interviews were decidedly mixed, with some regarding them as tasteless violations and others seeing them as vindicating the whole idea of in-depth interviewing, to which Clare was clearly attracted.[18]

By 1982, Clare felt that the time had come for a new series, on the basis that the public was now more knowledgeable about psychology, relationships, emotions and human behaviour.[19] Greater openness about people's inner lives meant that – in effect – the unconscious had shrunk since the time of Freud. The key task now, Clare argued, was not revealing the repressed and the forgotten, but processing and understanding what was already known. The purpose of the new series, he said, was to cast light on the sources of each guest's life and values. What motivates them? What sustains them through difficulties and crises? What fuels the notions of excellence that so many high-achievers appear to demonstrate? Above all, why do they do what they do? And how?

In pursuing these themes over the following years, Clare was unfailingly courteous and supportive with his guests, listening for the most part, rather than interrogating. He was also endlessly curious, often robust and, at times, remarkably and controversially persistent. Guests, chosen by Clare and Ember together, could expect a warm but penetrating conversation with the versatile, tenacious psychiatrist in the chair.

Finding its Feet

In a *Radio Times* interview on the eve of the first episode of *In the Psychiatrist's Chair* in 1982, Clare spoke about the curious position occupied by the profession of psychiatry in the United Kingdom compared to the United States, and he hoped that his series would make the science behind psychiatry more accessible.[20] Elsewhere, he bemoaned an over-emphasis on the flawed and the negative in psychiatry, and expressed a hope that the radio interviews would help shift attention to a more positive focus: while psychiatry was indeed concerned with the flawed and the negative, it was also concerned with values, strengths, survival and positive impulses.[21] What keeps a person from breaking down, he argued, is just as relevant as what pushes them to the brink.

The first interview in the series, with actress Glenda Jackson, was broadcast on BBC Radio 4 at 6.55 p.m. on Saturday, 31 July 1982. It started with a classic Clare theme: Why are you here, and how do you feel about doing this interview?

> CLARE: How do you feel, Glenda, about talking about yourself and revealing the private person as distinct from the public persona?
>
> JACKSON: I think I'm enough of an egomaniac to enjoy the idea of talking about myself. How much it will reveal I really don't know, because I don't think I've ever had a conversation like this before.

CLARE: Do you often reflect on what has brought you where you are?

JACKSON: Well, if I ever do reflect, it seems to have been a process of accident, and I don't know whether I actually accord any validity to the theory that there are no such things as accidents.[22]

The interview with Jackson was open, frank and fascinating, touching on her childhood, career in acting, and fears that she suffered 'a minor nervous breakdown':[23]

CLARE: Were you so low as to feel that life really had lost its purpose?

JACKSON: My prevailing sense was the most overwhelming panic and terror that life itself was going to end. It was at the time of the Cuban missile crisis, and I was absolutely convinced that every aeroplane that went over was carrying the first bomb that was going to be dropped. It actually took a concrete external fear form for me.

CLARE: Did you tell people that?

JACKSON: I don't think I did, no. I had one very bad night when I had this terrible shaking, and I went to see the doctor the next day, and I was given some form of tranquiliser. The effect was so horrendous, I threw the bottle into the dustbin and would never take anything like that again.

CLARE: Did you dream then?

JACKSON: If I did I can't remember what the dreams were. I can remember waking up in a cold sweat, but that happens to me still. I sometimes wake up with my teeth firmly clenched, covered in cold sweat – I've been in some nightmare.

CLARE: But you can't recall it?

JACKSON: Not directly. The most recurring nightmare is always of being chased – I take to the sky to avoid my pursuers, but they tend to be able to walk in the air too, so on it goes.[24]

The interview was fascinating and intense. Jackson admitted that having Clare's full attention was seductive.[25] Themes of seduction were to be a feature of the series: Clare later confessed to feeling seduced by Ann Widdecombe during his tempestuous 1997 interview with the outspoken politician.[26] The intimacy of the discussions undoubtedly heightened the emotional temperature in the small BBC studios where they were recorded.

Following the opening interview with Jackson in 1982, subsequent episodes of the series featured such figures as Buddhist judge Christmas Humphreys[27] and – most famously – comedian Spike Milligan, with whom Clare would later write a book titled *Depression and How to Survive It*.[28] While Clare's engaging style quickly became familiar to listeners, the content of the interviews varied considerably from episode to episode. Clare commonly asked why the interviewee had agreed to participate and enquired into their childhood, but beyond that there was considerable diversity, as Clare followed where the interviewee led and adapted his questions to the individual in the chair.

Reviewing the early episodes in *The Times* in August 1982, David Wade concluded that the degree to which Clare maintained a psychiatric distance varied between interviewees.[29] Wade also noted that Clare had recently lamented the generally low standard of celebrity interviewing,[30] and Wade concluded that *In the Psychiatrist's Chair* was doing something far more interesting than was usual in such interviews. The *Guardian* noted that Jackson found her interview with Clare 'delightful', but wondered if 'the title "Dr" gave [Clare] the right to ask *News of the World* questions in a middle-brow setting'.[31]

The first season of *In the Psychiatrist's Chair* proved a great success although it was clear early on that Clare revealed little of himself during the broadcasts. In 1984, Clare reflected that the series was intended to be more mutual than it turned out to be.[32] Indeed, a 1995 review of a book stemming from the series noted that many of Clare's brief contributions were as interesting as those of his guests.[33] In any case, regardless of Clare's initial reluctance to reveal much of himself, the early episodes generated a large and loyal following and ensured the continued survival of the programme over the following years.

Sebastian Cody interviewed Clare at the BBC for a British magazine in May 1984, two years after *In the Psychiatrist's Chair* commenced. Cody noted that Clare attacked the fantasy that the celebrated few have their molecules arranged in a different order to ours. Clare suggested that 'talking will go some way towards relieving neurotic feelings of inadequacy and insecurity that, at worst, can turn into destructive self-hatred'. Cody felt that Clare's clinical training shaped his interviewing style:

> Tough-minded – phone-ins were a 'mistake', the evidence for psychotherapy was 'unconvincing' – Clare looked slightly battered, a sense of 'I'm-too-busy-to-get-my-hair-cut-properly' … Clare's profession gives him the licence to ask questions denied other interviewers. In addition, his clinical training has given him a skill unique in journalism: often, towards the end of an interview, he will relate an answer back to something said much earlier.[34]

Clare pointed out that 'the paradox is that the way some people stay afloat costs something: some of my patients haven't exacted that price on others or themselves. There's something cannibalistic about the way some people survive: they do it at other people's expense or by virtue of a well-developed – even thick – ego.'[35] But would Clare 'answer his own questions?'

> Fear of cracking up, I would talk about. Latent homosexuality: there's not a great deal to say. First sexual experience: at 18, 19, but I won't tell you how. I wouldn't go on my own show …[36]

After the interview, as they walked to Oxford Circus tube, Cody asked why Clare's public work took the shape it did. Cody reasoned that Clare 'had worked hard to become a member of an elite group within medicine – psychiatry – but his response was to write *Psychiatry in Dissent'*, critiquing that profession. And although Clare 'now associated on radio with people who were all somehow exceptional – well-known, successful, intelligent, gifted and so on – his aim was to show their flaws, troubles and weaknesses, somehow to bring them down to size'. Clare brushed the question off with a smile and 'Oh I don't know, some kind of Irish darkness.'[37]

Cody's interview ended up not being published but Clare 'greatly enjoyed our conversation' and hoped 'that an opportunity may arise again in the future for us to get together'.[38] He added that his recent trip to the United States to interview subjects for *In the Psychiatrist's Chair* had gone 'reasonably well, although it is very hard to tell until these things are broadcast and I can never really decide on what is a good or not so good interview'.

Interestingly, reflecting in 1984 on both *In the Psychiatrist's Chair* and his television interviews in *Motives*, Clare commented that 'I'm better at destroying systems than I am at putting them together – I do rather look for people to interview who will not live up to the prediction; there's an element of destructiveness that's still in me':

On radio we record ninety minutes and edit that down to forty, sometimes sixty minutes down to forty; David Irving's interview took two-and-a-half hours but was also brought down to forty minutes. On television we recorded fifty minutes, edited down to forty, which didn't make the slightest difference.

I try to bring things said early in the interview back later, which is what medical notes are for – you have a look at the written notes before a clinical interview to remind oneself of what was said before. So, I try to get people to talk about themselves and then put some of that back to them in the same interview.

I am not John Freeman [host of *Face to Face*, the series of BBC television interviews from 1959 to 1962], letting so much go, interrupting; I am more fiery and more involved. Tears? I am not taken with the public expression of private grief. So, my interviews won't necessarily make as riveting television … If anything I am modest in my questioning.[39]

Musicians, Politicians and Others

By 1992, a decade after it started, more than sixty people had sat *In the Psychiatrist's Chair*, ranging from American tennis player Arthur Ashe to politician Edwina Currie, from film-maker Derek Jarman to pianist Vladimir Ashkenazy. Potential guests received a letter of invitation from Ember and a choice of three dates.[40] There was little socialising before or after the interviews, which took place in a very ordinary, drab little office in the BBC. Clare was skilled at putting his guests quickly at their ease. Ashkenazy, who, in 1986, spoke especially openly about his mother's contempt for his circus entertainer father and her ambitions for her son, later recalled 'a very professional interview, detailed and very warm'.[41]

Political activist Bruce Kent was interviewed in 1985 and remembers Clare as 'a decent man who had done his homework', 'with a direct but non-hostile and honest approach. I was well used by then to journalists who had their own knives to grind. He got me to talk openly and frankly. […] I remember leaving the BBC that day and thinking that I had got quite a lot off my chest.'[42]

Crime writer P.D. James was also interviewed in 1985, and Clare did not hesitate to explore areas of great personal sensitivity, as reported in the *Guardian*:

> This week's interview cut very deep. It was with Ms P.D. James, the crime writer, and went far beyond the familiar debate about why nicely-mannered, middle-class, middle-aged ladies write about horrid crimes. [Ms James] had a great tragedy in her life: her young husband came back from the war suffering from mental illness and, after being in and out of various mental hospitals, killed himself in 1964. When Dr Clare asked what happened, there was a long, almost unbearable moment of struggling silence before she replied: 'I found him dead.'[43]

Clare elicited genuine revelations from many of his guests.[44] Writer Carla Lane opened up quite unintentionally as she discussed her work, childhood, family and love of animals, stating that most people who have animals say that animals are better than humans.[45] Professor Wendy Savage, gynaecologist, 'had never met Anthony Clare before' her 1986 interview, but 'knew of him, respected his work, and found him an engaging personality. It was easy to talk to him and, being a doctor, I was probably less wary of him than non-medical journalists.'[46] The series was, in the words of one reviewer, 'great listening for the psycho-buffs'.[47]

In 1988, politician Edwina Currie gave a frank and moving interview, as Clare later recalled, telling him about the end of her relationship with her father, who never spoke to her again.[48] Reflecting back some thirty years later, Currie's recollection is that Clare 'wasn't able to delve very deep, as I was practised in revealing only what I wished to'.[49] Unlike most other guests, Currie knew Clare personally prior to the interview, from her time at the Department of Health, where she was Parliamentary Undersecretary of State for Health from 1986 to 1988:

> I [...] had met [Clare] several times and admired and liked him. To make psychiatry accessible to the general public, to talk through many issues that affect us all in a professional but popular way, was I thought entirely praiseworthy. We were trying at the time to improve services for people with mental illness and mental handicap, and to diminish the stigma attached to both. That's why I was glad to work with him. He sussed out motivations that his targets had no idea they held; he made his profession sound like a constant detective story.

Currie points out that Clare was 'deeply respected' in the United Kingdom and that he and Irish comedian Dave Allen 'were a reminder in the grim days of the IRA that Ireland was not all about politics'.

Like Currie, certain other politicians remember their interviews with Clare as being not very revealing. Nigel Lawson agreed to an interview with Clare in 1988 solely 'because I had enjoyed his previous programmes', even though Lawson emphatically considers himself 'a very private person'.[50] Lawson recalls that 'I told him very little and suspect that it was the most boring programme he ever made.' Lawson's was, in fact, a fascinating interview, as was Clare's 1997 interview with another politician, Ann Widdecombe, who, like Lawson and Currie, is skeptical about just how penetrating Clare was. Clare later described Widdecombe as a conviction politician with unmovable views on a range of issues, a theme that they explored in some depth in the interview:[51]

> CLARE: Are you someone who has doubts?
> WIDDECOMBE: About what?
> CLARE: About anything?
> WIDDECOMBE: I expect I've got doubts about some things, most people have.
> CLARE: Well, about important things. Do you ever think you might be wrong?
> WIDDECOMBE: No.[52]

The conversation with Widdecombe soon moved on to the nature of religious belief:

> WIDDECOMBE: ... I actually divide Christians up into two groups, if you like, on this. There are some who will say that it's a statement of belief and there are some who will say it is a statement of fact. Now when I say 'I believe', I am actually iterating in my view what is a statement of fact.
> CLARE: Absolute fact?
> WIDDECOMBE: Absolute fact.
> CLARE: Your life then has a number of rock-hard certainties in it, political certainties, religious certainties?
> WIDDECOMBE: Oh yes, oh yes, absolutely.
> CLARE: Personal certainties?
> WIDDECOMBE: Absolutely.
> CLARE: Does it surprise you that I'm surprised?
> WIDDECOMBE: Yes.

CLARE: Why?
WIDDECOMBE: Is your life sort of completely anchorless?
CLARE: No, no. Don't do that to me![53]

Towards the end, Clare asked, as he often did, why Widdecombe had agreed to the interview:

WIDDECOMBE: ... I looked forward to the duel and I think in many ways we've had one.
CLARE: That's what appealed?
WIDDECOMBE: Yup, we've had a duel.
CLARE: That's true, yes indeed.[54]

Curiously, Widdecombe, like Currie and Lawson, remembers the interview as being not very revealing of her:

In a way, there was a lack of originality to the interview. [Clare] went over ground that had already been covered extensively in press and media. Other than questions about if I would have been a good mother, he didn't really come up with anything original. He stuck with entirely predictable ground, which made for a very relaxed interview.[55]

The interview with Widdecombe might have been 'relaxed' for her but it was gripping for listeners. Clare, for his part, described the encounter as good-humoured, although he felt that Widdecombe was irked at having to discuss feelings and would have preferred to have an argument about sex on television or abortion.[56] Widdecombe recalls Clare as 'very personable':

It was remarkably straightforward. I went to a very small television studio, I think it was Broadcasting House. There was just the two of us in the studio. Unlike most political interviewers, he did at least give me time to answer. I'm naturally wary of people who go in for psychoanalysis but I enjoyed the interview. [Clare] was very personable. We chatted a bit before and a bit afterwards. He had a nice personality, and was somebody I could quite cheerfully have dinner with, despite his profession.

Widdecombe recalls that, after the interview was broadcast, one of her friends said that, 'listening to [Clare], she thought he simply didn't understand belief'. Another friend 'said she had been interested in him rather than me during the programme'. And a political colleague 'wasn't sure a practising psychiatrist should be doing this for entertainment'. When the first volume of interviews was published in 1984,[57] Dr Eimer Philbin Bowman, a psychiatrist, articulated similar concern in *The Irish Times*, noting that she was 'uneasy' when she first heard the programme's title:

> Why should a psychiatrist trained to deal with those who cannot cope either temporarily or permanently with the stresses of normal life, be particularly skilled at interviewing those who excel? Unless it is that people, believing that he has skills and insights not possessed by others, are thereby induced to lower their defences and allow access to their private world. It is clear from the opening responses in these interviews that most of Anthony Clare's subjects did feel this way. And I must admit that any listeners who commented to me on the series at the time were very enthusiastic about getting what they considered an 'inside view'. But my unease remained, and the subsequent interviews on television did not relieve it. The publication of this book has exacerbated it.[58]

Philbin Bowman pointed to a 'conflict underlying the whole series':

> Good psychiatry takes place in private, and only in public if the patient's interest is paramount. Good psychological interviewing is in the public interest and, as John Freeman [on *Face to Face*] has shown, it can be compelling viewing. Anthony Clare practises the first and could undoubtedly master the second, but he should not confuse one with the other.

Notwithstanding these concerns, Philbin Bowman 'liked and admired' Clare,[59] and two months after her 1984 book review appeared, a radio review published in *The Irish Times* found Clare's series 'fascinating' whilst noting tartly that Clare, an Irishman, described himself as 'a British psychiatrist'.[60] Like Philbin Bowman, Clare was keenly aware of potential criticism of the programme's title from the outset and worried that some listeners might think that the series was psychiatry being practised on the radio, with the guests as patients and the psychiatrist-presenter performing clinical analysis and possibly even therapy on the air.[61] In the end, however, Clare felt that no other title suited and that *In the Psychiatrist's Chair* was, at the very least, an honest title: after all, the interviews had a psychiatric flavour and the interviewer was undoubtedly a psychiatrist.

For the most part, Clare's gamble paid off richly. As Widdecombe notes, 'the programme had a very wide listenership. It was the sort of thing people would mention to me months later ... It was something that people remembered long after it took place which is always a tribute to the interviewer or interviewee or both.' In the interview with Widdecombe, certainly, both interviewer and interviewee performed with relish and aplomb, making the recording a memorable, if distinctly odd, classic of its genre.

Critics and Controversy

In the Psychiatrist's Chair was a general success with the listening public and most, but not all, radio reviewers.[62] Reviewing the first episode, Val Arnold-Forster in the *Guardian* described the idea as 'a poor one':

And an artificial one too, since presumably no psychiatrist, let alone his patient, would allow the broadcasting of anything approaching a clinical consultation. It seems more likely that someone had recognised the broadcasting talents of psychiatrist Dr Anthony Clare and had made a hapless and somewhat tasteless attempt to jazz up an interview series. And the interview with Glenda Jackson was no more than a rather personally directed show-biz interview ...[63]

But even the critics found much to enjoy and admire, with Arnold-Forster describing Jackson as 'both agreeable and intelligent', and Brian Sibley, writing critically in *The Times* in 1983, admitting that the series was widely praised.[64] And while the critics did not go away, they were in a small, dwindling minority, and did little to dent the popularity or growing prestige of the programme.[65]

By 1996, more than 100 people had taken their seat *In the Psychiatrist's Chair*.[66] In that year, violinist and conductor Yehudi Menuhin was Clare's 100th guest and the programme won a well-deserved Sony Broadcasting Award for Clare's interview with English long-distance walker Ffyona Campbell. Actress Joanna Lumley's appearance in 1994 was also widely heralded[67] and, after their sparkling interview, Clare duly described Lumley as delightful and very good at projecting herself.[68] Lumley was 'thrilled' to be invited and 'said YES at once. It was a great honour that he even knew who I was':

> It was immensely entertaining and fascinating. Sitting alone in a small recording booth could have been claustrophobic but Professor Clare was a great companion with whom to be shut into a small space. I thought he was awesome: wise, quiet, humorous, candid and wildly clever. I could have sat there all day [...] Clare was criticised for 'giving me an easy time' but to tell the truth I had nothing to hide and he liked me I think and we laughed a lot. People like Anthony Clare are few and far between and his presence was much needed and hugely treasured. He was a legend. I could not have liked him more.[69]

Not all interviewees, however, reported such positive experiences. In July 1988, Clare interviewed agony aunt Claire Rayner who became very upset during the discussion, causing considerable controversy afterwards.[70] Rayner worried that people would never trust her again. Reflecting on the interview, Clare acknowledged Rayner's distress, especially when he pointed out that time had not dulled her upsetting childhood memories.[71] But Clare also pointed out that most of Rayner's distress had been cut from the programme after he discussed it with Ember, the producer. They had no desire to broadcast such distress in its entirety. Clare felt that what remained was necessary in order to demonstrate the emotional intensity that reference to events that took place more than forty years earlier could still produce. Both Clare and Ember were surprised by the impact of the broadcast.

Clare's persistence in the interview despite Rayner's clear distress raised significant issues because Clare, of course, was not only a radio interviewer; he was also a medical doctor, bound by the dictum 'primum non nocere' (first do no harm). Did he cross the line here? In his defence, Clare wrote that those who questioned his persistence with his line of questioning did not realise that, in his view, Rayner expected these questions because this was not the first time that Clare had interviewed her.[72] He had spoken with her in 1982 as part of the television series *Motives*. The episode of *Motives* featuring Rayner was never broadcast, mainly for technical reasons, but Clare sensed in that interview that pain and darkness lay behind Rayner's jolly exterior. On that occasion, Clare did not get to the root of what happened.

Journalist and television presenter Dame Esther Rantzen, another Clare interviewee, felt that Clare's interview with Rayner on *In the Psychiatrist's Chair* added to Rayner's credibility, rather than undermining it:

> I remember talking to [Anthony Clare] about his interview with Claire Rayner which was really fascinating. I met her afterwards. She told me she was appalled by it as she'd never before talked about being abused as a child. She broke down during the interview, and thought that would destroy her credibility with the people she tried to help [...] I told her from my Childline experience how reassuring people told me they had found her interview on *In the Psychiatrist's Chair*. They found it very heartening. Far from destroying her reputation it increased her credibility and authority

[...] It was extremely positive in its impact on other survivors of abuse. Its impact on her was that she remembered it with real concern and distress as she didn't want the public to be aware that she was vulnerable.[73]

Rantzen 'remembered it because I'm very interested in Tony and his techniques and how he handled it. He was very skilful. He knew exactly where he was going with the interview.' Despite the controversy,[74] Clare agreed with Rantzen that the interview had a positive impact on public perceptions of Rayner. He wrote that responses to the programme, from both the listening public and the critics, bore out his reassurance to Rayner after the interview was recorded: the vast majority of listeners felt that she appeared as a more sympathetic, more rounded, less authoritarian and less bossy figure following the interview.[75] The only mystery to Clare was why anyone occupying the position that Rayner did could ever have believed it would be otherwise.

Esther Rantzen: 'The Series Was a Game-Changer'

Clare's interview with Esther Rantzen in 1993 was another classic of the genre that Clare was rapidly re-inventing with his *Chair*: warm, revelatory and frequently memorable.[76] Rantzen was and still is a very public figure who achieved great popularity as presenter of *That's Life*, a magazine-style television series between 1973 and 1994, and for her charity work. But she admitted to Clare that she had 'never felt attractive' and had changed her appearance:

CLARE: So in one sense, you have reconstructed yourself?

RANTZEN: I reconstructed my hair colour, that's right.

CLARE: What else did you change, if that's not too personal a question?

RANTZEN: No, it's not. I didn't think you minded about personal questions on this programme?

CLARE: Oh, there are boundaries to everything.

RANTZEN: Are there ... Another illusion shattered![77]

Rantzen spoke frankly about her experience of depression:

CLARE: Did you worry that you might lose absolute control?
RANTZEN: I worried that the depression would never lift.
CLARE: Did you worry that you might kill yourself?
RANTZEN: I worried that I would never be well again.[78]

For Rantzen, the interview with Clare 'was an interesting experience for me. Because the series was a game-changer, as an interviewer myself I was very interested in the whole process.'[79] Rantzen 'knew Tony because we both used to take part in *Start the Week* with Richard Baker. He was a regular on it and so was I':

We got to know each other quite well and I'd always been fascinated by his views. As a psychiatrist he was in an interesting trade. I remember many conversations I had with him about the books and authors we were discussing. I was a bit reluctant to do *In the Psychiatrist's Chair*. I took some persuading, because I knew it would be probing and revealing, and I am very bad at introspection.

Clare certainly probed, and Rantzen's answers were open and honest:

CLARE: You don't fear death?
RANTZEN: I fear a long-drawn, bad death. I fear a death of
   the mind before the body dies. I fear senility. I fear all those
   things that distort your family's memories and your friends'
   memories, that's what I fear.[80]

Rantzen was 'very accustomed to answering questions about what I do and campaigns I am associated with. That's normally what people talk to me about. I find that quite easy, if challenging. What I'm not used to are questions about who I am. Every time I tried to answer one of his questions about me with an answer about what I do, he wouldn't let me':

I'm very used to a radio studio full of microphones and pieces of random equipment, with a producer and technicians clearly on view through the window. But for *In the Psychiatrist's Chair* your chair was arranged so that the only person you could see was Tony. The producer and equipment were completely out of your sightline. It was low-lit and claustrophobic and he was sitting very close. He was inescapable.

When journalists interview you, they talk about things you've done but when you read their description, they've drawn conclusions (often unflattering in my case) about who you really are. But Tony was doing something quite other, getting you to describe yourself and analyse yourself – and that was quite a challenge.

Over time, certain aspects of the programme evolved.[81] Some of the emphasis shifted from the interviewee to the interviewer as the figure of Clare became more established in the public eye.[82] From a technical perspective, Ember used quite long silences in the final edits, which was very unusual on radio, and the interviewee had no editorial control over the final edit that was broadcast. It also became more difficult to get guests as time went on.[83]

But many features remained constant. Clare's wife Jane recalls that, after his return to Ireland in 1989, Clare would 'leave St Patrick's Hospital in Dublin with fifteen minutes to spare to catch the airplane to London. He'd run off the plane, do the interview, and come back that evening':

Different people elicited a different response from Tony. Tony was a debater and could be combative. He was very good at seeing where the chink was. Tony was very engaged and very focussed during the interviews but didn't remember anything about them afterwards. He was very good at completing something and then moving on to the next thing. Michael Ember, the producer, did the editing so Tony did not hear the final edit before broadcast. The programme was often first broadcast in the summer so we often listened to it on the car radio as we crossed France on holiday.

Jimmy Savile: Ducking and Weaving

In 1991, Clare interviewed Jimmy Savile, then noted as a disc jockey, compere for the first performance of *Top of the Pops* in 1964, former wrestler, successful charity worker and long-time presenter of *Jim'll Fix It*, which began on BBC 1 in 1975 and was still running at the time of Savile's appearance on *In the Psychiatrist's Chair*. The Savile interview was not one of Clare's easiest, he later recalled, as Savile reminded him of a boxer, constantly on his toes, extremely edgy, and ready to fend off any attacks.[84]

Despite these difficulties, the interview touched on familiar themes: Savile's childhood, early life, family relationships and financial success. Savile described himself as a 'pirate':

CLARE: Aren't you honest?

SAVILE: I'm 'dishonest' in inverted commas insofar as I'm a ducker and diver, and if I see an opportunity of getting something by only going halfway round the course I'll do it unfortunately! When you're well known like me you never get round to being like that because there's too many people watching you.[85]

Savile claimed to have no emotions:

CLARE: Now what about your feelings?

SAVILE: I haven't found them yet.

CLARE: Seriously.

SAVILE: No, I haven't found them yet.[86]

Discussing relationships, Savile said 'it doesn't matter to me if I've got people or I haven't got people'.[87] He was, however, at pains to point out that it's 'not that I'm funny or weird or anything like that':[88]

CLARE: What about children?

SAVILE: Yes, I couldn't eat a whole one.

CLARE: Do you like children?

SAVILE: Hate them.

CLARE: Really, seriously?

SAVILE: That's why I get on well with them [...] So if you said to
me 'What about kids?' I say basically I don't think I like them
particularly, but I get on well with them. Nothing wrong with
that is there?[89]

Savile asked if Clare thought Savile was 'weird' (Clare: 'I'll tell you at
the end')[90] and Savile insisted that, with him, 'what you see is what
there is':

CLARE: So what I see is what you are and in that sense everybody
who sees you knows you as much as they're ever likely to
know you?

SAVILE: But they know me very well 'cos that's all there is to
know. I mean I don't go away from here and indulge in
some wild fetishes or wild weirdo things or anything like
that. I mean, if you turned my stone over there ain't nothing
underneath it.[91]

Reflecting later on this sometimes frustrating interview, Clare
was struck by Savile's emphasis on two recurring themes: money and
denying his feelings.[92] In light of Savile's apparently non-existent love
life, Clare noted that other interviewers had speculated about possible
skeletons in Savile's closet.[93] Lynn Barber, in a newspaper interview
published just before Clare's programme, confronted Savile with a
rumour that he liked young girls. With Barber, Savile dismissed the
rumour in short order and, with Clare, he claimed that he did not like
children very much at all.

In some unusually judgmental comments, Clare concluded that
Savile was both calculating and materialistic, and Clare expressed a sense
of foreboding, suggesting that there was some profound psychological
disturbance in Savile, rooted in a deprived and emotionally indifferent
childhood.[94] While Clare was clearly intrigued by Savile, he was also
disturbed by him and, in the end, found Savile chilling.

Clare was right: there was something a lot more than chilling about Savile. Following Savile's death in 2011, hundreds of allegations of sexual abuse were made against him, leading to multiple enquiries. While it was noted that Savile was no longer alive to present a defence, a 2013 report by the National Society for the Prevention of Cruelty to Children (NSPCC) and the Metropolitan Police, entitled *Giving Victims a Voice*, was emphatic:

From the information provided by the hundreds of people who have come forward to Operation Yewtree, police and the NSPCC have concluded that Jimmy Savile was one of the UK's most prolific known sexual predators. Indeed the formal recording of allegations of crime on this scale is, to the best of our knowledge, unprecedented in the UK.[95]

It is now clear that Savile was hiding in plain sight and using his celebrity status and fundraising activity to gain uncontrolled access to vulnerable people across six decades. For a variety of reasons the vast majority of his victims did not feel they could speak out and it is apparent that some of the small number who did had their accounts dismissed by those in authority, including parents and carers.[96]

Reviewing Clare's 1991 interview with Savile in light of the 2013 report, it is striking that Savile repeatedly pre-emptively denied any wrong-doing, stating that 'I don't go away from here and indulge in some wild fetishes or wild weirdo things or anything like that.'[97] Savile also noted the transitory nature of the 'pop business' ('a flash game, a posing game, a candy-floss game, a phenomenon')[98] and even emphasised his vulnerability to 'scandal':

I can go skint in a day. I can be finished like that. If a scandal comes up or something like that or the people go off you, you're finished. I'd much rather go skint with a brand new Rolls Royce in the garage than one that's eight years old that I love, because I'll get more for it. So the day that I get finished by some whatever, then the bits and pieces that I've got, I'll make sure that they're all paid up, and they're all brand new because I could then go and be very unhappy in the south of France, covered in shame and sunshine and mad birds with bikinis on for a long time because there was a new Rolls Royce there and a new this and a new that.[99]

Savile added that with this 'ultimate freedom' brought by his vast wealth, 'it would be easy to be corrupted by many things, when you've got ultimate freedom, especially when you've got clout. I could be corrupted.'[100]

Was Clare right to refrain from confronting Savile directly with the rumours about young girls, as Lynn Barber had done in her earlier newspaper interview? Clare later regretted not exposing Savile.[101] But addressing specific allegations or staging confrontations were not usual features of *In the Psychiatrist's Chair* and Clare stuck with his trademark interview techniques with Savile: inquisitive rather than confrontational, incremental rather than dramatic, confessional rather than declamatory. Reflecting on the interview the following year, Clare mentioned the allegations against Savile and Savile's dismissal of them in his introduction to the published volume, and he also elaborated on his unusually judgmental, prescient appraisal of his chilling guest.

Rantzen, founder of the child protection charity ChildLine, remembers Clare's interview with Savile clearly, along with Savile's extraordinary 'cunning':

There are people whose very survival depends on their capacity to live a double life. If they're not good at it they come to grief. I think if Jimmy Savile had been Tony Clare's patient, Tony would have reflected on the creepiness, and perhaps uncovered the truth. But the last thing Savile would do is go to a psychiatrist. That mask was there for a purpose. As it turns out a good many people knew Savile was a child abuser because they had experienced it or witnessed it, and a few incidents were even reported to the police. But he evaded them all. Savile was extremely cunning.[102]

The Psychiatrist in the Chair

Clare clearly presented himself as a psychiatrist on *In the Psychiatrist's Chair*, not least in the title of the programme itself. Even so, not all of Clare's guests felt like they were talking with a psychiatrist. Widdecombe, interviewed in 1997, points out that 'if I hadn't known he was a psychiatrist, I wouldn't have guessed it. I would have thought he was just a particular kind of interviewer who was interested in motivation rather than an interviewer interested in political consequences. I didn't really relate to him as a psychiatrist.'[103]

Businesswoman Nicola Horlick, interviewed in 1998, had a contrasting experience during her particularly moving interview:

> I think the reason that the interview came across as being more intimate than most was because I was living in Great Ormond Street Hospital at the time with my daughter, who was having a bone marrow transplant with the hope of curing her leukaemia. We went into the hospital in December 1997 and stayed there until her death on 27 November 1998. As you can imagine, it was a very traumatic time for me and I found it incredibly beneficial talking to Anthony. It wasn't just a radio programme, it became an actual therapy session [...] Anthony could feel the pain that I was suffering and was extremely kind to me. After Georgie died, he wrote me a lovely letter saying that he felt he knew her, even though he had never met her, and how tragic her death at the age of 12 was.
>
> I thought he was a wonderful man. The two hours that I spent with him helped me to cope with the immense difficulties that I was facing at that time in my life and I was very grateful. It wasn't just that he was a psychiatrist, he was also a father and he felt a deep empathy for me as I watched my darling daughter battling for life.[104]

In a similar vein, writer Gillian Slovo, interviewed in 1997, remembers 'thinking what a relief it was to talk to someone who genuinely wanted to hear what I had to say and who had no agenda and no need to dwell in sensation'.[105] She recalls 'that there were tissues in the studio and when I commented on their presence Anthony said, "Oh, those aren't mine. Must have been left from the previous studio users."'

There were numerous other memorable, frequently emotional interviews with figures as diverse as Professor John Bayley, widower of Dame Iris Murdoch;[106] social activist Mary Whitehouse;[107] comedian Les Dawson, recorded just a week before his death in 1993; and politicians Tony Benn and Paddy Ashdown. Clare also conducted interviews in the United States and invited certain guests back for re-interviews, including writer P.D. James, his first guest Glenda Jackson, and even Claire Rayner. The programme transitioned from radio to television (receiving an enthusiastic review from Nigella Lawson in *The Spectator* in 1995),[108] but Clare preferred radio, feeling that seeing both him and his subject was a distraction and took away from what they were discussing.[109]

Over the years, the vast majority of guests were impressed by Clare's engagement with the process and genuine interest in their stories and motivations. Reporter Martin Bell commented that Clare had clearly done his homework before the interview.[110] Neuroscientist Baroness Susan Greenfield, interviewed in 2000, also recalls an enjoyable discussion with Clare. She was 'a fan of *In the Psychiatrist's Chair* so I was very pleased to be asked':

> The interview on *In the Psychiatrist's Chair* was different from usual media interviews. It was a more interesting and rewarding dialogue. Normally you are just asked to give sound bites and they overload the discussion with too many people. I enjoyed this interview very much and thought what a nice man Tony Clare was.[111]

The *Observer* reported that 'disappointingly, Greenfield came across as a well-balanced, confident woman who knows what she wants and plans to cram in as much as she can before she dies so she has no regrets at her moment of death'.[112] Greenfield relates this to her being 'grounded' and to her media experience:

I am grounded and also others would not have had as much media experience as I had. I don't feel I need to air my personal life as much as younger people. I'd like to think that although I'm involved in public activities, I'm still a private person.

Even so, the *Guardian* concluded that 'Clare delivered the revelatory goods as always', with Greenfield.[113] Like Widdecombe, however, not all interviewees felt that Clare penetrated their inner lives. Some, like explorer Ranulph Fiennes, found satisfaction in apparently eluding Clare's analysis.[114] Rantzen, while recognising that '*In the Psychiatrist's Chair* was compulsory listening if you were interested in people, or interviewing, or both,'[115] also felt that there was one guest whom Clare's gaze did not penetrate:

There was one interviewee who completely eluded him, for me: [comedian] Ken Dodd. Ken Dodd just defended himself against every question with a joke or something to distract Tony. I knew Ken Dodd was an extraordinary, brilliant talent but quite strange. I'm not sure how much of that strangeness emerged in the programme.[116]

Rantzen's own interview with Clare 'was an interview on a deeper level than many. There are many unscrupulous and superficial interviews done. It's nice to have experienced one that was actually skilful and insightful.' She adds that 'I think he said that Peter Hall [theatre, opera and film director] and I were the least introspective people he ever interviewed.' Introspective or not, Clare coaxed insight after insight from Rantzen and his other guests over many years, resulting in radio that was often riveting, always engrossing and certainly never dull.

Legacy

In the Psychiatrist's Chair ended in 2001, but its legacy has proven remarkably enduring. Episodes are frequently re-broadcast on the BBC and a CD set was released by BBC Worldwide in 2016. The four published volumes of interviews were generally well received.[117] Commenting on the 1992 volume[118] in *The Irish Times*, psychologist Maureen Gaffney noted that Clare 'pioneered a unique kind of psychological theatre' and, despite her questions about the addition of detailed commentaries in the book, concluded that Clare's 'use of psychiatry is always imaginative, sometimes brilliant':

> It is Anthony Clare's clinical skill [...] which makes these interviews unique. When a subject is obfuscating, the psychiatrist concludes, quite correctly, that this is revealing. The tools of the trade are masterfully used: the analysis of defences, the attention to seemingly unimportant details, the reading of unconscious cues. But as he acknowledges himself, making sense of an individual history is never conclusive. Essentially, it is a matter of plausibility. The listeners can make up their own minds.[119]

According to *The Times*, the final volume, published in 1998,[120] was compulsive reading owing both to its interviews with comedian Stephen Fry and musician Nigel Kennedy, among others, and to Clare's clear interviewing skills.[121]

In the Psychiatrist's Chair also fulfilled a need in Clare, of course. His friend David Knowles notes that 'Tony needed to find a place where he was valued. Once he discovered the BBC, it was clear that he was going to be a media star on his own terms. He was competitive and highly motivated, though I think that there was often a lack of confidence, a lack of self-esteem, that was underneath all of that.'[122]

As a result of the success of *In the Psychiatrist's Chair*, Clare received a great deal of correspondence and countless invitations to write, speak and chair events.[123] He even agreed to put lawyers 'in the psychiatrist's chair' at the Solicitors Law Festival in Disneyland Paris in 1999.[124] Clare also interviewed widely,[125] speaking especially memorably with biographer, historian and journalist Gitta Sereny at the Hay Festival in May 1998 (although it appears that Clare sold more books afterwards than Sereny did).[126] There was a particularly large postbag following Clare's 1994 *In The Psychiatrist's Chair* interview with forensic pathologist and crime writer Bernard Knight,[127] who admired Clare's 'tenacity and style, even when they reduced some of his subjects to tears':

> I was asked to submit myself to *The Chair* at about time of the Fred and Rosemary West murders in the 'House of Horror' in Gloucester in 1993 [...] I'm sure Anthony wanted to talk to me to discover what kind of a monster could dig up twelve decomposed corpses from the ground (thirteen if one counts the foetuses) [...] I recall going to an upper-storey room in central London, rather than a formal BBC studio [...] I certainly remember waiting in a room where some kind acolyte had placed a bottle of white wine and a glass. Though I am not much of a drinker, I availed myself of this luxury, which no doubt contributed to my unusual loquacity and injudicious opinions about religion and dislike of humanity, which stimulated one of the largest post-bags that Anthony had ever received![128]

Knight recalls Clare 'as a slight man with a great Irish accent and manner to match. I was reminded of a small terrier, as he had a persuasive, interrogative manner which never went beyond the bounds of polite enquiry.' Clare 'kept returning to his interest in my dreams, the only manifestation of my unease with my morbid profession':

> I felt that he was trying to prise open an admission of my dislike (during waking hours) of my horrible work – and he was somehow disconcerted by my stone-walling of his attempts to crack open a shell of assumed indifference to it.
>
> In fact, I was speaking the truth about my ability to compartmentalise my life in the mortuary or crime scene from my private life, but he kept returning to this theme in his inimitable way. He did not seem ready to accept this and I think I said at one point that I never thought about this potentially schizoid situation except when other people, including him, raised the subject!
>
> I know that this persuasive ability was part of his stock-in-trade that made the *Chair* series so popular over such a long period,

and I enjoyed sparring with him, as I always enjoyed fencing with opposing Counsel in the higher courts.

In the Psychiatrist's Chair was not unique in focusing on in-depth, somewhat tenacious interviewing, as it was preceded by John Freeman's *Face to Face* in the late 1950s and early 1960s, and followed by similar programmes featuring psychologists Oliver James[129] and Pamela Connolly.[130] James had clear views about the appeal of *In the Psychiatrist's Chair*, reported in the *Observer* in 2001:

> The programme's lack of psychoanalytic input is its greatest asset, says media rival Oliver James, the psychologist and author of *Britain on the Couch*. 'What most people are really enjoying is a quasi-tabloid revelation of the private life of a public figure,' James says. 'That we are none the wiser at the end about why this person is like they are is not important; all that matters is that we have witnessed the simulacrum of intimacy and heard a few biographical anecdotes.'[131]

Notwithstanding such views, Clare's work has richly outlasted that of virtually all other interviewers. Even several decades after their appearance in Clare's *Chair*, many interviewees still recall the particular impact of their interview with Clare both on them personally and on people they met soon afterwards. Clare did worry about his role in the media at times, commenting at one point that 'I don't want to become a kind of media shrink, but someday, somebody may make me an offer.'[132] Despite the ubiquity of his media involvement, however, Clare did not lose his professional gravitas or become over-exposed in the media in the manner of David Stafford-Clark.[133]

Magician and psychic Uri Geller recalls his 'amazing, in-depth' 1996 interview with Clare with deep fondness. He rates it well above the thousands of other interviews he has given over the course of his career:

> Ninety per cent of interviews are entirely superficial but Clare asked questions that I am usually not asked. He really went out

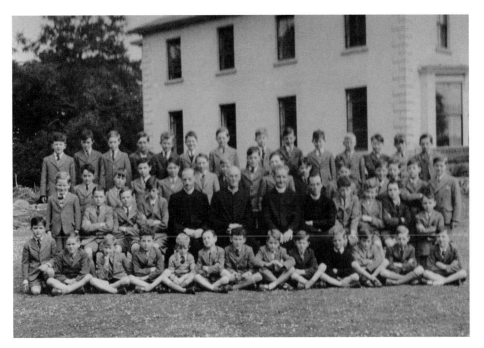

Class of 1950–51, Gonzaga College SJ, Ranelagh, Dublin. Anthony Clare is sixth from the left in the front row. (Reproduced by kind permission of Jane Clare.)

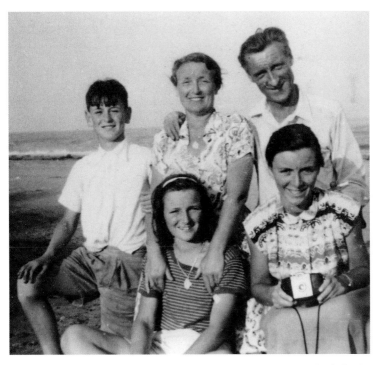

Family trip to Donabate Strand, County Dublin with Clare (on the left), his mother Agnes, his father Ben and his sisters Jeanne (in front of Agnes) and Wyn (in front of Ben). (Reproduced by kind permission of the Clare family.)

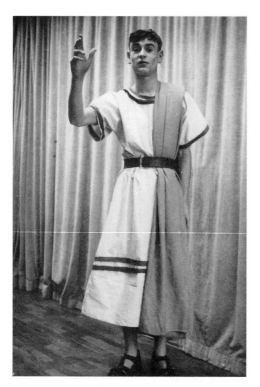

Clare, aged 17, plays the part of Felix in *The Comedian* by Henri Ghéon, the first play produced on the original stage at Gonzaga College SJ, Ranelagh, Dublin (4 February 1960). (Reproduced by kind permission of the Gonzaga College Archive.)

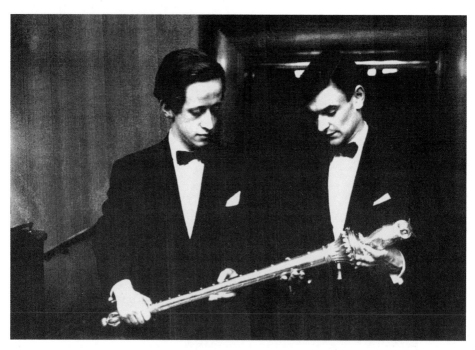

Clare was deeply involved in debating with the University College Dublin Literary and Historical Society and, with debating colleague Patrick Cosgrave, won the *Observer* Mace Trophy in 1964. (Reproduced by kind permission of *The Irish Times*.)

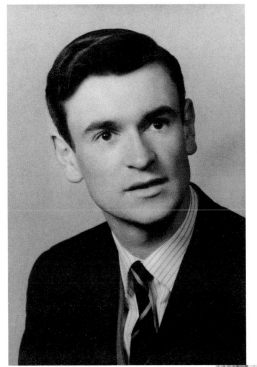

Clare in the early 1960s. (Reproduced by kind permission of Jane Clare.)

Clare and Jane on their wedding day, 4 October 1966, in Dublin. (Reproduced by kind permission of Jane Clare.)

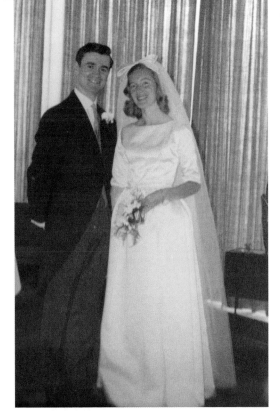

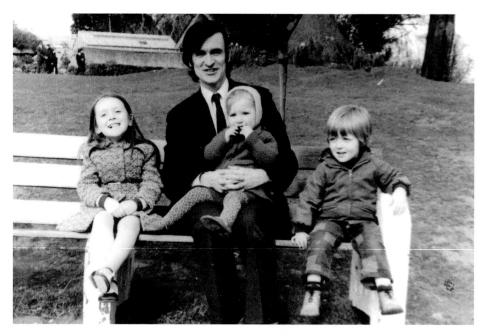

Clare with Rachel, Eleanor and Simon, in Herbert Park, Dublin in the early 1970s. The park was within walking distance of Jane's parents' house, 'Clogheen' on Shelbourne Road, near Lansdowne Road rugby stadium. (Reproduced by kind permission of Rachel Clare.)

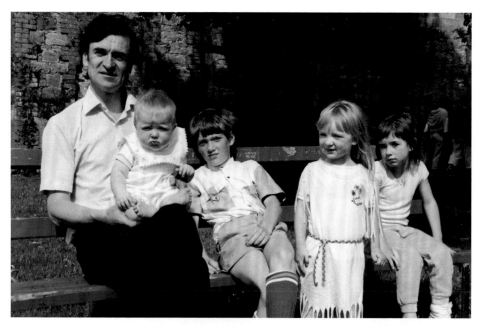

Clare with (from left) two of his sons, Sebastian and Peter, and two of his daughters, Justine and Sophie, on holiday in Stradbally, County Waterford in August 1985. (Photograph courtesy of Dr John O'Connell, reproduced by kind permission of the Clare family.)

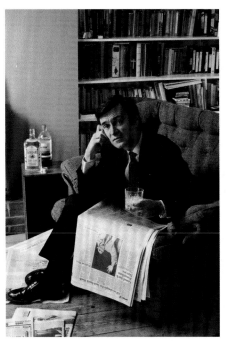

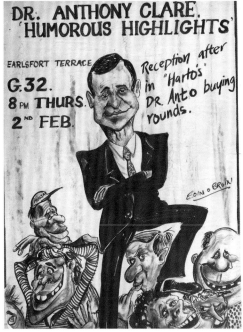

Clare at home in south London (1990). (Homer Sykes/Alamy Stock Photo)

A poster for 'Dr Anthony Clare: Humorous Highlights' at University College Dublin, Earlsfort Terrace, 2 February 1989. (Reproduced by kind permission of Mr Eoin Ó Broin and Dr Aidan Collins.)

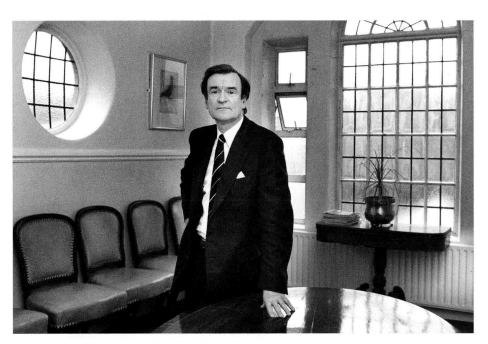

Clare outside his office in St Patrick's Hospital in July 2000. (Photograph: Brenda Fitzsimons. Reproduced by kind permission of *The Irish Times*.)

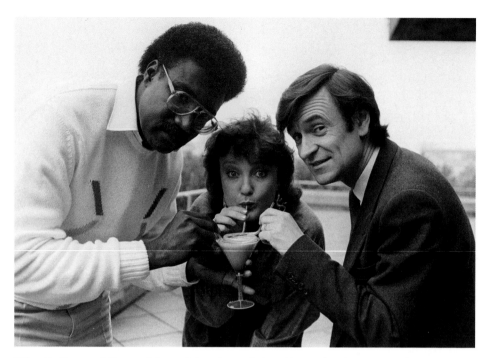

West Indies and Lancashire cricket legend Sir Clive Lloyd, BBC Radio One disc jockey Janice Long and Clare launched Drinkwise London, with the aid of an alcohol-free cocktail, at The National Theatre, London in September 1986. (PA Images/Alamy Stock Photo)

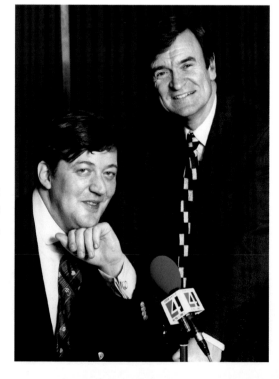

Clare interviewed actor and writer Stephen Fry on *In the Psychiatrist's Chair* on BBC Radio 4 in June 1997. (Jeff Overs/Getty Images)

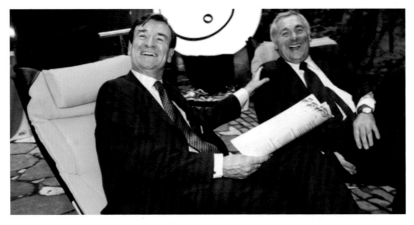

Clare with An Taoiseach Bertie Ahern on 11 September 2000. (Photograph: Cyril Byrne. Reproduced by kind permission of *The Irish Times*.)

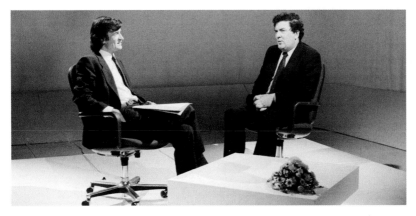

Clare interviewed John Hume, leader of Northern Ireland's Social Democratic and Labour Party (SDLP), on RTÉ Television's *Irish in Mind* in August 1988. (John Cooney/RTÉ)

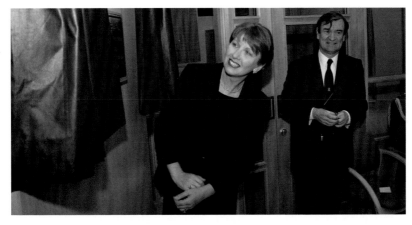

At Clare's invitation, President Mary McAleese visited St Patrick's Hospital on 6 November 2000. (Photograph: Frank Miller. Reproduced by kind permission of *The Irish Times*.)

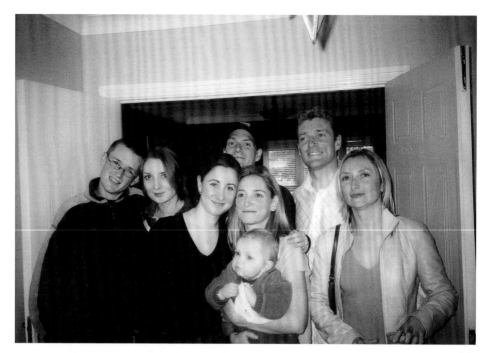

Clare and Jane's seven children (from left): Sebastian, Justine, Sophie, Peter, Eleanor, Simon and Rachel; Eleanor is holding her son, Sam Patterson. (Reproduced by kind permission of the Clare family.)

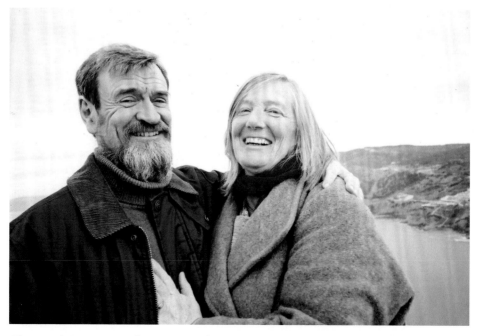

Clare and Jane in Sardinia, December 2003. (Reproduced by kind permission of Jane Clare.)

of the box. I know this was an excellent interview because it was really something that made a very major impression on other people who heard me answer his questions. Afterwards, a lot of individuals told me that they never knew these things about me. My mother comes from Sigmund Freud's family. My full name Uri Geller Freud, so maybe there was a subliminal connection between me and Clare.[134]

Rantzen links Clare's universally agreed charm with his Irishness:

Tony was charming. I always think the Irish have this very unfair advantage over the rest of the population with this thing called charm. I always enjoyed Tony's company. He was also extremely insightful so I remember our conversations with great affection.[135]

Rantzen is far from alone in recalling her interview with Clare with particular warmth. There was consistently similar feedback from the public too, commonly focusing on the value of seeing beyond the public persona of well-known figures.[136] Greenfield even sees a need for a similar programme today, over thirty-five years since the first episode of *In the Psychiatrist's Chair* was broadcast:

Given that mental health is now more centre stage and in the public eye, and given the rise in anxiety and depression among teenagers, I think we are now very aware of mental health as an issue [...] It would be interesting if the general public could again have a psychiatrist talking to people about these issues. Anything that empowers people is valuable. The brain is so poorly taught because it is perceived to be difficult, but the more you can talk about these things, the more you will empower people.[137]

David Hendy, in his history of BBC Radio 4, concludes that the striking message at the heart of *In the Psychiatrist's Chair* was simply that we are the people we are, and although we are shaped by our past, we need not be imprisoned by it.[138] This was Clare's key message not only on *In the Psychiatrist's Chair* but throughout much of his other work too: that we are all human beings, living and suffering as one, and we should take the time to listen and understand each other.

Clare's wife Jane is clear that Clare himself 'would never have gone on *In the Psychiatrist's Chair* as a guest. Not in a million years'.[139] She adds that Clare 'did what he did because he loved it'. That, too, is abundantly clear in his brilliant, sparkling broadcasts from his eponymous, timeless *Chair*.

6

Return to Ireland (1989)

• •

In January 1989, Clare returned to Dublin where he became medical director of St Patrick's Hospital and Clinical Professor at the Department of Psychiatry in Trinity College Dublin. Jane and the rest of the family returned in September. The three oldest children, Rachel, Simon and Eleanor, remained in London, living in the family home in Beckenham which remained the family's principal residence until 2001. Peter, one of Clare's other sons, who is now a qualified Doctor in Counselling Psychology (D.Couns.Psych, Trinity College Dublin), recalls the move:

> I was born in London and lived there until I was 12. I moved to boarding school in Ireland in 1988 before my father started his work as medical director at St Patrick's in 1989. I saw a lot of him at that time – that was the period when I had the most access to him.[1]

Peter points out that that his father 'was different within the four walls of the home. When he crossed that threshold, I can imagine his difficulty of leaving his professional persona at the door. Dad had a fantastic imagination. He would tell us stories at bedtime. He could create an extraordinary imaginary world':

> I have wonderful memories of playing football with my younger brother. There was a field beside our home, Delville, on the grounds of St Edmundsbury, which came with the medical directorship. We'd be kicking the ball around, the door would

open, and suddenly Dad would appear. He would be full of vim, vigour, activity and joy. We'd be there together, playing football with this great sense of togetherness. Then, suddenly, someone, my Mum perhaps, would yell out 'Tony, the phone!' He'd say, 'I'll be right back' and we wouldn't see him again. He'd be gone. There was this great sense of abandonment and we would wait for his return, which rarely if ever happened. Now, as an adult, I can realise how busy he was and how much of himself he gave to everyone.

All the family remained close. Rachel recalls that her parents 'kept coming back to London for Christmas and Easter. Mimi [the family cat] would travel with them too, over and back':

Dad left London for my mother, she was ready to 'go home'. But I don't think he saw himself growing old [in London] either. There was always a plan to go back, the question was when. It became very difficult practically too – the long commute was getting him down.[2]

Peter recalls that 'coming back to Ireland was challenging. Ireland was different to the UK; there was a sense of chaos; there was a need to compartmentalise':

Why did he come back to Ireland? Mum. He loved his wife. The oldest three, Rachel, Simon and Eleanor, all stayed on in England and studied there. There were the 'oldies', who stayed in England, and the 'youngies', who returned to Dublin in 1989. I was in the middle. There was parentification: we each looked after someone below us.[3]

Many moves were contemplated over the years, but they finally settled on a move to Dublin around 1989. Moving from the UK mental health system back to a large private psychiatric hospital in Dublin was a big change for Clare.[4] Following his arrival at his new place of work, Clare was clear that 'the main challenge facing St Patrick's

Hospital is posed by the move away from hospital-based treatment to community-based care':

> The fact that there will always be a need for high quality, multidisciplinary inpatient diagnosis and treatment means that there will always be a future for a hospital such as St Patrick's but if it is to survive in roughly the size and shape it currently manifests it will have to develop its therapeutic base. At present it is open to the criticism that it is somewhat excessively reliant on physical treatments (i.e. drugs and ECT) and insufficiently developed when it comes to psychotherapeutic interventions (i.e. family therapy, marital therapy, counselling) and social interventions (i.e. social work, community-based facilities, etc.).[5]

At that time, St Patrick's Hospital and St Edmundsbury Hospital in Lucan, which formed part of the same organisation, had around 2,500 admissions per year, a bed capacity of approximately 342 beds, and an average length of stay of 39 days. In 1990, Clare pointed out significant problems, especially with staffing.

Against this background, Clare introduced many changes at St Patrick's over the following years: additional facilities were built; a new intensive care unit was opened; psychological therapies were expanded; and Clare persuaded the hospital governors to fund research posts in psychiatry.[6] Professor James Lucey, a colleague of Clare and one of his successors as medical director of St Patrick's, 'arrived in St Patrick's in 1988 and then [Clare] arrived back to become medical director [the following year]. He transformed the place in so many ways. He came like a dynamo. No one could motivate people or channel the ideas of psychiatry like Tony':

> At St Patrick's, Tony found a hospital here that was very much reeling from the introduction of community psychiatry. He was now essentially running a private asylum and seeking to address the changes in the idiom. So, he led a programme of change. For

example, there were no shared clinical notes in St Patrick's at this time; patients' details were kept in the consultants' private rooms. Tony introduced multidisciplinary clinical notes into the hospital. He transformed the place, promoting multi-disciplinary teams and psychotherapy.

[Clare] was insistent that the hospital fund research and fund people to do research. So, Tony established the 'Norman Moore Fellowship', so titled to get the board's support and to acknowledge [Clare's mentor, Professor Norman] Moore. Dr Mary O'Hanlon was the worthy first recipient.[7]

When O'Hanlon moved on, Clare said to Lucey: 'I'm afraid I'll have to give the Fellowship to you.' Lucey accepted and recalls that 'that Fellowship made a big difference in my life; Ted Dinan provided a research paradigm and Tony provided the opportunity – my task was to synthesise the two'.

Over this period, Clare also made particular contributions to re-organising postgraduate training for junior doctors seeking to become psychiatrists and he attracted world leaders in psychiatry to speak at the annual 'Founder's Day' meeting in St Patrick's.[8] Dr Frank O'Donoghue, a consultant psychiatrist colleague and assistant medical director at the hospital, recalls that 'Tony was one of the smartest people I ever came across in my life':

I had come across him initially in UCD when he was auditor of the L&H. I didn't meet him again until he came to St Patrick's. Tony tended to look at things from a different perspective, but he was very reasonable. When he was appointed as clinical director, the general feeling was he had been appointed to raise the profile of the hospital because of his public persona.

Tony asked would I be his assistant clinical director in St Patrick's so I worked with him very closely. We used to go to the board meetings in the hospital and because he had so many commitments in the UK, I used to fill in for him quite a bit.[9]

Throughout much of this time, especially in the early years, Clare retained strong links with London and made frequent trips back and forth.[10] He was, as he put it in 1990, 'toing and froing at a great rate'.[11] One of the key reasons for this was Clare's continued involvement with the iconic television discussion programme, *After Dark*.

After Dark (1987–91)

Clare especially enjoyed hosting *After Dark*, a pioneering television discussion show developed by Sebastian Cody in the mid-1980s.[12] The show invited diverse guests who knew a lot about a topic in the news and talked freely for as long as they wished. *After Dark* ran for some ninety editions, first on the recently founded Channel 4 and, in 2003, on the BBC. Clare hosted twelve editions of the programme between 1987 and 1991, focused on such diverse themes as football, murder, sex, the death penalty and education.

Cody had interviewed Clare at the BBC in 1984, two years after *In the Psychiatrist's Chair* first aired and three years before *After Dark*, and 'was struck by his intelligence, his willingness to question himself, his confusion over the power of television and his own attraction to becoming a media star':

> From then on, I would occasionally phone Tony at Bart's, for reasons of a shared world view but also for entirely practical journalistic purposes (such as getting an off-the-record view of one of his interviewees or some contact details). I talked to him about *Club 2* [the Austrian forerunner of *After Dark*] and how this programme went a long way to dealing with the normally destructive workings of broadcast television; specifically, exactly those issues which had led his attempts to do *In the Psychiatrist's Chair* on TV [*Motives*] to fail.[13]

Cody formally approached Clare about *After Dark* in April 1986.[14] Clare suggested that they discuss the matter over champagne in Julie's Restaurant and Champagne Bar in Holland Park[15] 'which seemed astonishingly decadent' to Cody – not least because *After Dark* had not yet been formally commissioned by Channel 4. Cody and Clare agreed that *After Dark* would usually feature guests aged 40 years or over who were not just professional commentators but had lived a life (like *In the Psychiatrist's Chair*) and 'people of different class, region, age, experience but also psychological make-up; there was a priority to counteract the ubiquity and self-selection of narcissists'.[16]

By December 1986 they were in the early stages of production of a number of pilot episodes with Clare hosting the first one, devoted to the prison system. The eclectic line-up of guests included a friend of the Kray twins (notorious English criminals); a Conservative writer; a prison officer; a woman who had served a sentence for helping her mother to die; and John Stonehouse, a British politician whom Clare had already interviewed some time previously. After the recording, Clare opted to go to the crew room rather than the green room with the guests. Cody notes that Clare 'all but disapproved of the grand folk he interviewed. He was certainly rarely in touch with anyone he interviewed, never having anything to do with them once the interview was over'.

As Cody notes, 'the preconditions of *After Dark* (intimacy, no studio audience, uncensored, no obligation to show off, and, above all, open-ended) resolved most of the frustrations Tony felt with other formats including, indeed, *In the Psychiatrist's Chair* ... *After Dark* was also a programme guaranteed to feed someone so hungry for intellectual stimulus, so busy with ideas, as Tony'. In addition, '*After Dark* was better paid than radio or writing', which would have also appealed to Clare.

As with *In the Psychiatrist's Chair*, Clare generally arrived at the studio for *After Dark* at the very last moment, mastered his brief quickly, and handled any emergent legal complexities smoothly; the length and format of *After Dark* allowed apologies and retractions to occur before the programme ended, provided the host was assured in their role – as Clare invariably was. The role was far from simple, however, and was, at times, extravagantly complex. In June 1988, for example, Clare hosted an episode titled 'How Do You Survive a Murder' which Cody describes as 'a variously moving, thrilling and challenging encounter between a vicar who murdered his mother; Myra Hindley's best friend [Hindley was a notorious child murderer]; a woman who founded a self-help group for the parents of murdered children after one of her own was killed; the reclusive thriller writer Patricia Highsmith; a psychiatrist who married a killer; a senior detective policeman; and the daughter of Ruth Ellis, the last woman to be hanged in Britain'.[17] Widely discussed in the media, this and other episodes of *After Dark* invariably presented such a diverse range of opinions that Clare concluded, at the end of one episode in March 1991, concerning the teaching profession, that he had 'never seen any group of people less willing to listen to each other's point of view'.

That was the final episode of *After Dark* that Clare presented, despite Cody's repeated invitations for him to return to the programme: Clare 'was a magnificent chair and I broadly always wanted him'. But by 2001, Clare had largely withdrawn from all media work, telling Cody firmly that he would not return to television, 'not even for *After Dark*'.[18]

Back in Ireland

Following his return to Ireland in 1989, Clare initially continued his media involvements with the BBC and various other organisations, and saw patients in London on Friday afternoons,[19] but he clearly still missed the pace and excitement of the extraordinary life he had created for himself in London. So, why did he return to Ireland at all, given that he reported being happy in London and had plainly achieved so much there?

An interview in *The Irish Times* in December 1988, the month before Clare's return to Dublin, concluded that he was coming back because Ireland was *home*, and Clare felt a responsibility to *do something* about the place: to increase partnership in mental health care, to make a contribution, and to have a greater stake in the land of his birth.[20] The traffic congestion, cost of living and school fees in

London were other considerations.[21] Clare had also become unhappy at Bart's: the pettiness of medical politics had started to wear on his nerves.

Even so, Robin Murray reflects that Clare's return to Ireland was an unusual move:

> Why did he go back to Dublin? It would not have been an orthodox thing to do then, even though it is now. These were early days for academic research in Dublin and Tony's position was as a clinical director of St Patrick's Hospital. He didn't quite flourish quite so much when in Dublin. He ran a clinic in London after he had moved back to Dublin, returning every so often. He would return regularly to go to the BBC and he was still around in the media. But he was not quite the force in UK psychiatry that he had been before.
>
> Tony's most influential period was in the 1980s and on into the 1990s with things like *In The Psychiatrist's Chair* [Chapter 5]. After he went back to Ireland, he was invited to give speeches around the world. You wouldn't go to hear Tony talk about the latest biology, you'd go because he'd be funny, entertaining and stimulating.[22]

After his return to Dublin in 1989, Clare not only continued a clinic in London for some time and treated patients in St Patrick's, but also oversaw liaison psychiatry services to a number of general hospitals in Dublin where psychiatrists would visit to provide specialist opinions about medical or surgical inpatients with mental health problems. John Moriarty, then registrar in psychiatry in Dublin and later director of the Maudsley Training Programme in London, worked under Clare's supervision in a liaison psychiatry training post across several Dublin hospitals in 1991, shortly after Clare's return to Ireland. For Moriarty, Clare 'was an authoritative presence at weekly case presentations and teaching who was not afraid to challenge or quiz his senior colleagues on their assessments and management of cases, and I rather suspect we juniors enjoyed their discomfort as much as they may have mildly resented his role':

I worked specifically for Clare for my last six-month training rotation in liaison psychiatry, which was typically reserved for the more senior juniors, often immediately after their membership exams. This was a good post in which to develop and exercise autonomy. I met Clare for one hour weekly in which we could discuss all cases. One conversation I do remember (over lunch when he joined a group of us) was that he expressed the view that doctors' role in psychiatric practice was not a given and that the multidisciplinary nature of it was such that we needed to be clear, at least in our own minds, how medical knowledge and skills were important.

Clare remains well remembered and well regarded by those who are now very senior in their roles in psychiatry in London. His book *Psychiatry in Dissent* [Chapter 3] is still on many colleagues' 'Top Ten' lists and was again a featured book in our 'Maudsley Book Group' in 2018. It is still found relevant by trainees today.[23]

Throughout the 1990s, Clare not only travelled to London and elsewhere (to appear in media or give talks), treated patients in London and Dublin,[24] and developed services at St Patrick's, but he also deepened his media involvements in Ireland. He was a frequent guest on the iconic *Late Late Show* on RTÉ television, hosted a radio show on Lyric FM,[25] and presented *Irish in Mind*, a seven-part RTÉ television series in which he interviewed prominent Irish people such as journalist Nuala O'Faolain and barrister, former senator and future Supreme Court judge, Catherine McGuinness (1988–9). Clare particularly enjoyed his interview with John Hume, Irish politician and co-recipient (with David Trimble) of the 1998 Nobel Peace Prize.[26] Clare also continued to write prodigiously in popular and professional media,[27] and to contribute to the academic literature in medicine and psychiatry.

Clare had close working relationships with the Board of Governors of St Patrick's Hospital, which then included Gemma Hussey, a Fine Gael politician who served as a Senator for the National University of Ireland (1977–82) and *Teachta Dála* (TD) for Wicklow (1982–9), including periods as Minister for Education (1982–6), Social Welfare

(1986–7) and Labour (1987). Clare campaigned strongly for more women to be appointed to the St Patrick's Board: 'I sense', he wrote in 1993, 'that Gemma Hussey finds her position as the only woman on an all-male board not always that easy.'[28] Hussey presented certificates at the annual graduation day from the School of Nursing at St Patrick's in 1990 owing not only to her position on the board but also (as Clare wrote to her) 'your contribution to the debate about the quality and nature of education in Ireland, together with your achievements as a senior politician'.[29]

In 1990, Hussey published a book titled *At the Cutting Edge: Cabinet Diaries 1982–1987*[30] and Clare added a PS to his letter inviting her to graduation day that year: 'I read your book with fascination and have to confess that it certainly made one reader think again about the seduction of politics!' Clare was, however, fatally prone to seductions of this type and in 1993, four years after his return to Ireland, he ran for a seat in *Seanad Éireann* (the Senate), the upper house of the Irish *Oireachtas* (parliament).

Clare, a graduate of UCD, competed for a Senate seat in the National University of Ireland Senate constituency as part of the convoluted, controversial mechanism for allocating seats in the Senate.[31] Politically, Clare tended to vote for the Labour Party and had previously spoken with Labour TDs about extending a national health insurance scheme, giving private health insurance entitlements to people who could not afford it, rather than creating an 'Irish National Health Service'.[32] As Clare's friend David Knowles notes, 'Tony was left of centre in politics.'[33] But Clare's plans for health reform, like so many others visions for the Irish health service, never came to fruition.

Jane opposed Clare's 1993 Senate run as 'just one more thing on top of everything else'. She need not have worried too much: in the event, Clare polled 7.22 per cent of first preference votes and was eliminated in sixth position on the tenth count. Friends felt that Clare was naïve about Irish politics and that there was a resentful perception among some people that Clare saw himself as in a superior position, having returned from England apparently to solve Ireland's problems.[34] Whatever the reason, the outcome was a blow: Clare –

ever the competitor and debater – 'did not like to lose', according to Jane. As Rachel points out, 'I don't think he ever failed at anything significant before.'[35]

Murray, too, reflects that Clare's 'unfulfilled political ambitions were the major disappointment of his life':

> He stood to be a senator and didn't get in. That was very disappointing indeed for him. He had seen he could make a wide impact on the public through the media and he'd always been very interested in politics. He wasn't ideological. Politically, he was slightly left-ish although I don't think he had strong socialist principles.
>
> This was a big disappointment for him. I think Jane wanted to go back to Dublin and he thought he'd have a shot at politics as he was looking for something new. I'm not sure he felt running St Patrick's was the most fantastic job in the world.[36]

Jane agrees, pointing out that Clare 'became frustrated at meetings in St Patrick's, saying "nobody wants to reveal what they think"'.[37] Media work was Clare's release valve for many years as '*In the Psychiatrist's Chair* [Chapter 5] alleviated the tedium of his day job, but then personal interviews became mainstream' and Clare's once pioneering show was no longer unique. It was a victim of its own success and lost some of its excitement as a result. As Jane notes, 'initially, coming back to Ireland had no impact; he went back and forth to London frequently. Asked where he lived, he would respond: "in mid-air".' But Clare had become accustomed to the busy, buzzy life that characterised his London years and he struggled to settle in Ireland: 'He needed the energy, he was full of ideas, and like a coiled spring.' Dublin simply did not offer the same possibilities as London.

Psychiatrist Anthony Mann, like many of Clare's London colleagues, 'lost touch with Tony after his return to Ireland but I bumped into him several years later at a conference. He looked very different with his long beard, and at first glance I didn't know who it was. It seemed he was hiding behind his beard.'[38]

This prolonged period of transition back to Ireland, which, in truth, never really ended, was undoubtedly a difficult one for Clare. But, paradoxically, this difficulty might well account for Clare's extraordinary, almost frenzied rate of activity over many of these years: writing endlessly, teaching, researching, broadcasting and doing extensive clinical work – all with a view to advancing public education and debate about mental illness and improving psychological well-being.[39] As Jane recalls, Clare had a particular fondness for opinion articles which we wrote with a fluidity and eloquence that belied the speed at which he produced them: 'He didn't enjoy the book process. He preferred articles or opinion pieces. He was impatient. Speed was important. He was a quick man. He walked quickly. He talked quickly. He read quickly. He was very efficient at chairing meetings.'[40]

Following his return to Ireland, then, and despite the complexities of his very gradual readjustment, Clare remained actively concerned with a broad range of issues linking psychiatry, psychology and society, as well as more academic concerns about the nature and purpose of psychiatry. As a result, Clare's key outputs during this period included not only countless articles in popular and professional media, but also academic papers on a wide variety of themes and, perhaps most interestingly, in 2000, a fascinating if flawed book with a very telling title: *On Men: Masculinity in Crisis.*[41]

Writing and Research

Turning to Clare's research and academic writings first, it is notable that, despite his many commitments, Clare not only wrote academic papers and books, but was also generous in his support of the work of others, especially those engaged in public education about mental and physical illness. This was a recurring theme: understanding the links between mind and body, and improving the care of both.[42]

In 1991, Clare wrote a foreword to a book titled *Challenging Cancer: From Chaos to Control* by Nira Kfir and Maurice Slevin, which sought to inform and empower people with cancer.[43] Clare emphasised that facing cancer involved determination and commitment, rationality and common sense, precisely as the book's authors recommended. Ironically, Clare's short, punchy foreword was reprinted in the second edition eleven years later,[44] at which point it was joined by another foreword, this one written by Clare Rayner,[45] whom Clare had controversially interviewed on *In the Psychiatrist's Chair* in 1988 (Chapter 5). On this occasion Clare and Rayner found common cause in recommending the book's proactive approach to dealing with cancer.

Clare also found much to admire in a 2004 volume on *Men's Health*, edited by Roger Kirby, Culley Carson, Michael Kirby and Riad Farah.[46] In his foreword to this book, Clare discussed the apparent decline of patriarchy and increased recognition of men's fragility – themes that he explored in greater depth in his own book about men, *On Men: Masculinity in Crisis*

Most interestingly, Clare contributed an essay entitled 'The mad Irish?' to a 1991 book, *Mental Health in Ireland*, published by Gill and Macmillan and RTÉ, based on lectures delivered in the Thomas Davis Lecture series on RTÉ Radio One in the summer of 1990.[47] Other contributors included Dr Dermot Walsh of St Loman's Hospital in Dublin, Dr Charles Smith of the Central Mental Hospital in Dundrum, and Dr Margo Wrigley, then Consultant Psychiatrist in the Psychiatry of Old Age at James Connolly Memorial Hospital in Dublin and later National Clinical Adviser and Clinical Programme Group Lead for Mental Health with the Health Service Executive.

Clare, in his contribution, recounted how, when working in the United States, he told a senior colleague that he was returning to Ireland to become a psychiatrist and his colleague was astonished, stating that surely Ireland did not need psychiatrists?[48] Clare emphasised that Ireland did indeed need psychiatrists and went on to discuss Ireland's problem with alcohol, the stigma wrongly associated with mental illness, and a host of other themes. In his classic, eclectic style, Clare quoted the poetry of Yeats, referred to the comedy of Spike Milligan, and articulated the need for greater understanding of mental illness and its treatment. This was vintage Clare.[49]

Two years later, in the *Journal of Mental Health*, Clare reiterated the importance of demystifying psychiatry, especially in the media,[50] and in September 1992 he devoted the Jansson Memorial Lecture at Trinity College Dublin to 'communication in medicine', suggesting that medical students should be tested on how well they can explain some aspect of medicine to lay people.[51] This later became a standard feature of undergraduate medical education in many universities, including Trinity.

Clare continued with the theme of public understanding of mental illness in 1994 with a coruscating lecture on 'violence, mental illness and society' at the Royal Society of Medicine in London.[52] Clare's contribution was the twenty-third in the series of the Stevens Lectures for the Laity; previous lecturers included Professor Sir Richard Doll (the epidemiologist who linked smoking with health problems) and Sir Ludovic Kennedy (a journalist and campaigner whom Clare interviewed on *In the Psychiatrist's Chair*). In his 1994 lecture, Clare noted that 'society yearns for simple solutions to complicated problems':[53]

> Anxious voices have been raised concerning the possible relationship between psychiatric illness and violence, the anxiety nourished by a series of dramatic, well-publicised and highly disturbing events – of which the most recent and tragic was the murder of an innocent bystander, Jonathan Zeto, by Christopher Clunis, a patient suffering from schizophrenia.

After a brisk and rather bleak run-through of the history of mental hospitals, Clare turned to the contemporary situation and noted that recently (in the 1990s), owing to a lack of psychiatric services, 'only when patients deteriorated to the point of violence were they being admitted. This is a truly dismal state of affairs and it is not new – I recall it well during my period working as a psychiatrist in Hackney in the early 1980s.'[54] After considering the relevant research, Clare concluded that the risk of violence associated with mental illness was 'low',[55] but problems of perception remained:

> The combined effect of the deployment of persistently inadequate community resources and the growing proliferation of media

accounts of violence and mental illness has been to increase public misperceptions and the stereotyping and stigmatisation of the psychiatrically ill. What is urgently needed now is corrective action [including] the appropriate and adequate provision of a quality and quantity of care for psychiatrically ill people that stands comparison with what we provide for the physically sick.[56]

It was also necessary 'to ensure that the psychiatrically ill enjoy the same public treatment, respect, understanding and tolerance as have been gained by other minority groups'.[57] Clare recommended greater engagement with the media to ensure that this occurred. Overall, Clare's 1994 lecture was an impassioned plea for understanding, tolerance and practical positive action in order to dispel negative myths about mental illness and provide better care to those who need it, thus reducing the risk of rare, unfortunate outcomes such as violence by the mentally ill.

Clare returned to this theme in the sixth series of Linacre Lectures (1995/6), a high-profile public lecture series focused on issues of environment and cross-disciplinary research, at Linacre College, a graduate college of the University of Oxford.[58] Clare's contribution, entitled 'Meeting of minds: the import of family and society', combined psychology with sociology, and – this being Clare – Sigmund Freud with poet Philip Larkin. Clare emphasised the importance of family relationships in maintaining mental health and the need for economic and legal policies to support family stability. Above all, he pointed to the fundamental inter-connectedness of all aspects of human life and the centrality of family relationships to individual flourishing.

In addition to his many lectures, Clare's research work in Dublin from 1989 onward involved a broad range of projects, many of which mapped onto themes of long-standing interest since the late 1960s and early 1970s. In 1976, Clare had bemoaned the false dichotomy between 'functional' (mental) and 'organic' (physical) disorders in *Psychiatry in Dissent*,[59] and in the 1990s he returned to this theme with gusto, co-authoring a series of papers seeking to better elucidate relationships between mental illness and physical health and function, focusing chiefly on the roles of hormones such as growth hormone,[60] progesterone,[61] prolactin,[62] cortisol[63] and thyrotropin-releasing hormone,[64] all of which have complex links with both mental and physical wellbeing. For Clare, the brain was clearly integrated with the rest of the body and neither part of the whole could be ignored.

A deep acknowledgement of these links was also apparent in Clare's writings about complex, contested conditions such as irritable bowel syndrome[65] and fatigue syndromes, such as the syndrome that can follow glandular fever.[66] Clare played a key role as chairman in the nuanced task of writing consensus 'guidelines for research' regarding chronic fatigue syndrome in 1991.[67] As medical director at St Patrick's he oversaw the development of a clinic dealing with chronic fatigue[68] which was based on the 'very good treatment model' developed by 'Dr Simon Wessely at King's College Hospital' in London.[69] Some of these activities were not without controversy. In 1999, Dr Fionnuala Lynch and Clare co-wrote an article about chronic fatigue syndrome in *Modern Medicine of Ireland* (Clare was on the journal's editorial board)[70] which elicited a strong, reasoned response from Dr Ellen Goudsmit, an archivist specialising in chronic fatigue syndrome.[71] This was certainly a controversial theme, but Clare was irresistibly drawn to robust dialogue and to topics that generated discussion, debate and dissent. He simply could not stay away.

Clare had a keen interest in alcohol dependence syndrome since the late 1960s and this was duly reflected in his later collaborative work with Dr Conor Farren and Professor Ted Dinan, among others.[72] He also continued to publish in the areas of depression and its treatment,[73] and wrote extensively about suicide and self-harm,[74] co-authoring a book with Caroline Smyth and Malcolm MacLachlan in 2003, titled *Cultivating Suicide? Destruction of Self in a Changing Ireland.*[75] MacLachlan, then Associate Professor of Psychology at Trinity and later Professor of Psychology and Social Inclusion at Maynooth University, recalls Clare's inclusive, reflective approach to their theme:

I first encountered Tony at a lecture he gave at the Institute of Psychiatry in London in 1988; the air of hushed excitement prior to his talk anticipated the personal, purposeful and reflective insights he went on to share. Some fifteen years later I co-authored a book with Tony, and with Caroline Smyth, when all three of us were living in Ireland. My sense was that Tony acknowledged more than most psychiatrists, the psychogenic component of psychological problems/mental illness. For instance, I recall him being very enthusiastic to learn from the experience of people who had clearly made genuine attempts to end their lives, but had failed to do so. He recognised that, at least for some people, there was a rationale for suicide, it was not just a compulsive, thoughtless or isolated act stimulated by brain chemistry imbalance. While recognising the value of biological psychiatry, he was far from the 'orange a day keeps depression away' type of psychiatrist, with whom I was then more familiar; and I believe he foreshadowed a closer and more respectful collaboration between psychiatry and cognate disciplines.[76]

Clare's involvement with the book followed on from a paper he co-wrote six years earlier, in 1997, with Dr (later Professor) Gregory Swanwick examining suicide in Ireland between 1945 and 1992, concluding that there was a true rise in suicide over this period, possibly linked with changing societal values.[77]

Clare also co-wrote papers about inpatient psychiatric care,[78] involuntary admission and treatment[79] (another long-standing concern),[80] and psychiatric liaison services to general hospitals,[81] including two further papers with Swanwick on this theme.[82] Swanwick, then registrar in psychiatry and later Dean of Education with the College of Psychiatrists of Ireland, recalls that his first publication, a review article on insomnia,[83] was also co-authored by Clare: 'For me, as a junior trainee, Anthony Clare's support and guidance provided significant encouragement.'[84]

Clare was unstoppable. He wrote and co-wrote papers about virtually every mental illness and psychological condition imaginable, ranging from obsessive compulsive disorder[85] and anxiety[86] to personality disorder,[87] and from the consequences of sexual abuse[88] to the psychiatric sequelae of termination of pregnancy[89] and abortion.[90] There was also a steady stream of articles in mainstream and medical media, as well as book reviews in publications as diverse as the *Literary Review*,[91] the *Irish Journal of Psychological Medicine*[92] and *Social Policy and Administration*,[93] as well as the *American Journal of Psychiatry*, in which he reviewed a study of portrayals of mental illness in the theatre (which, predictably, intrigued him),[94] a psycho-historical examination of British Prime Minister William Gladstone (who was, it seems, disturbingly obsessional)[95] and, in 2001, a volume on the relationship between violence and mental illness[96] – a topic that Clare had addressed seven years earlier in his lecture on 'violence, mental illness and society' at the Royal Society of Medicine.[97]

Teaching, Talking, Thinking

In addition to all of his other activities, Clare not only taught medical students at Trinity College, Dublin and overhauled postgraduate training for early career doctors seeking to become psychiatrists, but also published educational texts and papers for undergraduate and postgraduate training. For undergraduate medical students, he wrote, in 1987 at Bart's, a superbly clear chapter on 'psychological medicine' for the medical text book of that time, *Clinical Medicine: A Textbook for Medical Students and Doctors*, edited by Parveen Kumar and Michael Clark (also at Bart's).[98] From St Patrick's, Clare contributed to the second,[99] third[100] and fourth editions of that book,[101] and Peter White of Bart's joined as co-author for the fifth,[102] sixth[103] and seventh editions of the text.[104] The seventh appeared in 2009, two years after Clare's death, and acknowledged the extreme sadness of the editors to lose a colleague who had contributed so well to the now classic volume, ever since its first edition. To this day, Clare's chapter remains an excellent guide to a complex field.

Clare also published extensively on various aspects of postgraduate psychiatric training, which was another long-standing concern of his ever since he co-founded the Association of Psychiatrists in Training (APIT) in the United Kingdom in the early 1970s. At St Patrick's, Clare wrote about training in psychodynamic psychotherapy for postgraduate trainees,[105] alcohol use among medical students and doctors,[106] the future of postgraduate psychiatry training in Ireland,[107] the role of the Royal College of Psychiatrists in the twenty-first century,[108] and proposals for a national body to advance psychiatric research in Ireland, which, sadly, never came to pass.[109] Clare also narrated *Safety in Psychiatry: The Mind's Eye*, an audiovisual and written training pack for postgraduate psychiatry trainees published by the Royal College of Psychiatrists and Gaskell in 2000, which was very well received.[110]

Over his time at St Patrick's (1989–2001) and at St Edmundsbury (2001–7), Clare also kept himself wildly busy with the administrative, clinical and academic affairs of the two hospitals, in addition to his other work. He devoted particular attention to his voluminous correspondence with colleagues, managers, politicians, patients and members of the public who wrote to him in great numbers after hearing his broadcasts or reading his articles in newspapers. In 1994, when the Royal College of Psychiatrists in London forwarded him yet another letter from a member of the public, Clare ruefully admitted that 'I don't have a standard letter' of response to such queries.[111] As a result, each of the thousands of letters that Clare wrote in response to queries from the public was unique and, as often as not, filled with warmth and personality.

Clare also devoted a great deal of time to lectures for the general public. The 'All in the Mind' biennial lecture series, for example, was running at St Patrick's before Clare's return to Dublin in 1989, and Clare visited from London to speak about 'psychiatry and the media' in 1985[112] and 'the concept of care in mental illness' in 1987, while also contributing a chapter of that title to the book that accompanied the 1986 lecture series.[113] After he returned as medical director, Clare spoke about the 'stigma' of mental illness in 1989 and 1991, and about 'attitudes to psychiatric illness' as part of the 'somewhat more modest' 1993 lecture series that he now organised, retitled 'Mental Health: The Way Forward'.[114]

Clare also organised the St Patrick's Hospital 'Founder's Day Lectures' held on or around 30 November each year, the anniversary of the birth of the hospital's founder, Jonathan Swift. The 1989 meeting saw Clare's good friend and colleague Robin Murray of the Institute of Psychiatry deliver a 'splendid lecture'[115] on 'the maddening causes of schizophrenia', and celebrated that year's launch of *Swift's Hospital: A History of St Patrick's Hospital, Dublin, 1746–1989* by Elizabeth Malcolm.[116] Clare continued to invite world leaders to deliver the Annual Jonathan Swift Lecture over subsequent years: Norman Sartorius, Director of the Division of Mental Health of the WHO (1990), Nancy Andreasen of the University of Iowa (1991), George Vaillant of Dartmouth Medical School and Harvard University Health Services (1992), Joseph Coyle also from Harvard (1993) and A.C. Robin Skynner, family therapist and author (1994), who spoke about a theme of long-standing interest to Clare: 'social change and family adjustments'.

The 250th anniversary of St Patrick's Hospital was in 1995 so Clare, as medical director, organised a much larger conference over two days (Friday and Saturday, 20 and 21 October) at the nearby Royal Hospital Kilmainham (Irish Museum of Modern Art), including a 'major buffet' on the Friday evening.[117] Key speakers included David Goldberg of the Institute of Psychiatry in London, Leon Eisenberg of Harvard University and the WHO, an old friend and colleague, Lesley Rees of Bart's and Kay Redfield Jamison of Johns Hopkins School of Medicine in Baltimore, who appeared on *In the Psychiatrist's Chair* in July 1996 and whose 1993 book *Touched with Fire: Manic Depressive Illness and the Artistic Temperament*[118] Clare positively reviewed in the *British Journal of Psychiatry* in 1997.[119] The 1995 meeting was a great success: 'There has never been a more exciting nor a more demanding time to be in psychiatry,' Clare declared – just as generations of psychiatrists had declared before him, and many more would do again.[120]

Clare continued to attract leading figures to speak at Founder's Day in subsequent years, including Isaac Marks of the Institute of Psychiatry and the Bethlem-Maudsley Hospital, a world expert in anxiety disorders, in 1996, when the meeting was moved from November to

October to facilitate Clare's scheduled trip to Goa in India,[121] Trey
Sutherland from the Institute of Mental Health in Maryland in 1997,
and Kenneth Kendler from Virginia Commonwealth University in
1998, speaking on another topic of long-standing interest to Clare:
'The genetics of alcoholism'.

Friends, Politicians and a Globe-Trotting Psychiatrist

Clare gathered support for his various endeavours from a range of
sources including medical and other colleagues within St Patrick's
and the 'Friends of St Patrick's Hospital', an organisation founded in
1978 to fund research and amenities for patients and staff, through
events such as tea parties, balls, gardening seminars and an annual golf
classic. The society's supporters were many, varied and very dedicated:
Peter Sutherland, for example, businessman, barrister, politician and
friend of Clare, could not attend the 1999 ball owing to a previous
commitment, but sent a generous financial donation instead.[122]
Sutherland, like Clare, had been greatly influenced by Father Joe Veale
at Gonzaga College, which he also attended.[123] Clare was clearly an
effective fundraiser and networker for the association and the hospital,
often donating payments, such as the one he received for an article he
wrote in *Cara*, Aer Lingus's in-flight magazine in 1999, to the academic
bank account in St Patrick's.[124]

In 1992, the Friends of St Patrick's Hospital organised a particularly
memorable dinner in St Edmundsbury Hospital in Lucan, which Clare
hailed as 'marvellous' in a subsequent letter thanking Darina Allen,
Ireland's leading chef, for her 'splendid generosity' on the occasion:

> You know from the response of everybody present how much your
> efforts and those of your colleagues were appreciated. I cannot
> say how delighted I was to see St Edmundsbury used in such an
> aesthetically attractive and gastronomically satisfying way![125]

The Friends of St Patrick's, with Clare's guidance, duly supported
a range of educational and research projects at the hospitals. They

were also willing to fund a hospital newsletter so, in 1991, Clare found
a printer 'who can put together a very acceptable and economic six-
page A4-style two-tone production, including photographs'.[126] The
first edition of *Swift Times*, published at Christmas 1991, reported
on the official visit of President Mary Robinson to St Patrick's on
19 November 1991 as part of Mental Health Week, and the formal
opening of the Martha Whiteway Psychiatric Day Hospital for the
Elderly:

> President Robinson delivered a short, impromptu and clearly
> heartfelt address. She was delighted to visit the hospital, expressed
> her approval at the philosophy of 'empowerment' of patients
> reflected in the treatment programmes, the hospital policy and the
> outreach community services managed by St Patrick's on behalf of
> the Eastern Health Board.[127]

Initially edited by Rolande Anderson,[128] *Swift Times* reported on
a wide range of hospital activities, including staff changes, sporting
events, research, examination results, academic promotions and the
annual Founder's Day Conference. At Christmas 1996, Clare wrote a
moving tribute to Norman Moore, one of Clare's early mentors who
had died the previous May,[129] and whom Clare also obituarised in the
Psychiatric Bulletin[130] and in *The Irish Times*:[131]

> [Moore] loved this hospital and believed it to be a treasure of
> the nation bequeathed to us by the beneficence and foresight of
> Swift to provide succor, support, relief and care for generations
> of psychiatrically ill [...] We who work in the modern St Patrick's
> owe Norman Moore an incalculable debt. His single-minded
> dedication to the relief of psychological pain and suffering was
> inspirational.

Clare also spoke at Moore's funeral in St Patrick's Cathedral,
highlighting how Moore had moved St Patrick's out of 'a time-warp of
Victorian rigidity':

He was, from the outset, a therapeutic enthusiast. He took to using the newly developed major tranquillisers and antidepressants with relish. He exuded optimism. For him, psychiatric illness was, for the most part, eminently treatable. What was needed was appropriate knowledge, a healing atmosphere, an optimistic therapist and time.[132]

Moore's family deeply appreciated Clare's 'moving tribute to a great man'.[133] In his address, Clare openly acknowledged that Moore's influence was always with him:

In St Patrick's, at his old house Delville where I now reside, on the banks of his beloved Liffey and in the grounds of St Edmundsbury, I, in common with others who were so crucially influenced by him, still anticipate that he will materialise, grip me gently but firmly by the elbow and calmly suggest that a little more patience or a change in therapy will transform an incorrigible problem into a therapeutic triumph. He was one of the great figures of Irish medicine in this century and his legacy in the shape of the hospital he so magnificently served and the generations of young men and women he so cardinally influenced is incomparable.

Like Moore, Clare assumed myriad roles within the hospital and beyond: he participated in the St Patrick's Hospital Research Ethics Committee,[134] sought to expand the hospital's research programme in various ways,[135] led proposals for a national body to advance psychiatric research in Ireland (which never actually happened in the end),[136] and was unfailingly supportive to individual researchers who came to him with specific requests.[137] Clare also accumulated a dizzying array of roles outside of the hospital including a visiting professorship at the School of Health Sciences at Birmingham University and memberships of the Council of the Royal College of Psychiatrists (from 1989), Comhairle na nOspideal (the Department of Health body regulating hospital consultant appointments in Ireland, from 1992), the General Council of the King's Fund (an English health charity, from 2000)[138] and various editorial boards (e.g. *Journal of Medical Ethics* and *Modern Medicine of Ireland*). In 1990, he received an Evian Health Award for his work promoting good health[139] and in 1996 he was awarded an honourary DSc (*Scientiae Doctor*; Doctor of Science) degree by the University of East Anglia and *In the Psychiatrist's Chair* won a Sony Broadcasting Award.

Clare was politically well connected, attending, for example, a dinner for 'friends of Mary McAleese' at the Davenport Hotel in Dublin on 25 October 1997.[140] Five days later, McAleese was elected President of Ireland. Clare and Jane were duly invited by the Taoiseach (prime minister) Bertie Ahern, TD to a reception in Dublin Castle following McAleese's inauguration on 11 November. They were also commonly invited to all kinds of other events, both in Ireland and England, including, for example, a reception at the Irish Embassy in London in June 1996 when Mary Robinson, then President of Ireland, was visiting. The Clares were regular visitors to the Irish Embassy in London.

In 1995, Dick Spring, Minister for Foreign Affairs and friend of Clare,[141] and Joan Burton, Minister for Overseas Development, invited Clare to chair the semi-state Agency for Personal Service Overseas (APSO), the 'Irish national agency which enables Irish men and women to exchange skills and knowledge with people in the developing world'.[142] Ever the networker, Clare noted that 'the advantage of the chairmanship of APSO is that it does keep me in touch with a number of senior Ministers'. To take up the post, Clare resigned from the chairmanship of the Public Education Committee of the Royal College of Psychiatrists ('a post which actually did involve me in a fair amount of rather pointless work') and the Prince of Wales Advisory Group on Disability, which the Prince established following the International Year of Disabled Persons (1981). Clare already knew the Prince of Wales 'through my work on the King's Fund and SANE, the schizophrenia charity' and when invited to join the Prince's Advisory Group on Disability in 1991, Clare accepted 'although quite what help I can be to the man I just don't know'.[143]

All of these involvements led to Clare travelling a great deal to speak at events and venues as diverse as – to take random examples –

the BUPA 'Doctor of the year' Luncheon (London, 1989), the Institute
for the Study of Alcoholism and Addiction (London, 1990), the Grand
Committee Room of the House of Commons (London, 1993), the
launch of the 'Defeat Depression' campaign at the Royal College of
Psychiatrists (London, 1994), the Harvard Graduates' Club and Johns
Hopkins Medical School (Baltimore, 1995), Southampton Medical
School (for its twenty-fifth anniversary in 1997) and the World Council
of Enterostomal Therapists in Copenhagen (1999).

Other far-flung locations included Australia in 1989 (where he
delivered a scintillating lecture just hours after landing in Sydney,
despite jet lag and loss of luggage),[144] Goa in India in 1996 ('Stress
and patients; stress and doctors'), Cancun in Mexico in 1998 ('Stress'
and the 'Role of personality in the presentation of illness') and Hong
Kong in 1998 ('Postgraduate medical education: biopsychosocial
approach').[145] In Hong Kong, Clare gave an interview to the *Hong
Kong Sunday Post* which, when published, he found 'reasonably
accurate' although 'some of it is not exactly as I remember it when
I gave the interview'.[146] This is, perhaps, little wonder, given Clare's
hectic work and travel schedules, which also, over the years, included
Thailand, Malaysia, Jamaica, Bermuda and Barbados – sometimes for
work, sometimes with family, and sometimes both.

Clare's local speaking engagements were equally diverse and,
in a sense, undisciplined. A random sample from his years at St
Patrick's (1989–2001) includes the Gilmartin Lecture at the College of
Anaesthesiologists of Ireland (Dublin, 1990), the Irish Division of the
Royal College of Psychiatrists (Dundrum, 1991), Ireland's Management
Institute (Dublin, 1991),[147] the Annual General Meeting of the Irish
Hospital Consultants' Association (Kilkenny, 1992), the launch of the
Mental Health Association's 'Mindful of Art' exhibition (Dublin, 1993),
the World Association for Psychosocial Rehabilitation (Dublin, 1993),
the launch of 'Women for Sobriety (Ireland)' (St Edmundsbury, 1994), a
conference on drug addiction in general practice (St Patrick's, 1996), the
Annual Conference of the Institute of Personnel Development (Tralee,
2000) and the International Meeting of the Association of Healthcare
Human Resource Management (Trinity College Dublin, 2000).

Maureen Browne, a health analyst and commentator whom Clare met at the *Irish Medical Times* was in awe of Clare's ability to multitask:

> Spending time with Jane and their children, running a major hospital and a leading medical academic department, pursuing research, going over and back to London for his television work, writing books and articles, dabbling in politics – he seemed to have discovered how to cram forty-eight hours into half that time.[148]

Clare's diary was, however, usually uncomfortably full, despite him rejecting as many invitations as he accepted.[149] In 1995, for example, he declined an invitation to write a text for an exhibition of paintings for the Irish Museum of Modern Art (IMMA). Clare 'thought long and hard about it' but was 'terribly overcommitted as it is':

> But the most potent reason for turning down your invitation is that I just have to confess that I do not think I would be up to it! I have tried to do this kind of thing once or twice before and I think I have to conclude that it is just too much for me.[150]

Notwithstanding his globetrotting ways, Clare remained doggedly concerned with training the next generation of psychiatrists in Ireland, vigorously pursuing a plan for trainees to take up research jobs[151] and continuously improving and expanding the postgraduate training programme in psychiatry that he initiated across St Patrick's and other hospitals.[152] Lucey recalls:

> Around 1990, the trainees in St Patrick's asked why Tony wasn't teaching them more. They wrote to him asking for more teaching. Tony wrote back saying he would teach them on a question-and-answer basis. This led to the most memorable seminars I have ever attended, answering questions like: 'How should we relate to our patients?' 'Should we allow our patients call us by our first name?' In response to the latter, Clare said: 'I tell them my name is Dr

Clare; I don't practise as Tony. But sometimes', he added, 'it isn't the way.'[153]

Clare was also concerned with a wide variety of educational matters such as 'journal clubs' for trainees,[154] the availability of food for doctors 'on-call' at night-time[155] and the acquisition of a new photocopier,[156] among other items, for the St Patrick's Hospital library, to be sourced from hospital management: 'We also need new shelving as we are running out of space for both books and journals. Any chance of a clock?'[157]

In August 1999, Dr Tom McMonagle, a registrar in psychiatry in St Patrick's, suggested that the hospital subscribe to the 'Cochrane Library', an evolving collection of 'systematic reviews' of various treatments.[158] 'I have been involved in two of these which may explain my enthusiasm for the process,' wrote McMonagle. Clare – predictably – supported McMonagle's 'very good suggestion' and authorised the necessary spending.[159] Twenty years later, McMonagle, now a consultant psychiatrist, recalls Clare 'inspiring a generation of psychiatrists, myself included, with intellectual fascination and the glamour of the media replacing the dreary corridors of the asylums'.[160]

Campaigns, Networks, Celebrities

Clare kept up a lively correspondence with all kinds of prominent figures over his years at St Patrick's and St Edmundsbury, including Taoiseach Charles Haughey, (inviting him as guest of honour at a book launch in St Patrick's in 1989);[161] Barry Desmond, Member of the European Parliament (seeking support for research on the mental health of Irish women);[162] Vincent Browne, editor of the *Sunday Tribune* (Clare: 'I greatly admire your editorial position on Northern Ireland');[163] Joan Burton, Minister of State at the Department of Social Welfare (inviting her as guest of honour at a 1994 meeting on the effects of family break-up; she accepted);[164] Rory O'Hanlon, TD (thanking Deputy O'Hanlon for the 'kindness and concern and consideration which you showed at all times in your dealings with me since I returned from the

UK');[165] and Mary O'Rourke, Minister for Health (inviting her to the Annual Swift Psychiatric Lecture in 1991; she declined).[166]

In the mid-1990s Clare embarked on a particularly intense campaign of lobbying and letter-writing to politicians and others, following suggestions that new regulations would result in private health insurers reducing the level of benefit provided for psychiatric care but not medical care – a move that would impact severely on St Patrick's. In August 1994, Clare pointed out to the Department of Health that 'the average weekly average cost of a private psychiatric bed is substantially lower than its equivalent in the public sector' and asked 'why psychiatric care is being singled out for such adverse and damaging treatment':

> I have often argued that for psychiatric patients time is the only high-tech treatment. Where highly expensive diagnostic and treatment interventions are the rule rather than the exception in most areas of modern acute medicine, time, together with some relatively inexpensive drug and psychotherapeutic interventions, are the hallmarks of good acute psychiatric care. The savage reduction in [private health insurance] benefit [...] to my mind constitutes a particularly unattractive example of discrimination against sufferers from psychiatric illness, a group already in receipt of considerable public discrimination and stereotyping.[167]

This controversy raged on for quite some time, with Clare and Dr Conall Larkin of St John of God Hospital in Stillorgan both objecting strongly to the proposal that health insurers offer a statutory minimum of only forty days inpatient treatment for psychiatric patients compared to 180 days for medical inpatient treatment.[168] Clare argued that the minimum would likely become the norm, resulting in 30 per cent of private psychiatry patients being transferred to the public sector. The government argued that the change was an EU requirement in order to create an open market for health insurance[169] but an *Irish Times* editorial in July 1995 strongly backed Clare and Larkin, praising their stance and bemoaning this apparent discrimination against the mentally ill.[170]

In August, Dr Dermot Walsh, a prominent psychiatrist,[171] recommended, also in *The Irish Times*, that private hospitals such as St Patrick's should maximise the reduced insurance cover likely to be available by reducing their length of stay, developing centralised inpatient care aimed at meeting niche needs that local public psychiatric services could not cost-effectively meet, and developing community-based, geographically accessible alternatives to hospitalisation.[172] In a private letter to Walsh later that month, Clare expressed particular disappointment at Walsh's public remarks regarding 'hospitalisation for alcohol abuse' which came 'during a rather difficult time in our negotiations with the Minister for Health concerning the draft health insurance regulations'.[173] Clare pointed out that 'a smaller proportion of our patients [at St Patrick's] are admitted with this diagnosis [alcohol abuse] than are currently admitted to public psychiatric hospitals':

> I am glad to say that in general Irish psychiatrists have been exceedingly supportive of the role and value of St Patrick's and have been likewise exceedingly supportive in helping us battle to ensure that any health insurance regulations that are implemented in Ireland do not discriminate against psychiatric patients.[174] I am hopeful that the Minister has taken on board these concerns and is making a determined effort to ensure that the original draft regulations are modified to take account of our legitimate concerns.

Clare mounted an extraordinary (even for him) campaign of letter-writing to public representatives on this issue: TDs, Senators, Members of the European Parliament. In the face of considerable subsequent pressure from these representatives, Minister for Health Michael Noonan met with representatives of St Patrick's and St John of God Hospitals and subsequently discussed the issue with the EU Commission in an attempt to reach agreement for parity of psychiatric cover with medical cover. The pressure exerted by Clare, Larkin and others paid off and, following negotiation, the eventual regulations increased the minimum cover for psychiatric patients to 100 days as opposed to the 40 days originally proposed. It was a partial victory, but a significant one.

On 1 May 1996, *Seanad Éireann* (the Senate) held a debate on the matter, tellingly titled 'Discrimination against psychiatric patients', and sought to overturn the new regulations which still fell short of the 180 days cover provided for medical patients. Senator David Norris, among others, quoted from Clare's correspondence in the Seanad debate, but in the end the Fianna Fáil motion to upturn the regulations did not succeed.[175] The relevant minister continued to strongly defend the measures,[176] which also stipulated a statutory minimum of 20 days per year for psychiatric day-patient care. Clare appreciated this innovation but – with tireless zeal – requested that Minister Noonan increase this to '30 or even 40 day-patient days'.[177] But these were, as Clare noted to one Senator, 'very difficult and indeed unpredictable times'[178] and, on the substantive issue, Clare and colleagues had to make do with their partial victory on inpatient days. Notwithstanding their disagreement, it was, as Clare pointed out to Noonan, a 'major advance'. And the assertive actions of Clare, Larkin and colleagues had ultimately helped ensure 'that health insurers continue to respect Ireland's admirable record in the provision of extensive insurance protection against the cost of serious illness – psychiatric as well as physical'.[179]

Over the following years, Clare remained both active and vocal in relation to insurance cover, writing to Noonan in 1996 in support of 'community rating, lifetime cover and equal treatment of psychiatrically ill and physically ill patients',[180] and writing in the *Sunday Independent* in 1997 that competition in health insurance was generally good but not if it resulted in discrimination.[181]

Clare's contacts with politicians also extended well beyond insurance matters during this period. A patron of the Eating Disorders Association for many years,[182] Clare wrote to his long-standing friend Minister for Health John O'Connell in 1992, proposing St Patrick's as a 'national referral centre' for eating disorders, a suggestion that eventually came to pass.[183]

Clare also commented to O'Connell about the Department of Health's 1992 Green Paper on Mental Health with which he was generally 'very impressed', but he felt it displayed excess enthusiasm for 'sectorisation' of mental health services and should say more about 'further collaboration between the public and private services',[184] a theme that was close to Clare's heart.[185] Clare also made various suggestions to the minister concerning involuntary psychiatric admission which was another issue of long-standing concern to Clare.[186] Involuntary admission (or 'sectioning') remained 'a regrettable necessity', as Clare pointed out in 1992 in *Forum* (journal of the Irish College of General Practitioners):

A good psychiatric service working with a good primary care service will doubtless reduce the need for compulsory intervention by dint of earlier intervention and better monitoring. A better educated and informed media and public will ensure that more people will come for help earlier and more willingly. But the nature of psychiatric illness is such that there will always be a few who by virtue of their disturbance are unable to make a rational judgement and who need help. For them compulsory intervention is a regrettable necessity. Hence the need for legislation which is fair, feasible and respects the conflicting rights and duties involved.[187]

There was essentially no end to Clare's networking activities through personal communications, official letters, organising events, holding meetings and issuing invitations to St Patrick's for activities ranging from broadcasting the Gay Byrne RTÉ radio show in 1995[188] to inviting Chief Justice Ronan Keane to lunch in 2000.[189] Clare also helped organise the annual graduation day from the School of Nursing at St Patrick's, inviting guests of honour including Dr John O'Connell, TD (Minister for Health, 1992), Her Excellency Dame Veronica Sutherland (British Ambassador to Ireland, 1998) and, again, Chief Justice Keane (2000).

Clare's ability to attract both high-level visitors and visiting academic groups[190] to St Patrick's was rooted in both his ongoing industriousness as a public ambassador for psychiatry and his long-standing celebrity links from his time in the United Kingdom. In 1999, Clare highlighted to

St Patrick's Hospital management an article in the *Guardian* newspaper concerning a private psychiatric facility in the United Kingdom, which was known for caring for celebrities.[191] Clare wrote:

> Of course it is doubtful that publicising celebrities who go to a hospital does that hospital any good. Many of these people are only too delighted to get publicity but many others are not, as I know to our cost. When I think of St Patrick's and St Edmundsbury, I realise that we have built up quite a list of 'celebrities' as well, but as you can imagine our main selling point is our confidentiality.[192]

Some 'celebrities' did, however, speak out about their visits to Clare. In 2013, for example, six years after Clare's death, singer-songwriter Morrissey provided an evocative description of a consultation with Clare in 1994.[193]

Clare's hectic work rate was not without personal cost and Clare seemed to understand this to a certain extent, although he felt helpless to rein it in. After his return to Ireland, Clare still sought the advice and support of his old mentor, Michael Shepherd of the Institute of Psychiatry. They met for lunch at the Garrick Club in London, but it is unclear to what extent this actually helped.[194] Clearly, Clare was still in need of a mentor, a father figure, a person to look up to – someone, perhaps, to help him take control of a professional life that was increasingly spinning at an entirely unsustainable rate.

7

Work, Life and the Crisis in Masculinity (1989–2007)

· ·

Clare's period in Dublin after his return to Ireland in 1989 was a time of increasingly intense, progressively unmanageable professional engagements, covering everything from writing academic papers to speaking in the media, supervising research projects to judging *The Irish Times* Literature Prizes.[1] All of this rather frenzied activity was in addition to his family commitments, clinical work and medical directorship of St Patrick's Hospital, which involved a dizzying range of routine and non-routine activities.

In 1996, Clare presented and narrated a promotional DVD about St Patrick's and St Edmundsbury Hospitals, titled 'Swift's Hospital, 1745–1995'.[2] In this fascinating twenty-five-minute film, Clare provided a crisp account of the history of St Patrick's, noting proudly that it opened its doors in 1757 and had functioned on the same Dublin city centre site ever since then. The DVD explored the subsequent history in some detail, with a contribution by psychiatrist Dr Anthony O'Flaherty, and brought the story right up to 1995, with features on current treatments, the hospital laboratory, its art collection and the hospital archive, which was opened in 1995 by President Mary Robinson. The film also included contributions from a wide range of multi-disciplinary staff and a warm tribute by Clare to Professor Norman Moore.

Despite being put together 'within a very confined timescale', Clare felt 'the final result reflects well on what we do'.[3] And Clare was undoubtedly the star: measured, urbane and ever so convincing. But the truth was that over the course of the 1990s, Clare became ever more pressured, distracted and stressed. And, with all of his positions and achievements, there inevitably came a range of further additional responsibilities and involvements, compounded by Clare's own deeply held principles of engagement and collegiality – all of which added to his burden and fuelled his endless sense of self-expectation.

'A Great Sense of Justice'

In early 1996, Professor Ivor Browne, former Chief Psychiatrist of the Eastern Health Board (1965–94), Professor of Psychiatry at UCD (1967–94) and one of Ireland's leading reforming psychiatrists, was the subject of a 'fitness to practise' hearing at the Irish Medical Council.[4] The story was this. Browne's patient, Phyllis Hamilton, had a son by Fr Michael Cleary, a well-known priest. Cleary died in 1993 and in 1995 Hamilton decided to make details of the relationship public. Both Hamilton and her son, Ross, were deeply stressed by the thought of the publicity, denials and accusations that likely lay ahead. They both wanted Browne to speak out publicly in support of them because he knew the truth about the relationship.

This placed Browne in a dilemma. On the one hand, Browne was concerned that, without such support, Hamilton and Ross would be unable to withstand the pressure. On the other hand, speaking out would involve disclosing information about Cleary without Cleary's permission, because the priest was now deceased. But Browne was deeply concerned about Hamilton and Ross and, after consulting the relevant ethical guidelines, he concluded that his duties to his patient (Hamilton) and to Ross were greater than his duty to the deceased Cleary. Browne then spoke to the media in support of Hamilton and Ross.[5]

Following this, Browne was alleged to have committed a serious breach of medical ethical standards by disclosing information given to him in confidence (by Cleary), failing to act in the best interests of his patient (Hamilton), and acting in a manner derogatory to the reputation of the medical profession (by speaking to the media about the case). In ethical terms, the issue centred on medical confidentiality and whether or not Browne was right to reveal information about Cleary in the media for the purpose of assisting and supporting Hamilton and her son during this uniquely difficult period for them.

At the Medical Council hearing in October 1996, Hamilton and her son spoke in strong support of Browne. However, despite the clear medical ethical dilemma Browne had faced, he could find no doctor to support him – except for Clare. Browne and Clare were an unlikely pairing in many ways. Browne worked in the public sector, Clare in the private. Browne was towards the unorthodox end of the psychiatry spectrum, Clare was firmly at the orthodox end – he was, after all, the medical director of St Patrick's. And, as Clare pointed out to the Fitness to Practise Committee, he and Browne 'would stand on very different terrain on modern psychiatry, so even our professional sympathies are cool rather than warm'.[6]

Even so, Clare did not hesitate to support Browne and he told the hearing that he 'would not have any doubt about [Browne's] professional integrity or serious purpose in the practise of his profession'. The issue in the case was, Clare felt, 'what happens when there is a conflict between duties of confidentiality on the one hand to a patient [Hamilton] and on the other hand to third parties [Cleary]'. Clare had 'never in twenty-five years been in a situation where the conflict was quite as sharp' as this. When asked if a doctor in such a situation familiarises themselves with relevant ethical principles, considers the clinical and ethical issues raised, and the facts, and makes an 'honest decision', is there anything else the doctor should do, Clare was unequivocal: 'I don't believe there is anything more a doctor can do as long as those things are done.'

Notwithstanding Clare's evidence, the Fitness to Practise Committee found that Browne was guilty of professional misconduct because, it concluded, his disclosure to the media was not the minimum possible disclosure in the circumstances. It also found that Browne had acted in a manner derogatory to the reputation of the medical profession and the committee recommended to the full Medical

Council that Browne engage in a one-to-one course on ethical issues relevant to psychiatric practice. Considering the recommendations of the Fitness to Practise Committee, the full Medical Council censured Browne for the breach of confidentiality and admonished him for damaging the reputation of the medical profession, but dropped the requirement for the course on ethical issues. At all times, Browne had acted in the interests of his patient and her son, and Browne rightly remains, to this day, a respected and admired figure in Irish public life.

Clare's evidence to the 1996 enquiry was tremendously interesting because it showed him strongly supporting a colleague whom he held in high professional regard even though their 'professional sympathies [were] cool rather than warm', as he put it. Reflecting on the matter in 2018, Browne still appreciates Clare's sense of justice and supportiveness:

> Tony was very ethical and had a great sense of justice. When I was in front of the Medical Council in 1996, Tony came down to support me. Even though he said we had very different views about many aspects of psychiatry, he supported me very strongly. I got no support from any of my other colleagues at the time. Tony had no particular personal reason to support me. It was after that I got to know him. At that time, I didn't know Tony had such a strong sense of justice. He had no personal reason to bother to support me, but he did. I was very grateful to him.[7]

Clare's principled stand did not go unnoticed or unadmired. Professor James Lucey recalls the 1996 inquiry clearly:

> Tony gave evidence at the 1996 Medical Council inquiry into Ivor Browne. Tony said he was speaking in favour of a man whose view of mental health he did not share, but at that time no one in Ireland was practising with a true understanding of confidentiality. Tony undermined truths all the time; he was a truth teller. Tony said there is a limit to confidentiality but no one understood the

limits. It was not good enough for a person to say they failed to disclose on the grounds of confidentiality – there must be limits; people can't just use the lie of confidentiality. The Medical Council censured Browne and initially recommended he do training in this area. All of the profession was on one side and Tony – with no reason to gain – stood by Browne. And Tony did this because Tony was a very special man.[8]

In addition to his collegiality, Clare's 1996 evidence also reflected a nuanced understanding of medical confidentiality that was entirely consistent with his long-standing engagement with this and other ethical issues in psychiatric practice. Almost two decades earlier, in 1979, Clare had explored a range of issues relating to ethical professional obligations and confidentiality in a 'special report' in the medical journal *The Practitioner*, where Clare pointed to not only the importance of confidentiality but also its complexity.[9] All of that complexity was in plentiful evidence at the 1996 Medical Council enquiry and, most of all, in the clear, logical and measured evidence that Clare provided in support of Browne.

The Seven Secrets of Happiness

While much of Clare's activity in the 1990s was of a very focused, professional nature – treating patients, running St Patrick's, engaging with important ethical and political issues – there was also a playful, impish side to Clare that came readily to the fore when the situation presented itself. On 5 November 1999, Gyles Brandreth, English writer, broadcaster, actor and former Conservative Member of Parliament (1992–7), visited Clare in St Patrick's in search of nothing less than the secrets of happiness.[10] Paradoxically, perhaps, he had come to the right place.

Brandreth and Clare spoke for three hours about the science and psychology of happiness, Freud, Jung and Laing, among many other topics. Clare was clearly at his most seductive on the day: Brandreth found him charming, intelligent, gossipy and irresistible.

Toward the end of the encounter, Brandreth asked for something that he and his readers could stick on the fridge door – the seven steps to happiness, perhaps? Clare sighed, closed his eyes, and pondered, before finally obliging Brandreth and his readers with some sound advice. First, Clare advised, cultivate a passion (to get you through the bad times); second, be like a leaf on a tree (be part of something bigger); third, avoid introspection (which puts other people off); fourth, do not resist change (change is both vital and inevitable); fifth, live in the moment (if you like going to the movies, go to the movies; if you dislike opera, avoid it); sixth, audit your happiness (check out if you're happy more than half of the time; if not, change); and, seventh, be happy: act the part and that alone can trigger change.

In fact, Clare had earlier planned to write a book about happiness with Jane, at Jane's suggestion. Clare's advice delighted Brandreth who headed back to London filled with new-found wisdom. Brandreth had a very broad interest in happiness and he spoke about it widely, soon finding that audiences showed particular interest in the 'seven secrets' he gleaned from Clare. Brandreth went on to publish his own wonderful book about happiness in 2013, titled *The 7 Secrets of Happiness: An Optimist's Journey*.[11] Brandreth wrote warmly of Clare, and Clare's advice is central to the book's message about achieving and attaining greater wellbeing.

Ironically, it is far from clear that Clare himself experienced increasing happiness throughout the 1990s, despite following much of his own advice, at least to a certain extent. Looking at the 'seven secrets' in turn, it is clear that Clare cultivated passions (literature, cinema, opera, tennis), was a leaf on many trees (his family, the BBC, the media more generally, St Patrick's, the medical profession) and generally avoided negative introspection (chiefly through his extraordinary ability to focus on other people). But it is also clear that Clare experienced a sense of sustained and deepening disappointment during this period: he was no longer central to London media life, he failed in his bid for a Senate seat, and the routines of hospital administration eventually ground him down. *In the Psychiatrist's Chair* was coming to an end, and – perhaps most of all – he never re-experienced the euphoric high of his student debating years. The absence of a guiding figure or mentor in these later years was also a problem for Clare, who continually sought the approval of strong, distant men.

As a result, Clare's ability to live in the moment and to act happy (two of his 'seven secrets') was both diminished and increasingly limited to the fleeting moments of joy he experienced when an audience applauded (as they invariably did). The solutions, however, appeared to lie in the two remaining secrets that Clare shared with Brandreth in 1999: audit your happiness and do not resist change. In 1999, Clare announced his intention to step down as medical director of St Patrick's at the end of 2000, although he would remain on as a consultant psychiatrist.[12] Clare had made his contribution to St Patrick's – and it was a huge one, of which he was justifiably proud – but it was now time to move on and embark on one final reinvention, a final phase in what everyone except Clare could see was a remarkable lifetime's journey, bringing his deeply compassionate, humane version of psychiatry to patients, colleagues, the media and the world in general. After his time at St Patrick's, the plan was to focus more on private and family life, which is also central to happiness.

In November 1999, Clare wrote to Her Excellency, Mary McAleese, President of Ireland, whom he knew personally,[13] and invited her to St Patrick's to open its new 'state of the art, thirty-bed intensive care and acute admission facility' during the following year:

> I step down at the end of the year 2000 as Medial Director of St Patrick's.[14] I will have served for 12 years. It would give me enormous pleasure and satisfaction if one of the last tasks I performed as Medical Director was to welcome yourself and Martin [President McAleese's husband] to the hospital. I would so much enjoy showing you what has happened to Swift's extraordinary idea over 250 years on.[15]

President McAleese accepted Clare's invitation and the event took place on 6 November 2000. It was a fitting occasion in the lead-up to

Clare's departure as medical director. In August 1999 he commented to *The Irish Times* that, over his period as medical director since 1989, St Patrick's had reduced costs, reduced readmissions and increased first admissions – a state of affairs that Clare regarded as a healthy one.[16] He added that people were now more forthcoming about psychological distress, but admitted that even he got stressed at times. He said that he intended to continue his media work in future years and, most importantly, finish writing a book about men by the end of 1999.

That book, eventually titled *On Men: Masculinity in Crisis*, had a difficult gestation but it duly appeared in 2000 and was widely seen as the most revealing and personal of Clare's writings to date. While it is not Clare's best book, *On Men* nonetheless remains an intensely interesting volume for all kinds of different reasons. And while Clare later regretted that he had never written anything better than *Psychiatry in Dissent* (1976), he could take solace from the fact that no one else had either and that *On Men*, despite its weaknesses, was still a fine contribution to an evolving debate about the nature of masculinity in modern societies.

On Men: Masculinity in Crisis (2000)

What would Clare have made of the cacophonies and chaos of the online world, the arrival of 'fake news', and the emasculation of expertise during the 2010s? There are references in *On Men* that suggest he might struggle with the naked hatred that accompanies much online dialogue today.[17] Certainly, the conflicts of gender politics – so prominent now – caused Clare considerable disquiet during his life.[18] And it is for this reason, along with several others, that Clare's *On Men* still rewards close reading, some two decades after it was written.

Behind *On Men* and the radio series *Men in Crisis*[19] lay the idea that Clare found the entrenched animosities on both sides of the gender debate fundamentally distasteful. In his 2000 *Guardian* review of the book, Andrew Rissik, made this point forcefully:

These hatreds, whether rooted in gender, sexual orientation or ideological cause, are little more than psychological strategies to allow groups of people to feel for the 'enemy' group a contempt or loathing of which they would be morally ashamed if they applied it to themselves or their associates.

Seeking an accommodation, a healing therapy of mutual respect capable of resolving these long-entrenched divisions, [Clare] argues powerfully against the purely chemical or biological determinism that holds that men are the helpless, testosterone-fuelled prisoners of their genes.[20]

It is clear from *On Men*, and indeed other aspects of his public life, that Clare was a natural conciliator and a populist. He made his points with clarity, but he also often strove hard not to offend, a characteristic that runs consistently through *In the Psychiatrist's Chair* and is apparent in *On Men*. Clare declares at the outset of the book that he knows what it is like to be a man, but he immediately follows this with a series of doubts: was he effective as a part-time father? Was he a good husband? Had he allowed work to overshadow the rest of his life?[21]

Clare crystallises these doubts into the concept of the dying phallus. Unlike the anatomical term 'penis', the phallus is an anthropological and theological term referring to the male organ's image, as well as being a symbol of male power. Clare argues that authoritative, dominant, assertive, controlling, phallic man is starting to die, and he wonders whether a new man will emerge in his place.[22] Or will men become redundant?

Clare posed this question almost two decades ago. Has a new man emerged in the interim, or are the ashes of 'turn of the millennium man' still blowing in the wind? Almost twenty years after *On Men* was published, there are certainly signs of change but these are still interspersed with signs of struggle noted by Clare, as evidenced in ongoing media discussions of the nature of male sex drive,[23] male violence,[24] reported (and disputed) differences between male and female brains,[25] men's apparent struggles in a post-feminist world,[26] and a seemingly perpetual 'crisis' in masculinity, as, in the words of writer Pankaj Mishra, the 'hunt for manliness continues to contaminate politics and culture across the world in the twenty-first century'.[27]

One notable feature of Clare's *On Men* is its extensive use of endocrine research in a bid to nail down the role of testosterone in this whole melee. The book was originally to be co-authored by consultant endocrinologist, Professor Lesley Rees, a friend and colleague of Clare at Bart's, and Clare acknowledges her input in focusing his attention on the relevant literature about the hormonal basis of gender difference. Clare also acknowledges the research base for a link between testosterone and dominant behaviour, but asserts that testosterone is not necessarily the main culprit here.[28] He concludes that testosterone, rather than being the core cause of aggression in men, aggravates the aggression that is already there. He is drawn to research that supports the hypothesis that men can tame their aggression while still being men. And, in accepting that the roots of male aggression lie in an interaction between man and society, he argues that we must analyse both in order to find solutions.[29]

Having dismissed the Y chromosome and testosterone as sole culprits, Clare moves on to ask what, then, is the ultimate source of man's predilection to violence? He dismisses the notion of a single biological factor – the so-called aggressive instinct – as an explanation. Rather, he asks us to consider how the average male is encouraged to deny feelings of frailty, helplessness, uncertainty, empathy and sensitivity.[30] Clare suggests that this makes it easy for men to disguise their feelings and this, in turn, makes it easier for men to be converted into terrorists (to take an extreme example). Less overtly, it means that men resort to violence when their power is threatened – as it can be when women threaten male single-mindedness. Most research shows that violence is multi-factorial in origin, so, as well as biological factors, social factors such as deprivation, inequality, injustice, overcrowding and poverty appear to play a role.[31]

In her review of *On Men*, doctor-columnist with *Medicine Weekly* Juliet Bressan posited the view that Clare believed men fundamentally fear women and, as a result, seek to control and dominate women but, as patriarchal society crumbles in the western world, men are now in crisis.[32] In the *Sunday Times*, David Quinn argued that Clare did not pay sufficient attention to the idea that women were in crisis too, as twice as many women as men suffer from depression, twice as many women attempt suicide, and ten times as many have eating disorders.[33]

In a major interview in *The Irish Times*, journalist Kathryn Holmquist noted that Clare 'does his own ironing and regrets having smacked his children':

> I know he likes women and prefers them as friends. But what I don't know is this: why is this 57-year-old media-savvy psychiatrist so afraid of women's power? [...] He seems so passionate in his arguments that one wonders if the book is actually a metaphor for something deeper – Clare's own late mid-life crisis, perhaps?[34]

Clare described himself to Holmquist as 'a typical confused male'. Confused about what?

> What's the point of an awful lot of what I do. I'm in my 50s. I think one should be spending a good deal of your time doing things you want to do ... and what is that? I want to see much more of my family and friends. I want to continue making a contribution, but how can I best do that?

Holmquist hints that something of a public school reserve would not allow Clare to cross certain personal boundaries in the book. He tells her that he has always loved women with fight. His wife, Jane, whom he met at UCD aged 19, was the family 'rock'. And his mother was combative and passionate, he says – just like him.

Holmquist acknowledges Clare's apology for his criticism of her in *On Men*, but says she still considers his comments possibly 'patriarchal'. Clare himself acknowledges that 'I am contaminated by patriarchy; there is no man who isn't':

There is hope for men only if they 'acknowledge the end of patriarchal power and participate in the discussion of how the post-patriarchal age is to be negotiated,' Clare believes. He is dissatisfied with the conclusion of the book, but he was under a lot of pressure to finish it, on top of all his other work. At least he's starting the discussion.

Addressing the issue of masculinity in the book, Clare refers to the stories of many of his interviewees on *In the Psychiatrist's Chair* who, he says, spontaneously referenced their childhood and adolescence as a time of trial when denial of feelings such as sadness, loss, pain and fear signalled their status as men.[35] Fathers were commonly distant and aloof, and this created a model of masculinity marked by independence, emotional control, self-reliance and suspicion of intimacy.[36]

Is there a way out of this cul-de-sac? Clare suggests that men could join with women to reassert and revitalise a system of values in which the personal and the intimate take precedence over the pursuit of power and the generation of wealth. Even today, two decades after *On Men*, has society explored this avenue to the fullest extent? Or, as Clare opined, is it still the case that, if men do not reconsider and re-evaluate their roles, they will soon be entirely irrelevant as social beings?[37]

So, What Next for Men?

Clare enters reflective mode when considering a likely farewell to the family man, noting that the decline of the nuclear family presents a particular challenge to male dominance.[38] Clare acknowledges the emergence of a 'new man' in the 1980s and 90s, but argues that while many men did indeed discover new sides to themselves during this period, most did not.[39] At this point, Clare comes close to (reluctantly) admitting that critics of fatherhood might be right and men might indeed become redundant in the modern family.[40]

But not wanting to give up just yet, Clare says that if men still have a role, then it is high time that they explained what that role is and started to fulfil it. A chapter on men and fatherhood follows, looking in depth at fathers as providers and protectors. Significantly, Clare writes that if men are to negotiate a move away from patriarchy and towards gender equality, they need to make radical changes to the current imbalance between their public and private lives.[41] He nails his own colours firmly to the mast on this one, arguing that the value of fathers now lies less in income generation and more in cultivating involvement, awareness, consistency and caring.

But the chapter finishes with yet more doubt. Clare asks: if men's commitment is so important to the health of their families, why aren't they so committed? And what does male dominance mean any more if women increasingly find that loving men and living with men is more hassle than it's worth?[42]

The final chapter of *On Men* is duly devoted to men and love. Clare notes that men commonly fear and marginalise women and therefore cannot rely on women to save them from their present dilemma.[43] Later, he writes that men are not just fearful of, and angry with, women, but men also repudiate the feminine in themselves.[44]

So, what next for men? They must, it seems, firmly acknowledge the end of patriarchal power and participate actively in the negotiation of a post-patriarchal age. And they can learn from women who have consistently analysed the unbalanced relationship between the public political world, from which women were largely excluded for so long, and the private domestic world, in which they were largely immersed.[45] Man can be redeemed, Clare argues, but much work is needed.

Reviewing *On Men* in the *Sunday Times*, Liam Fay concluded that the book was significant because of its general coherence, dispelling of various senseless nostrums often trotted out on this theme, psychological insight and elegance.[46] But Fay disagreed with the author's assessment of a terminal decline in the role of the male. In *The Irish Times*, Harry Ferguson, Professor of Social Policy at UCD, was impressed by Clare's research, courage and deep engagement with his theme.[47] Ferguson was disappointed, however, that Clare presented relatively few proposals for advancing change[48] and that Clare excluded gay men from his analysis.

The latter decision is especially interesting because, ten years earlier, in 1990, the year in which the WHO finally declared that homosexuality was not a mental illness,[49] Clare had written about homosexuality in *The Irish Times*, objecting to intolerance and repression:

> I take consolation from the fact that wherever repressive and intolerant regimes seize power and set about persecuting and intimidating minority and opposition groups they invariably include amongst these groups – homosexuals *and* psychiatrists. We must be doing something right.[50]

In the *Guardian*, Madeleine Bunting noted Clare's worries about the future of men, but also his hopes for salvation:

> In the conclusion to his book, *On Men*, Anthony Clare quotes scary predictions of what faces men. Rising suicide rates, one in three men living alone and 1.5m men excluded from the workforce either because of early retirement or because they don't have the education and skills for employment. Perhaps, Clare hopes, women will find a compassionate awareness of men's insecurities, while not compromising their own legitimate self-assertion [...] as Clare argues vigorously, winning brings only isolation and insecurity.[51]

Many readers and reviewers found Clare's calls for change powerful and compelling,[52] and some even recognised themselves in Clare's text. Kevin Courtney in *The Irish Times* wrote about reading an interview with the supermodel Caprice and noted that 'Prof. Anthony Clare laid out the whole male malaise in his book, *On Men: Masculinity in Crisis*, and it makes for scarier reading than the entire output of Stephen King':

> As I reached the end of my riveting Caprice interview, I began to acknowledge that Prof. Clare's assertions about men were all too true, and that I was a near-perfect example of masculinity in crisis. Of course, I've always suspected as much – after all, the symptoms were there. But I also suspect that women are in crisis too – except

now it's their turn to hide it all behind a facade of financial success, family stability and macho behaviour. It's our turn to do the girly thing and admit to being weak, lonely and in need of support.[53]

Overall, and despite its uneven structure and pacing, *On Men* was impeccably researched, written with greater personal passion than many realised, and played an important role in a debate about gender that prefigured much of the media discussion triggered by #MeToo almost two decades later. But have matters really moved on since *On Men* appeared in 2000?

Interestingly, recent discussions about gender have tended to focus on transcending binary gender divisions rather than trying to resolve the age-old debates about male and female genders that Clare explored so elegantly in *On Men*. Richard Godwin, writing in the *Guardian* in 2018, wondered 'if viewing everything through the prism of masculinity really helps men to be better men'.[54] It probably does not, as Clare would undoubtedly agree.

And, certainly, recognising male uncertainty and perceived impotence, as recommended by Clare in 2000, remains an important step today, as Godwin concludes after attending 'men's groups' in 2018:

Not one of us has a clue what he's doing. I think it's one reason many men are finding this moment so hard: we are perceived to have the power, yet most of us feel powerless in relation to our own lives, emotions, relations. You get a real rush when you admit that in front of another man, and another rush when you hear pretty much the same thing echoed back. It may not be much to work with, but it's a start.

Personal Life

Not uncommonly, journalists sought to relate aspects of Clare's personal life to his work, especially when *On Men* appeared in 2000.[55] In *The Irish Times*, Kathryn Holmquist noted that Clare's 'publishers were "uneasy", he says, because they felt the book was too heavily researched and referenced and did not contain enough personal material':

> In the battle between the sexes, Clare has always been on the front line in his personal life, enjoying a combative relationship with Jane, even to the point of arguing publicly – albeit in the refined media of print – over divorce [see below]. The couple have seven children: Rachel (33) who works for the Henley Centre, social forecasters; Simon (30) media director with Coral, the gambling and leisure group; Eleanor (29) nurse in Crumlin, and getting married next year; Peter (24), studying acting at TCD; Sophie (20) doing English at TCD; Justine (17) who has just completed the Leaving Cert and intends to do equine studies and Sebastian (15) who has just done the Junior Cert.
>
> Guiding all their lives has been Jane, whom Clare calls 'the rock'. Jane is a 'truculent, feminist in domestic clothing', he says, but after a few seconds' consideration takes back the words 'truculent' and 'feminist'. In fact, he tells me, of all the words he used, 'feminist' was the one his wife would find 'most insulting'. Throughout her life, Jane has passionately believed that her place has been as a full-time wife and mother in the home, and that the feminist movement got it all wrong by encouraging women into the workplace at the expense of family life. Clare admits to being utterly dependent on his wife.[56]

Perhaps the most outstanding feature of Clare's relationships with women was the enduring depth of his relationship with Jane, who 'married Tony because he was so witty, so funny, a brilliant speaker'.[57] But as Clare became steadily busier throughout the 1980s and 1990s, there were times when he and Jane had less time for each other: she at home minding everyone, and he out earning money and, increasingly, appearing in media.

Ann Buckley, a family therapist who worked closely with Clare at St Edmundsbury from 1990 until 2007, confirms that, 'in many ways,

Jane kept the show on the road. In the days before mobile phones, Tony was travelling around the world and Jane was doing everything at home. In later years, Tony felt he owed it to Jane to spend more time with Jane, the family and the grandchildren. Tony was very lucky with the woman he married.'[58] Jane notes that 'a relationship is two people, but the audience was a third person in this relationship'.

Consistent with this, Clare was, in later life, drawn to the concept of 'performance-based self-worth' in men, chiefly through the work of Terrence Real, a family therapist, speaker and author whom Clare admired.[59] Clare's son Peter recalls that Clare became interested in the work of psychotherapist Terry Real in Boston 'for the love of his marriage, the love of his wife'.[60] In 2005, Clare wrote about the impact of Real on his thinking in relation to clinical practice:

> I was trained to bring little or nothing of myself, my humanity as a person, my experience of life to the therapeutic situation. As a young man this mattered little – in that I had not an awful lot to bring! As an older man, however, someone who has experienced much more of life's highs and disappointments, I disregard that original exhortation and speak much more 'from the I', as a favourite psychotherapist of mine, Terry Real from Boston, describes it.
>
> But not until I experienced a major, near-catastrophic life event myself and saw Terry Real being open, frank and sharing with patients did I see what a simplistic and barren proscription that is – a proscription endorsed in the main by heavily defended but somewhat grandiose practitioners implicitly behaving as if in possession of some superior experience of health and life. I am not really very surprised that so many doctors are reluctant to admit to stresses, strains, breakdown and despair when the whole professional edifice rests on an implicit dichotomous assumption of health/doctors on the one hand and sick/patients on the other. Such a model works well enough in physical medicine (though even here it has its limitations) but I believe it to be seriously limited in the area of psychological health and illness.[61]

This realisation brought Clare to the work of Real, the risks of 'performance-based self-worth' in men, and many of the themes of *On Men*. As the consummate performer, Clare undoubtedly saw his own addiction to performance and to the adulation of the audience as a significant issue in his personal life.

The impact of the audience as a 'third person' in Clare's relationship with Jane was certainly very real, very complex and, on occasion, very public. On 24 November 1995, Ireland held a referendum on the 'Fifteenth Amendment of the Constitution Act 1995' to remove Ireland's constitutional prohibition on divorce and allow for the dissolution of a marriage provided specified conditions were satisfied. The change was narrowly approved by a majority of 50.28 per cent and signed into law on 17 June 1996.

Clare, in his own words, 'supported the introduction of divorce as the lesser of two evils but made plain the need for society to devote much more resources to marriage guidance and mediation'.[62] The country was, however, very evenly divided on the issue and so were Clare and Jane. On 26 November 1995, two days after the referendum, Clare[63] and Jane[64] each wrote articles side-by-side in the *Sunday Independent* outlining their contrasting positions. Jane recalls that while Clare supported the introduction of divorce, Jane felt the question was more complex than a simple Yes or No permitted.[65] And – critically – she felt that Clare should have discussed the matter with her before taking a public position; they were, after all, a married couple. Why should the audience come first?

They were also an exceptionally busy married couple with a large family and myriad activities and commitments. Clare was continuously and impossibly occupied with his medical and media work, and, in 1995, Jane, with Madeleine Keane, published her own best-selling book, *What Will I Be?*, a guide to the daily routines of occupations as diverse as nursing, teaching, law, police work and art.[66] They did not discuss psychiatrists.

Clare took clear and often controversial public positions on all of the topical issues of the day, supporting, for example, the legalisation of abortion in certain circumstances following a highly controversial court case in 1992 (the 'X case'), but later supporting the unsuccessful 2002 amendment to the Irish constitution to limit the impact of the 'X case', arguing against allowing abortion on psychiatric grounds.[67] These complex issues, and how they impacted on individuals and families, were of great interest to Clare.

He had a particular interest in families: how they work, how they support people and how they can cause conflict. In 1997, Clare produced a play on the theme of family, Eugene O'Neill's *Long Day's Journey into Night*. This, just the second Irish production of O'Neill's play since its first production in 1957, took place at the Crypt Theatre, Dublin in August 1997. In his 'Producer's Note' in the programme, Clare highlighted the centrality of 'family' to O'Neill's tale:

> It has been called the nucleus of civilisation. Our own Constitution enshrines it as 'a moral institution possessing inalienable and imprescriptible rights'.[68] For Simone de Beauvoir, however, it was the means whereby women are oppressed, while the psychiatrist R.D. Laing accused it of being the factory wherein madness is produced. The family is emotionally potent and extraordinarily destructive, liberating and imprisoning, enriching and malevolent. It is the psychological crucible of intense altruism and paralysing selfishness.[69]

Clare described 'guilt and blame' as 'the gothic horrors that stalk many an Irish family, turning the crucible of love into a maelstrom of persecution. Relationships metamorphose into ritualistic and recurrent games of pass the parcel, where the participants are the family members, the parcel a parcel of blame.' Clare let his full rhetorical gifts run riot in his praise for O'Neill's play:

> Forty years on from the appearance of this magnificent play, we could do worse than ponder its revelations, the sometimes fixed, sometimes changing affections of parent–child relationships, the murderousness of human love, the corrosiveness of sibling rivalry, the undervalued importance of constitution and of temperament

... O'Neill's towering achievement is that as the curtain falls on a misery, an agony that we, the audience, know full well continues in a terrible dance of death, we are purged, we are exorcised and we are privileged to be reminded once again of the truth which eludes the four protagonists – namely that human beings can do better than this and that it is understanding not blame, forgiveness not accusations which truly make men and women free.

St Edmundsbury Hospital, Lucan (2001–7)

After he stepped down as medical director of St Patrick's, Clare moved more of his clinical activity to St Edmundsbury Hospital in Lucan in 2001. While he soon ceased most media work and undoubtedly had periods of personal difficulty over these years, this was – paradoxically – a time of growth for Clare as a clinician and therapist. From the moment he returned to Ireland, Clare always liked St Edmundsbury, a more suburban location than St Patrick's, which is located in Dublin's city centre.

Ann Buckley, family therapist at St Edmundsbury, recalls that 'when Tony Clare returned to Ireland in 1989, he saw patients mostly in St Edmundsbury Hospital in Lucan, rather than St Patrick's, admitted patients to St Edmundsbury, and held weekly team meetings there':

The team meetings were like workshops – you learned so much. Tony shared his love of psychiatry with us. I was doing training in psychotherapy at that time and Tony was very interested in that. I got great experience in St Edmundsbury because Tony Clare did a lot of therapeutic family work there. Early on, Tony decided he would have a nurse-therapist on his team and I applied. It was fabulous to have a job where I could give such time to patients [...]

Tony felt very comfortable in St Edmundsbury. Everyone loved the changes he introduced there. He made work more interesting for everybody. He encouraged taking very detailed case-histories from patients, for example, and this made work so much more interesting. He loved peoples' stories. Tony also drew a distinction between a person's illness and their behaviour. He was never afraid to challenge his patients about their behaviour and did not want his patients to be over-dependent on him or anyone else.[70]

Dr Michael DelMonte, clinical psychologist, recalls that 'Tony was very hard working and passionately driven.'[71] He was 'fascinated by family dynamics' and was 'eloquent and convincing. With Tony, there was never a dull moment.' In addition, 'Tony would always stand by his staff during difficult times. He was very loyal to his staff, his team and to struggling junior doctors.'

Dr Frank O'Donoghue, a colleague, recalls that 'When Tony moved from St Patrick's to St Edmundsbury in 2001, I had to say a few words to mark the occasion':

So, I asked: 'What is the difference between Tony Clare and God? God is everywhere but Tony Clare is everywhere but here.' Tony laughed at that. He could always laugh at himself.

Tony had a great capacity to talk you around. He'd always get around me. And he was very supportive as a clinical director. There are times when you need to make tough calls and he would back you up fully. I can't recall any resentment against Tony. We found him an entertaining character and very helpful. He was very even-handed at senior staff meetings, listening to everyone's view and taking them into account. He would incorporate any suggestions that were made.[72]

Dr Noel Kennedy, consultant psychiatrist at St Edmundsbury, points to Clare's continued 'generosity towards trainees' and recalls 'reading Tony's books and hearing him speak passionately at case conferences usually expounding a more holistic and family-oriented view of psychiatric disorder than would have been conventional at the time'.[73]

Kennedy also recalls Clare's willingness to support young psychiatrists in their research and clinical work, an activity that nourished Clare more and more as the years passed:

I got to know Tony well when I returned to Ireland in April 2004, working alongside him in St Edmundsbury until his untimely death. From a personal point of view, he was extremely warm and inviting, and took an almost paternal interest in my welfare and how I was settling in, regularly advising me about limiting workloads and taking regular holidays. He was very supportive regarding clinical work, research and teaching. I got the impression that he was happy supporting and mentoring younger consultants to achieve their potential. He was also very generous in sharing limited clinical resources to allow me to develop a functioning multi-disciplinary team.

From a clinical perspective, Tony put the holistic view he had of medicine into practice in St Edmundsbury and had a broader multi-disciplinary team than any other team within St Patrick's or St Edmundsbury, including psychodynamic psychology, cognitive behaviour therapy, family therapy, physiotherapy and even a masseuse. All were encouraged to give their opinion at team meetings which therefore lasted at least three or four hours!

Buckley recalls Clare's open, interactive style with both patients and colleagues:

Tony wrote lovely notes and lovely letters to patients. He wasn't materialistic at all. He did not charge patients very much. He never turned anyone away because they could not pay. He would write to colleagues at Christmas and express himself very well on paper. [At work,] he was more a snacker rather than sitting down to eat. He would sit down and have cup of tea with nurses and a chat. He was very open.[74]

Dr Frank O'Donoghue confirms that 'Tony was also very good to his patients and gave them lots of time. He charged them well below what he could have charged.'[75]

Kennedy points out that Clare's clinical 'team were very loyal and he treated them with the utmost courtesy and respect. He had a particular interest in family/couple therapy, and two or three-hour couple or family meetings were common, in conjunction with his family therapist, Ann Buckley.'[76] He was 'hugely perceptive and unafraid of challenging patients' or families' dysfunctional modes of behaviour while being very kind at the same time. He also continued to teach and inspire students and registrars with intellect and charisma.'

Outside of work, Clare was deeply charitable, serving with Jane on the board of Plan Ireland, a charity that promotes child rights in order to end child poverty.[77] He was chairperson of the Prince of Wales's Advisory Group on Disability from 1991 to 1997.[78] In his personal life, Clare enjoyed tennis, opera and cinema.[79] He loved to read. Rachel recalls that '*Middlemarch* was one of his favourite books. *The Great Gatsby* another':

> He enjoyed a good read, good conversation, a great newspaper article. He was a great communicator, it was always fun to talk to him, he made such interesting connections, and always challenged a received point of view.
>
> Dad would have loved the 2012 Olympics coming to London; as a family we used to watch the athletics – the classic Seb Coe and Steve Ovett years – and dip in and out of the Olympics' on holiday. He was genuinely really into sport. He played tennis as an adult.[80]

As Kennedy recalls, Clare socialised with colleagues but, deep down, might have preferred the more formal role of orator:

> Despite being quite a shy man behind his persona, Tony took time out of his very packed schedule to socialise with and get to know all the team, from consultants to domestic workers. I always got the feeling that these events were much more difficult for him than making an impromptu speech in front of several hundred people, but he made a huge effort to get to know staff and their families.

Buckley agrees that this world-famous psychiatrist 'would have been very uncomfortable with having admirers. He was quite a shy person':

Tony used to say that he was 'over-stretched' or 'on a merry-go-round'. To most people he came across as very confident and self-assured, but he was always concerned about the next talk, the next lecture, the next event. He didn't worry clinically as a psychiatrist, but would be anxious about the next event, and this surprised us.[81]

The renewed fulfilment that Clare found in his clinical work at St Edmundsbury from 2001 onwards was linked in no small part to his very conscious and by no means easy decision to step back from media work and various other commitments around this time. Psychiatrist Ivor Browne recalls talking things over with Clare during this period, pointing to Clare's tendency to over-commit professionally and its negative consequences on decision-making in other areas of Clare's personal and professional lives:

> I knew Tony vaguely over many years but only got to know him personally around 2000. He talked things over with me on a number of occasions and I also met his wife Jane at this time. Tony had got over-extended as a result of *In the Psychiatrist's Chair* [Chapter 5] and I guided him to withdraw down from some of that. He followed this advice and went to work in St Edmundsbury Hospital. He was working too much. I had influence on him drawing back from his over-exposure because Jane was very worried about him.[82]

Jane confirms that when Clare stepped back from the public arena in 2001 'there were no half measures; he got Bernie Butler (his secretary in St Patrick's) to say "No" to everything'.[83] Clare and Jane spent more time at their homes in Waterville, County Kerry and Sardinia, and Clare grew a beard. While he continued to see patients at St Edmundsbury, Clare eliminated all his other professional commitments. This was, in any case, a busy time in the Clares' family lives, as their children were now young adults and there were weddings and babies aplenty during these years. This was a time of great energy, focus and creativeness.

Robin Murray, as an especially long-standing friend and colleague, recalls that he 'never had a conversation with Tony when he talked about regretting things, except in his very last days when he seemed depressed':

> For several years he didn't come to London and wouldn't see anyone from UK psychiatry or media. I kept contacting him and trying to get to see him. Eventually when I was in Dublin I managed to meet him. I was shocked by what he looked like.
>
> His glory days were the 1960s as a student debater and the 1970s and 80s; he was a celebrity. He was disappointed that even though he had this fame, he hadn't revolutionised psychiatry in Ireland or got into politics, and he remained most admired for his first book [*Psychiatry in Dissent*; Chapter 3]. He kept refusing the College's honourary fellowship in later life. He said he wasn't worthy of it and declined it for four years. I kept urging the College to offer it again and he eventually accepted it.[84]

The Royal College of Psychiatrists, when Clare finally accepted its fellowship in 2007, shortly before his death, emphasised Clare's insight and empathy, along with his clinical, research and media work, and his unique, invaluable contribution to the profession. Clare had refused the College's offer of fellowship for so long because he felt that honours should not be heaped upon people who are doing their job – especially if they are rewarded in other ways such as financially or with general acclaim. In the end, Clare accepted the fellowship but did not attend the meeting to receive it in person.

Ruth Dudley Edwards recalls that 'Tony was lively, funny, irreverent and brave', and 'would have been a wonderful senator', but suggests that his return to Ireland in 1989 was a 'fatal mistake':

> Tony thought he was going to be well received in Dublin. But he was stunned at how people had turned on him. In Ireland, there is a resentment of someone who went away and became famous. He was desperately upset by the vicious response to his

television programme with Paul Cusack and his rejection for the Senate where he would have been a powerful voice for reform. Returning to Ireland was a fatal mistake. I can still see Tony's crushed expression.

… Tony grew a long beard and castigated himself as a bad, selfish person which was utterly untrue. In those years, Tony was filled with self-abnegation and self-hatred. At Patrick Cosgrave's funeral [24 September 2001], he made a speech about how Patrick had been a much better person than Tony, with his selfishness and desire for fame. In fact, Patrick had crashed and burned in his 40s and was a failure with few friends and Tony had had a stellar career and was much loved. Tony was a wonderful person.[85]

One of Clare's successors at St Patrick's, Professor James Lucey, recalls that 'Tony had an extraordinary decline. He got depressed between 2002 and 2006' and 'had feelings of unworthiness about the Fellowship offered by the Royal College of Psychiatrists':

For most of his life, Tony's energy was phenomenal and his recession from that life was equally phenomenal. During this period, I bumped into a dishevelled old man with a beard in a toyshop and scarcely recognised him as Tony. We picked out a gift together for my son – a red fire engine.[86]

Clare's son Peter recalls that, 'in later life, he became stressed, depressed, withdrawn, harried'.[87] Clare also grieved the loss of his friend Liam Hourican, who had died in August 1993.[88] Colm de Barra recalls that 'when Liam Hourican died suddenly while holidaying in Kerry, Tony arrived that afternoon with his own family to offer support and sympathy to Liam's family. That morning he had attended the funeral of his own mother. However, he made the nearly five-hour drive out of loyalty.'[89]

This was just one of a number of difficult events that Clare faced over this period, which also included the critical panning of his Irish television series *Irish in Mind* (1989), his failed bid for a Senate seat

(1993) and, in 2000, legal action by nuns regarding allegations of abuse on a programme in TV3's *20/20: Stolen Lives* series introduced by Clare.[90] Clare was also dogged by the nagging sense that he could have done more, written more and achieved more in his life.

But it would be wrong to present these later years as a time of inexorable decline or depression for Clare. This period also reflected a new-found balance for him, interpreted by some as depression but also resembling a period of sobriety after a prolonged addiction to adrenaline. Not only did Clare operate an effective, expansive clinical team at St Edmundsbury during this period, but his time there, away from the demands of his previous roles, eventually paid off more generally. As Lucey notes, 'Tony came back to life in 2007, in the months before his death':

> He was a magnificent thorn in the side of management during this time, opposing the closure of St Edmundsbury. He promoted the idea of an almost Langian centre for therapy there. He had energy and fluency again.[91]

Buckley confirms that 'at one point, plans were made to change St Edmundsbury into a treatment centre for young adults. Tony spent an entire night writing to management to encourage them to change their minds. He was in such shock after hearing the plan that he didn't sleep at all that night.'[92] Much to his relief, Clare prevailed.

Clare's years in St Edmundsbury, from 2001 until his death in 2007, also saw changes in his attitude towards religion. Murray 'never knew [Clare] to have a belief in God until the last few years of his life. He came back to his Jesuit faith.' In a 2000 interview about *On Men* in *The Times*, Clare admitted that, despite serving Mass as an altar boy and being involved in pilgrimages to Lourdes and Croagh Patrick in his youth, his Roman Catholic faith had slipped away over many years, as he struggled to believe in a God who permitted natural disasters and genocide to occur in an apparently haphazard fashion.[93] Clare also felt that the Church turned a blind eye to drinking problems in Ireland and that many priests set a bad example.[94]

But in spite of all of his rational thought and logical reasoning, Clare – like many others – found that his loss of faith left him with an emptiness that he struggled to fill and, as Murray and others noted, he developed a renewed affinity for Roman Catholicism in his later years.[95] God, it seemed, returned to Clare, just as Clare himself was winding down towards retirement – a retirement that was scheduled, tragically, for December 2007.

8

The Psychiatrist in the Chair

· ·

In September 1989, Anthony Clare received a letter from a schoolgirl in the United Kingdom, seeking his advice:

> Dear Dr Clare,
>
> I am a 17-year old schoolgirl who regularly listens to your radio programme *In the Psychiatrist's Chair*. Through listening to you for the past eight years, I have decided to become a psychiatrist. I will be applying for medicine later this month and to tell the truth, I'm extremely apprehensive about it all ... I'm dreading the interview. I was wondering whether you could share some of your experience and give me any advice on how to fulfil my lifelong ambition of becoming a doctor. I would be very grateful for your help.
>
> In a recent interview you said that psychiatry was the 'most relevant branch of medicine'. What do you mean by that? As your radio show has been successful, have you ever considered doing a television version? Would you ever consider sitting in the psychiatrist's chair yourself?[1]

As was his way, Clare wrote a lengthy letter in response, advising his correspondent that medical schools look for 'people with a wide range of interests because in practice such people cope with the demands of medical training best, certainly better than people with a very narrow range of interests and a very single-minded approach to life':

You should approach the interview much more with a view to
the fact that it is their loss if they do not select you than that it
is yours! It is very important what kind of frame of mind you are
in coming into the interview and believe you me the student who
is confident without being brash does start with a considerable
advantage.[2]

Clare advised his correspondent to read up on 'the sorts of
controversies that you know rage in medicine' such as AIDS, smoking
and 'issues relating to the way in which money is spent on health and
disease'. In a description that applied quite precisely to himself, Clare
advised his correspondent 'to sell yourself to these people as someone
who is interested in medicine, curious about people, anxious to learn
and able to get on with various people of all shapes and sorts!'

Thirty years later, Clare's letter-writer still vividly recalls receiving
Clare's response to her letter and its impact on her:

I used to avidly listen to *In the Psychiatrist's Chair* on my radio,
and the show and Anthony Clare really did lead to an interest in
the mind and its effect on the way we think, feel and behave, and
ultimately, the way we shape our own lives and the lives of those
around us. I wanted to become a psychiatrist and it was an honour
to receive such a detailed response from such an eminent gentleman.[3]

The aspiring medical student cherished her letter from Clare,
and while she went on to work in education rather than health, her
daughter, interestingly, decided on a career in psychiatry:

[My daughter] has made it to one of the top medical schools in the
country. I absolutely believe that Dr Clare's wise words have stayed
with me and helped me to raise a confident, sociable young lady with
a wide range of interests, curious about people, anxious to learn,
great at working in a team and able to get on with people from all
sorts of backgrounds. She really did go into her university interviews
believing that it would be their loss if they didn't select her.

Clare continually wrote letters such as this, published thousands of articles, and participated in countless media broadcasts over the course of his life. While it is impossible to calculate how many people his words and thoughts reached, it is clear that he had a substantial impact on people from all walks of life, in all corners of the globe, and in many different ways, both directly and indirectly. Never was this more apparent than in the outpouring of grief that followed Clare's untimely death in October 2007, just two months before he was due to retire from his post in St Edmundsbury.

October 2007

Clare commenced private clinical work in the Hermitage Clinic in Dublin in June 2007 and had intended seeing patients part-time after his retirement, which was scheduled for December 2007. But Clare's plans were cut tragically short when he died suddenly of a heart attack in Paris, on 28 October 2007, as he and Jane were travelling home from Sardinia, *en route* to see their latest grandchild, Simon's son Ollie.[4] Peter recalls that his father 'was stressed. There's a reason why he died at 64. His shoulders were broad but there was a lot on them.' After his death, his general practitioner wondered: 'why didn't he come to see me?'[5]

Rachel recalls that 'Dad was a terrible coward about medical interventions':

He was a bit hypochondriacal. He would catastrophise a headache into a brain tumour. He never saw himself in a hospital, or being treated by another doctor. Illness happened to other people [...] Like many in medicine, Dad had quite a functional attitude to diet and the body, and he was tough on himself physically, living in the way that he did, on adrenaline.[6]

The irony is that while the ever-active Clare, in what turned out to be his final days, told Jane that he wished he could have given more to psychiatry, he had finally started to look forward to retirement, only to have it denied him at the last moment. Ann Buckley confirms that while 'at times, Tony regretted coming back to Ireland, in later years he and Jane spent a lot of time in Kerry and he loved that. Coming towards retirement, Tony was really enjoying his life. He was planning his retirement well, intending to spend two days per week seeing patients even after he retired':

> Tony could be a bit gloomy but it was easy to distract him; he always reacted to patients' stories. Tony could also have a short fuse when he was under pressure but, again, he was the easiest person in the world to distract from that ... Why was Tony so popular? He had great time for everybody. He treated everyone as equals. He was a modest man, kind, caring, empathetic. His famous patients did not get treatment different to anyone else. His empathy was such that patients felt that he too could feel their sadness.[7]

Clare was widely mourned.[8] The *Guardian* described him as 'elfin and nimble' and argued that his 'lasting legacy will be his books' and his media work:

> Professor Anthony Clare, who has died aged 64 of a heart attack while in Paris, did more than anyone of his generation to improve the public understanding of psychiatry and to raise it from its former outcast status. His several series of BBC radio programmes, *In the Psychiatrist's Chair*, reached a wide audience and spawned four books. He was respected by both his public and his peers, and his book *Psychiatry in Dissent* in 1976 inspired many young doctors to train in psychiatry.[9]

A broad range of colleagues acknowledged Clare's undoubted intellectual brilliance, deep sense of compassion and profound supportiveness towards colleagues.[10] The *Times* and *Financial Times* highlighted his interviewing skills;[11] the *BMJ* emphasised his role in demystifying psychiatry;[12] and the *Irish Journal of Psychological*

Medicine both mourned his loss and celebrated his enormous contribution to the profession of psychiatry.[13]

The Irish Times noted Clare's many book reviews for the newspaper over the years,[14] including a superb essay about neurologist Oliver Sacks's 1995 book *An Anthropologist on Mars*,[15] and summarised the general sense of loss that followed Clare's abrupt death:

> Prof Anthony Clare's contribution to medicine and the media was truly immense. Following his sudden and untimely death in Paris last weekend, he has variously been described as 'the leading psychiatrist of his generation', 'coruscatingly intelligent ... a broadcasting star' and a 'gentle and caring man'.
>
> After the publication of his book *Psychiatry in Dissent* in 1976, he became a regular broadcaster and commentator while also working at the Institute of Psychiatry in London.
>
> Incisive contributions to BBC Radio 4's discussion programme *Stop the Week*, led to a steadfast partnership with the producer Michael Ember. Together they came up with the formula for *In the Psychiatrist's Chair*, the radio series which made him famous and which ran from 1982 until 2001. The programme is widely credited with helping to demystify psychiatry in Britain.[16]

Ruth Dudley Edwards recalled Clare's charm, brilliance and energy, but also wrote that he was naïve about Irish politics and that her doubts about his return to Dublin in 1989 were borne out when he was, she argued, eventually torn apart by envious onlookers.[17] But it was Clare's laughter and mischief that Dudley Edwards missed the most, and Clare's achievements were uncontestable.

At the hospital he loved, Ann Buckley and other colleagues 'wanted to do something at St Edmundsbury, so we created a garden in his memory. We wrote to President Mary McAleese to come and open it. She accepted within a week. President McAleese was wonderful on the occasion, speaking with even the most depressed of patients. She said that when you buy a dozen plants, ten will do well and grow on their own, but two will need more nurturing and minding – just like the patients who come to the hospital.'[18]

Clare is buried in Coad burial ground in the parish of Caherdaniel on a hillside looking out over the Kenmare River. His funeral mass was held in the Church of Mary Immaculate, Lohar in the parish of Caherdaniel, just above the Clares' home in Rineen, Waterville, where they attended mass every Sunday with their neighbours. Clare's gravestone carries a quotation from William Shakespeare's *Hamlet*:

> There's a divinity that shapes our ends,
> Rough-hew them how we will.[19]

The epitaph by Jane Clare describes Clare as a 'loving and beloved husband, father and grandfather, orator, physician, writer and broadcaster'. The order in which Clare's roles are presented is an accurate and insightful reflection of his priorities. First and foremost, and despite the extraordinary pace and complexity of his life, Clare's commitment as a 'husband, father and grandfather' was never in doubt. Robin Murray, a particular friend and colleague, notes that Clare 'was a great father. He doted. He was very attentive to his children.'[20] Rachel Jenkins recalls that 'he was very much a family man, devoted to his wife and children throughout his immensely busy working life'.[21]

After Clare's family roles, 'orator' is next on the list, appearing before 'physician', let alone psychiatrist (a term that does not appear at all).

James Lucey also highlights Clare's particular talent for public speaking, discussion and argumentation, and it was this oratorical gift that formed the deepest root of Clare's broadcasting, writing and various other achievements:

> Tony had the capacity to make an argument either way. He was the most compelling debater for either side. In the end, you didn't know where he stood on anything. I enjoyed working with him enormously. The degree to which he could master language was an enormous skill for a psychiatrist [...] Tony was constantly asking: 'What's the truth?' Everything was debatable. Tony believed that

the whole thrust of civilisation was about the assembly of cities, the assembly of people in collectives. Our momentum must go forward. We cannot regress to the cave. The apical question was, 'What is the progress of man?' At any point, Tony could lift the thrust of the conversation from the study of detail to the bigger questions. He was a free thinker, a meritocrat.[22]

Physician

Following his family priorities and his role as 'orator', it is Clare's profession as a 'physician' that is given pride of place on his headstone. Doctor–patient relationships are, however, quintessentially private, confidential matters so it can be difficult in a biography such as this to gain an accurate impression in retrospect and from the outside. Lucey, however, has 'seen hundreds of Tony's patients since his death and he [Clare] was completely himself with them'.[23] Murray notes that Clare's 'funeral service in Dublin was full of patients … I sat next to a lady who had been a patient who cried furiously and said he had been very good to her'.[24]

Medical journalist June Shannon recalls being treated by Clare in St Edmundsbury Hospital in Dublin in 2005. Her vivid account bears quoting in full in order to paint a picture of Clare the psychiatrist. Shannon notes that Clare 'was much smaller than I imagined, with very kind eyes':

> I had read a lot of his work, listened to his voice on the radio and seen him on television. He was the great Professor Anthony Clare, a renowned psychiatrist, credited as one of the first psychiatrists to break down the walls between psychiatry and the public in an effort to normalise and de-stigmatise mental illness. He was one of my mental health heroes and perhaps like we tend to do with all heroes, I imagined he would be taller and larger in real life. I had always wanted to meet Professor Clare in person but never imagined it would be in an acute psychiatric hospital as one of his patients.[25]

By the time Shannon was admitted to St Edmundsbury with 'an acute episode of depression and anxiety', she was 'broken, terrified, sick, weak, confused, too tired to fight, too exhausted to care. I just wanted it to stop':

On learning that I was a medical journalist, Professor Clare came laden down with studies and research papers on the link between chronic pain and depression in an effort to help me better understand my condition. He also presented me with independent information on the drugs he was proposing to prescribe and the rationale behind them. He took the time to listen to my crippling concerns about the physical pain I was in and never dismissed it or me. Instead he found answers in a way I could understand.

The drugs worked and continue to work to this day. When I was very ill, I was on two different antidepressants – a combination worked out by Professor Clare that worked very well. I have since been able to drop one of them but there have been times in the recent past when I had a recurrence of my illness and adding in the second 'Professor Clare' antidepressant always works. I am still very grateful to him today knowing that if I get sick again that 'Professor Clare' add-on is available.

When I was well enough to go home and back to work, I still visited Professor Clare on an outpatient basis. Over time as I slowly recovered back to my full health, my appointments were less about me and my illness and more about the various issues facing the health service, what needed to be done around mental health stigma and various health topics of the day. I always enjoyed my appointments and looked forward to them as I saw them as a golden opportunity to discuss topical areas in mental health and psychiatry with the master himself.

One day as I entered his room for my regular appointment before I had opened my mouth, he said, 'Hello June I see you are feeling good today.' I was, but I replied 'How did you know that today was a good day without even asking me?' He explained that his office at the time overlooked the car park and he would regularly watch his patients getting out of their cars in an effort to assess their mood. He said if they got out slowly or carefully and walked bent down or shakily to their appointment, he knew they were not doing so good. He explained that he had seen me hop out of the car and walk purposefully towards his office, leading him to correctly deduce that day was a good day.

I got a call from Professor Clare one day asking me if I could do him a favour. This man had saved my life, so of course I agreed without hesitation. He explained that one of his patients was having a very difficult time and he thought it would help if they could talk to me, as their case was similar to mine and I had been where they were now. I arranged to visit the patient in hospital and we met up a number of times afterwards. I don't know if it helped the patient. I like to think it did but I realise now that Professor Clare was the first person to introduce me to peer support and its importance in recovery. In asking me this one favour, unbeknown to him, he also inspired me to talk and write openly about my experience, which I hope has helped others and in some small way helped to break down stigma.

Lucey recalls that, as a psychiatrist, Clare 'had no allegiance for no one particular school, but if anything, he was a social psychiatrist',[26] who returned to Ireland in order to make a real contribution in his native land:

He was a stellar character who chose to come back to Ireland. Did he waste his time at St Patrick's and St Edmundsbury? Not at all. Why did he come back and what did he achieve? One of the things of which he was most proud was establishing the Dublin University Psychiatry Training Scheme, educating an entire generation of Irish psychiatrists. Had Tony not established this commitment to training, the College of Psychiatrists of Ireland would not exist. He regretted not collecting more data about what was achieved by the training scheme.

Clare promoted the idea of an 'Irish Association of Psychiatrists' to exist alongside the Irish Division of the London-based Royal College of Psychiatrists; the latter would have a particular remit for 'education, training and research', while the new 'Irish Association of Psychiatrists' would focus on improving services:

> Surely we can arrive at a situation whereby psychiatrists of a sovereign country, the Republic of Ireland, can have a body representing them in their negotiations with the Government of that state and in their meetings with other national bodies while maintaining the present admirable arrangement whereby Irish psychiatrists together with psychiatrists in Northern Ireland, England, Scotland and Wales share resources and skills in the organisation of postgraduate education, research and the accreditation of training establishments and facilities? My own view is that we could arrive at such a situation and the result would be of benefit to all of us.[27]

It was to take many more years and much more discussion before this issue was resolved in Ireland. In the event, the College of Psychiatry of Ireland was founded in 2009, two years after Clare's death, and took over both the training and representative roles that Clare described. (It was retitled College of Psychiatrists of Ireland in 2013.) The 2009 development represented a much greater break from the Royal College of Psychiatrists in London than envisaged by Clare, who was a dedicated internationalist: not only did his own career have a particularly international flavour, but he also promoted further international exchanges, supporting, for example, delegates from the developing world to attend the World Congress of the World Federation for Mental Health when it was held in Ireland in 1995.[28]

From an academic perspective, Clare tirelessly supported the development of links between the clinical and academic worlds (especially Trinity College Dublin),[29] as well as links between private and public psychiatry for both adults and children.[30] He spoke out publicly again and again about understaffing in the Irish health service, low bed numbers and the lack of proper education and career structures for doctors.[31] He was deeply involved in the development of a 'Patient's Charter' in St Patrick's in the mid-1990s[32] and, for the industrial relations dimension of his medical directorship, his guiding values were clear: 'What psychiatry needs more urgently than ever is a united front fighting for the rights of patients and staff and for a just and fair deal comparable to that received by other patients and staff in the health services, public and private.'[33]

But, in the end, it is the testimony of Clare's patient June Shannon, the sorrow of the patient who wept bitterly beside Murray at Clare's funeral service and the untold stories of Clare's thousands of other patients that provide the most compelling evidence that, despite all of his involvements and other achievements, Clare was first and foremost a physician, seeking to relate to individual patients and to heal their pain. More often than not, he succeeded.

Writer

Ruth Dudley Edwards, in her appreciation of Clare, noted how multi-talented he was and how he proved in time to be a fine writer of prose.[34] This is certainly true of Clare's apparently effortless journalism and his finest book, *Psychiatry in Dissent* (1976), which was both lucid and brilliant. Some of his other writings, most notably *On Men* (2000), were less well organised and could have benefitted from further reflection and reorganisation, but for the most part he was clear, compelling and a pleasure to read.

Clare had a particular love for journalism and wrote prodigiously for a wide range of local, national and international publications, aimed at both the public and healthcare professionals. Most of his contributions were signed but some were not. Geraldine Meagan, journalist with the *Irish Medical Times* in the early 1980s and now chief executive officer of MedMedia Group, recalls Clare's many editorials for the *Irish Medical Times*:

Tony used to write the editorials and he sometimes came over to Ireland and would sit with us in the office, chatting away in his wonderful animated style and flicking back his lovely hair. He was a fascinating character and would have you enthralled with the stories. That was when John O'Connell [later Minister for Health] owned the *Irish Medical Times* and it was the medical newspaper that you had to read.[35]

Maureen Browne recalls Clare's 'limitless energy, great kindness and wonderful fun' during this period:

I first met him when he literally bounded into the offices of the *Irish Medical Times*, where I then worked. It was the late 1980s and [Clare] came back to an Ireland torn apart by what we euphemistically called 'The Troubles' in Northern Ireland … Tony Clare brought optimism, positivity, glamour and great fun. We were impressed and a little nationally flattered that he had given up his celebrity television status and prestigious job in London to return to his native city.

At a time when most Irish doctors viewed the media with deep suspicion and no little distrust, Tony loved us. He dropped into the *Irish Medical Times* to meet us, his celebrity status sitting very lightly on him. He was one of us; he would be delighted to write for the paper. And, so it began: he worked with us, socialised with us, introduced us to Jane, met my journalist husband and through him reporters all over town. He laughed with and at us and made us laugh at ourselves.[36]

Clare 'wrote a weekly column for the *Irish Medical Times*, startling even us hardened hacks by the speed with which he churned it out, and went on to write the paper's editorials, challenging accepted conservative mores and pushing for social and medical changes. His philosophy was that we needed these changes and the world would not stop if we introduced them and sent a few sacred cows on their unhappy way. Erudite, sociable and funny, he held a high view of medicine and psychiatry, of the responsibilities of psychiatrists and the standards to which they must adhere at all times.'

It helped that Clare was an avid reader, capable of digesting books and writing about them in bewilderingly short periods of time. He was also deeply interested in creativity and the links between writing, the mind and mental illness. He brought this interest to bear in many aspects of his work.[37] In July 1996, for example, *In the Psychiatrist's Chair* featured Kay Redfield Jamison who is, as Clare noted, a very remarkable person: professor of psychiatry at Johns Hopkins in Baltimore; author of a superb book on the relationship between manic-depressive illness and the artistic temperament, titled *Touched with Fire*;[38] and a person with manic-depressive illness herself.[39]

In the 1996 interview with Clare, Jamison spoke openly about her mental illness, its treatment and her suicidal ideation, stating 'that there's a reason why people kill themselves who have this kind of illness. The pain is simply unbearable. You also think you are unbearable to other people.'[40] Jamison was equally forthright about the role of different forms of treatment and the importance of the therapeutic relationship as the foundation of creative care:

JAMISON: Well, clearly without medication I would be dead or insane so medication is central in keeping me alive.

CLARE: You'd put it that strongly?

JAMISON: Unquestionably. It is unquestionably true. But having a doctor who had the sense not to equivocate on my diagnosis, not to equivocate on the fact that I needed medication, who didn't buy into all of my discussions of why I didn't need to be on medication, who was compassionate, deeply compassionate, humanistic, who knew my love for the arts and my concerns about losing the edge, and who never for a second doubted that I ultimately would be able to get out there and compete again ... He never gave up on me.[41]

In 1997, the year after the interview, Clare reviewed Jamison's book *Touched with Fire* very positively in the *British Journal of Psychiatry*.[42] Jamison went on to write a similarly themed book about

American poet Robert Lowell (1917–77) in 2017, titled *Setting the River on Fire: A Study of Genius, Mania and Character*.[43] Highly praised by novelist John Banville in *The Irish Times*,[44] *Setting the River on Fire* did not shy away from the complexity of the links between mental illness and creativity: mania can inspire but it can also disable. Jamison quoted Lowell writing to poet Elizabeth Bishop in the late 1960s about the benefits of treatment with lithium, which greatly reduced Lowell's symptoms and his need for hospitalisation, and made Lowell finally feel free, moving out from the shadow of his bipolar disorder.[45]

These themes and views accorded precisely with Clare's informed, nuanced understanding of how mental illness can nourish creativity, quench it, or – over time – do both. In *Depression and How to Survive It*, co-written with manic-depressive comedian Spike Milligan (1918–2002), Clare noted that Milligan's creative work and mental illness raised the ancient issue about possible connections between creativity and psychiatric illness.[46] After a brisk run-through of the research, supporting links between creativity and manic-depression (but not schizophrenia), Clare concluded that while the nature of Milligan's humour suggested a link between manic-depression and comic genius, Milligan doubted that this was the case, pointing out that many people with manic-depression were not especially creative. In addition, Milligan was certain that, even if there was a link, comic genius was not worth the agony of manic-depression.[47]

As both Milligan and Lowell experienced, and Clare understood, serious mental illness involves very great suffering. This sense of understanding and compassion infused Clare's extraordinary interview with Jamison in 1996 and much of the rest of his work. Over two decades later, Jamison remembers Clare as 'immensely imaginative, full of curiosity and life, and a doctor who approached his clinical work with a wonderful blend of clinical knowledge and humanism. He was, as he said of writers he admired, a voyager.'[48] And Clare was also a writer himself, ever ready to explore new ways of describing the relationships between the written and spoken word, the workings of the human mind, and what happens when the mind loses its way.

Broadcaster

The final role specified on Clare's headstone in Rineen is 'broadcaster', listed after his family roles and his pursuits as 'orator', 'physician' and 'writer'. But it is, ironically, Clare's broadcasting that probably linked him with his greatest and most enduring audience, as *In the Psychiatrist's Chair* remains available on the BBC Radio 4 Extra website even today, several decades after it was first broadcast.[49] Twelve interviews were released on CD by BBC Worldwide as recently as 2016. The reason for this longevity is simple: Clare's programme changed the nature of broadcast interviews forever, exploring people's inner lives in depth and in public while maintaining a dignity and gravitas that is sorely lacking in so many similar programmes today.

Clare was also willing to use his interviewing and broadcasting skills for other causes, such as recording an audio-cassette for the Royal College of Psychiatrists on the subject of stress in the 1990s,[50] and participating in the College's 'Defeat Depression' campaign, which he felt had a real impact on stigma: 'I am impressed at the steady increase of public awareness of and public interest in psychological ill-health. There is an enormous constituency of support out there for us.'[51] He even recorded interviews for the Irish Rugby Football Union for their historical records, with figures such as Jack Coffey and Eugene Davy, an Ireland international rugby union fly-half.[52]

Today, over a decade after Clare's death, it is clear that appreciation of Clare's broadcasts and various other elements of his work has only grown with time. Psychologist Maureen Gaffney, who positively reviewed the 1992 volume of *In the Psychiatrist's Chair*[53] in *The Irish Times*,[54] draws particular attention to Clare's warmth and engagement:

> I liked Tony and was always struck by his warmth. He was engaging, interested, very entertaining and not at all pretentious, given his celebrity at that time in the United Kingdom. I recall noting at the time that he was sometimes the object of a kind of disparaging envy by some people. It was kind of mean-minded I always thought. And he was probably perceptive enough to have picked that up.[55]

Psychiatrist Anthony Mann emphasises Clare's popularity with colleagues and his contribution to the field of psychiatry, not only in the media:

> Tony was very popular with our peer group at the Institute of Psychiatry. People knew he had this special talent and weren't remotely envious of him at all. Tony was so charming that everyone was so pleased for him. He was greatly liked; there was no one I knew who didn't like him.
>
> Tony made a vast contribution to promoting psychiatry in an intelligent and articulate way. He never pretended to be a great researcher, but he was able to assemble facts and stories. Tony's talents were in the media, lecturing, writing and broadcasting – and he was brilliant at all of that.[56]

For Rachel Jenkins, Clare's 'greatest talent and achievement was his public education role via his media work and writing ... his book *Psychiatry in Dissent* was a brilliant exposition of the key issues then pre-occupying the psychiatric field, many of which remain relevant today; and his media work brought psychiatric concepts to the wider public ensuring justice to the subject matter without over-simplification. His untimely death has been an enormous loss.'[57]

Ivor Browne describes Clare as 'a very fine person'[58] and Robin Murray says he was 'the most amazing psychiatrist I've ever met':

> He was always full of plans. Whenever you went to talk with Tony you were always entertained and provoked and went away with your head reeling with different ways of looking at things. Tony knew literature, philosophy, Byron and the classics. I would listen with wonder. I was star-struck by Tony.[59]

So were many others, and Clare is remembered through his writings, broadcasts, clinical care and the example he set for other psychiatrists and workers in mental health. In the year following his death, Clare was formally remembered by colleagues in St Edmundsbury who made a commemorative donation to Plan Ireland, the charity which Jane chaired.[60] In November 2009, Murray delivered the Founder's Day Lecture at St Patrick's in Clare's honour.[61]

A decade later, in June 2018, the inaugural Amergin Solstice Poetry Gathering was held in Waterville, county Kerry, sponsored by Jane, to celebrate contemporary Irish poetry and honour her husband's memory.[62] The successful festival concluded with the 'Anthony Clare Memorial Session' featuring talks, music and drama on the theme of mental ill-health and recovery from a diverse range of contributors – precisely as Clare would have wished. Ponc Press in An Daingean published a limited edition commemorative volume featuring poetry by Eiléan Ní Chuilleanáin, Harry Clifton, Michael Longley, Nuala Ní Dhomhnaill and Paula Meehan, and an introduction by Paddy Bushe.[63]

'What Was His Goal? It Was Never Clear'

Anthony Clare was not perfect. He described himself as easily bored, impatient, explosive and a bit abrasive, especially when his children were younger.[64] At the height of his fame, personal details of his family life essentially became public property, often through interviews Clare himself gave to journalists.[65] He was prone to irritation and could suddenly become angry,[66] chiefly if he felt his time was being wasted. Rachel recalls that 'he misplaced things like keys, or lost them altogether. He would leave things behind on planes, trains: his speech notes, gloves, scarves, sunglasses. He could be irritable, quite short-tempered.'[67]

Clare was also very, very busy, both at work and at home. His son Peter recalls that, 'as a child growing up in a family of seven, we individually needed to fight for our father's attention':

We all sought my father's approval and he had such high standards. I remember I did my Leaving Certificate [final second-level school examination in Ireland] twice. The first time around I didn't fail, but I needed to repeat it and get a better result to get into college. I got a C1 in English first time round and the second time round I got an A2. When I got my results, Dad was at work in the hospital and my mother said: 'Ring your father! Ring him! Ring him! He will be so proud!' I was hesitant, I remember, my instinct warned me not to phone, but I relented and I phoned and when I told him my A2 result over the phone he responded: 'What stopped you from getting an A1?' It was an impulsive answer and I was told by others, but not by my father, that he regretted saying it. It was a crushing response to hear from my father. It was as if he could not help himself but be critical. He had such high standards for both himself and others.[68]

Much of this was both understood and forgiven by those around him: Lucey remembers what another of Clare's colleagues said about him: 'You know, great men get a different licence.'[69] Clare had, as Lucey notes, 'tremendous capacity and tremendous frustration in his life',[70] so allowances were generally made. He was so charming and eloquent anyway that it was impossible to be angry with him for very long.

In retrospect, it can be argued that Clare made some debatable choices in his professional career. Following his return to Ireland in 1989, for example, his decision to focus on private rather than public psychiatry can be partially understood in light of his training in St Patrick's and the limited alternative options at his level at that time, but it was still regrettable that Clare did not devote more of his energies directly to building Ireland's public mental health system: it desperately needed someone like Clare in the 1980s and 1990s and – arguably – still does.[71]

So, while Clare's decision to return to Ireland in 1989 was correct and probably inevitable (he had clear reasons for it and, like most people, wanted to come 'home'),[72] Clare might have reconsidered the position of medical director of St Patrick's Hospital after his first term in the post. It was certainly a job that he did well, and the hospital and its patients benefitted greatly from his industry and imagination, but there were other things that Clare might well have done even better and with greater impact: writing a follow-up to *Psychiatry in Dissent*, for example, or linking his psychiatric expertise with his philanthropic impulses to work at global level to improve mental healthcare around the world, through the World Psychiatric Association or WHO (with which he worked a little).[73] Clare was capable of all of these things and much, much more; time spent on very local administrative matters could, perhaps, have been better devoted to greater issues more suited to his extraordinary, expansive talents.[74]

Clare also came in for criticism, sometimes in the media (from, for example, a chronically disgruntled Bernard Levin in *The Times*)[75] and sometimes from within his own profession. Noël Browne (1915–97), one-time politician and psychiatrist, was especially scathing and wrote in 1989 of 'Anthony Clare's old fashioned, establishment style of voodoo psychiatry'.[76] But Browne's real criticism was of conventional psychiatry as a whole rather than Clare himself; Clare had simply and inevitably come to represent establishment values, a development that baffled and bothered Clare in equal measure: 'I've become part of the establishment,' he would moan, dismayed.[77] The firebrand debater of the 1960s had become a pillar of convention by the late 1980s. It had been a roller coaster couple of decades, but the final outcome forever puzzled Clare, much as he enjoyed the ride.

Rachel emphasises her father's mix of professional commitment, benign opportunism and personal kindness:

Dad contributed significantly to a change in UK culture by engaging with the world and being in the world. His patients were convinced that 'successful' people, whether rich or famous, didn't face the same challenges, didn't struggle with difficult family issues, with depression, with anxiety. He and Michael Ember (through *In the Psychiatrist's Chair*) were motivated by a desire to challenge that, to explore the extent to which 'the successful' share common experiences with the rest of us, that they may not be as happy and well-adjusted as they seem on the surface.

What was [my father] trying to do? He was just enjoying himself, finding fulfilment from whatever life presented. He was making the most of opportunity. And, of course, he was trying to pay the bills. In many ways, my father lived in the present and the future.

Rather than a core set of beliefs, he had a moral compass. He understood shades of grey. He was a very humane, kind person. He believed in doing for others what you would want done for yourself.[78]

Jane's assessment of her husband's life and work is understandably complex. She notes that Clare's career and activities were not strategically planned in advance but were 'largely opportunistic'.[79] Peter points out that 'he spontaneously made choices, almost impulsively. He liked to be in control but was surrounded by chaos':

Reflecting on my father, I realise how much I don't know about him. And I realise how much I've learned about 'Professor Anthony Clare'. People say I resemble him and that's a little strange – they all know a different man to me. I had a terrible feeling that I was never good enough, and I strived to be good enough. I struggle with that. He had unrelenting standards. If it was in wartime and he wasn't a psychiatrist, he would have been a very good leader of men. He lived and led by example. As he approached retirement, he was very proud of the fact that he only took thirteen sick days over the course of his entire career.[80]

Peter asks: 'Who was he? Who was Professor Anthony Clare? He was both selfless and selfish – always demanding of himself. Why? What drives us? Our character, our upbringing? Selfish is not quite the right word. There was an element of thoughtlessness, impulsiveness. In sight, in mind; out of sight, out of mind. What drove him? Acclaim, praise. What was he trying to achieve? Approval. He had broad shoulders, but whatever void he was trying to fill, nothing was enough.'

Despite his relentless work rate, many of Clare's plans did not come to fruition, including a worldwide programme about religious faiths that would have been so big, he said, it would have required him to leave psychiatry. Like many other grand visions, this one never happened, which is a real pity. What emerged instead was that, far too often, Clare was over-scheduled, heavily reliant on last-minute preparations, and utterly dependent on Bernie Butler, his secretary in St Patrick's, who was a beacon of quiet organisation in Clare's frenetic world.

Over the years, in response to the ceaseless, often petty demands of others, Clare let his imaginative canvas shrink rather than expand, and that was his tragedy. But while Clare was occasionally overwhelmed by the whirlwind that surrounded him, he also thrived on it from day to day. This was oxygen to him. This was the life he loved. This was the life he *chose* to build: filled with action, movement, energy and – above all else – words. Jane wonders: 'What was Tony trying to do? What was his goal? It was never clear.'

There is, perhaps, a hint in the epitaph on his grave in Rineen where the role of 'orator' appears first on the list immediately after Clare's family roles. And no one can deny that words, spoken and written, literally gushed out of Anthony Clare. They could not be stopped. *He* could not be stopped.

But Clare's words did not build a proud stone edifice in a desert, Ozymandias-style, declaring vainly that it would last forever. Clare's words were more like the incoming tide, sweeping up the strand, making their way over stones, reviving rock pools, lifting plants, flowing fluently in and around and over and under, taking the shape of the other but remaining of themselves, gentle but persistent, irresistible and ultimately all powerful.

Anthony Clare *lived* through words.

And his ultimate message was a simple one: that we must engage with each person as an individual, speaking, listening, relating. He would have agreed heartily with the American Buddhist psychiatrist, Mark Epstein, who says that being right is not the point in the profession of psychiatry; being *useful* is.[81] And Anthony Clare was very useful indeed. Most of all, he knew the usefulness of words and he deployed them to superb effect in public, in private, and in all of the contexts in between.

Italian physicist Carlo Rovelli writes that words, literature and, especially, poetry might be one of science's deepest roots – the ability to see beyond what is visible.[82] Clare had a gift for using words to move beyond the visible, be it in his exploration of creativity in the book with Spike Milligan; in his interviews with well-known but private figures who opened up to millions on *In the Psychiatrist's Chair*; in his book *Psychiatry in Dissent*; or even in *On Men* which, in 2000, prefigured much of the media discussion about gender in recent years.

And, returning to Jamison's description of Clare as a 'voyager',[83] looking back on Clare's life and work, there really *is* a sense of voyage. Where to? Who knows? Lucey recalls entering Clare's office one day just as Clare finished a phone call 'and he said to me: "Someday, I will tell you what's going on, but not now".'[84] As with all lives, there is much that is unknowable about Clare's.

Perhaps there never was to be a final destination for Clare, only a continuous voyage. And what a voyage it was. A restlessness for more. A profound thirst for relationality. And at all times, Clare's clever, impassioned voice stating the logical, the reasonable, the insightful and often the lyrical, regardless of the capricious, prevailing winds that swept around him. He was a paradoxical still point in the midst of a tempest that he created for himself, a bundle of passion and brilliance in a world increasingly devoid of both.

Endnotes

INTRODUCTION:
WHO WAS ANTHONY CLARE?

1 A. Clare, *In the Psychiatrist's Chair III* (London: Chatto & Windus/Random House, 1998), p. 160.
2 Ibid., p. 177.
3 Personal communication: U. Geller, interview with BK (8 May 2018).
4 A. Clare, 'Triumph of the will', *The Listener*, 26 July 1984.
5 Personal communication: N. Lawson, email to BK (9 May 2018).
6 Personal communication: N. Horlick, email to BK (8 May 2018).
7 Clare, *In the Psychiatrist's Chair III*, p. 453.
8 Ibid., p. 455.
9 Ibid., p. 435.
10 A.W. Clare, 'Diazepam, alcohol, and barbiturate abuse', *British Medical Journal*, 4, 5783 (6 November 1971), p. 340.
11 A. Clare, *Psychiatry in Dissent: Controversial Issues in Thought and Practice* (London: Tavistock Publications, 1976).
12 B.D. Kelly, *Hearing Voices: The History of Psychiatry in Ireland* (Dublin: Irish Academic Press, 2016), pp. 229–32.
13 R.M. Murray, 'Obituary: Professor Anthony Clare', *Psychiatric Bulletin*, 32, 3 (1 March 2008), pp. 118–19.

1. BACKGROUND AND EDUCATION (1942–66)

1 R. Geoghegan, *Tony Clare (Private Memoir)*, 4 November 2007.
2 Kelly, *Hearing Voices: The History of Psychiatry in Ireland*, pp. 229–32; A. Crane, 'Radio psychiatrist who quizzed the famous', *Financial Times*, 31 October 2007.
3 Personal communication: R. Clare, interview with BK (7 March 2019).

4 S. Monick and O.E.F. Baker, 'Mega, February 1941: The role of the 1st South African Irish Regiment', *Scientia Militaria: South African Journal of Military Studies*, 20, 4 (1990), 27–53.
5 R. Geoghegan, *Tony Clare (Private Memoir)*, 4 November 2007.
6 Personal communication: J. Clare, interview with BK (10 May 2018).
7 P. Coleman and A. Clare, 'Me and my family', *Daily Telegraph*, 8 January 1993.
8 M. Proops, 'What's your problem with agony aunts like me?', *Daily Mirror*, 24 April 1995.
9 For more on Clare's thoughts about motherhood, see: A. Clare, 'Mother or someone', *The Listener*, 18 February 1982.
10 L. France, 'I was never good enough for my mother', *Daily Mail*, 22 July 1995; S. Vincent, 'The elusive self', *Guardian*, 23 September 1995.
11 Personal communication: R. Dudley Edwards, interview with BK (14 June 2019).
12 Personal communication: J. Clare, interview with BK (10 May 2018).
13 Personal communication: P. Clare, interview with BK (9 February 2019).
14 P. Lewis, 'What drives people to the top?', *Daily Mail*, 19 September 1995.
15 G. Bridgstock and A. Clare, 'Stress sense', *Evening Standard*, 28 July 1989.
16 S. Vincent, 'The elusive self', *Guardian*, 23 September 1995.
17 Personal communication: R. Clare, interview with BK (7 March 2019).
18 A. Clare, 'Off the air, on the couch: a life in the day of Anthony Clare', *Sunday Times*, 8 July 1984.
19 Personal communication: J. Campbell (nee Clare), interview with MH (8 May 2019).
20 For more on An Comhdháil, see: C. Lysaght, 'Memories of the 1950s', in M. Bevan (ed.), *Gonzaga At Sixty: A Work in*

Progress (Dublin: Messenger Publications, 2010), 46–55.

21 Personal communication: J. Clare, interview with BK (10 May 2018).

22 R. Geoghegan, 'Remembering Joseph Veale', *Interfuse*, 114 (Christmas 2002), 4–9; extracts from this memoir were printed in the *Gonzaga Record, 1950–1959*. See also: R. Geoghegan, 'Joseph Veale, SJ', *Irish Times*, 4 November 2002.

23 Gonzaga College website: www.gonzaga. ie/about (Accessed 8 June 2019).

24 A. Clare, 'Truths my Father told me', *Sunday Independent*, 23 July 2000.

25 J. Veale, 'Men speechless', *Studies: An Irish Quarterly Review*, 46, 183 (Autumn 1957), 322–39. See also: C. Lysaght, 'Memories of the 1950s', in M. Bevan (ed.), *Gonzaga At Sixty: A Work in Progress* (Dublin: Messenger Publications, 2010), 46–55.

26 Personal communication: M. Bevan, emails to BK (24 June and 4 October 2019)

27 G. Bridgstock and A. Clare, 'Stress sense', *Evening Standard*, 28 July 1989.

28 C. Richmond, 'Obituary: Anthony Clare', *Guardian*, 31 October 2007.

29 Personal communication: R.M. Murray, interview with BK (25 February 2018).

30 E.J. Dickson, 'Hometown: Anthony Clare, Dublin', *The Times*, 14 October 1995.

31 E. Delaney, 'Where politics and culture collide', *Irish Times*, 30 March 2004; T. Weekes, 'Sitting and waiting', in F. Callanan (ed.), *The Literary and Historical Society, 1955–2005* (Dublin: A&A Farmar, 2005), 46–7; A. O'Brien, 'Did the mirth move for you? How it was for me', in F. Callanan (ed.), *The Literary and Historical Society, 1955–2005* (Dublin: A&A Farmar, 2005), 84–6; M. McDowell, 'Braving the cockpit of controversy', *Irish Times*, 12 March 2005; D. McCartney, 'The L&H – windbag factory for Ireland's gilded youth?', *Irish Independent*, 24 July 2005; K. Holmquist, 'Where the sharpest pit their wits', *Irish Times*, 19 February 2010.

32 C. Lysaght, 'First stirring of dissent, 1958–62', in F. Callanan (ed.), *The Literary and Historical Society, 1955–2005* (Dublin: A&A Farmar, 2005), 50–63.

33 L. Hourican, 'Louis Courtney and Flann O'Connor take America by storm', in F. Callanan (ed.), *The Literary and Historical Society, 1955–2005* (Dublin: A&A Farmar, 2005), 90–2; P. Hourican,

'The audience howled for blood', in F. Callanan (ed.), *The Literary and Historical Society, 1955–2005* (Dublin: A&A Farmar, 2005), 93–4.

34 Anonymous, 'Sees Ireland as fount of labour for Europe', *Irish Times*, 20 November 1962.

35 Anonymous, 'School curriculum "deplored"', *Irish Times*, 28 November 1960.

36 Anonymous, 'Students look at Irish parents', *Irish Times*, 10 December 1962.

37 Anonymous, '*Irish Times* trophy won by UCD', *Irish Times*, 15 February 1963.

38 Anonymous, 'The winning team', *Irish Times*, 16 February 1963.

39 *Irish Times* Reporter, 'UCD reach final of *Observer* tournament', *Irish Times*, 18 March 1963.

40 *Irish Times* Reporter, 'Glasgow students win debating tournament', *Irish Times*, 8 May 1963.

41 R. Dudley Edwards, 'Patrick Cosgrave – Tory rebel', in F. Callanan (ed.), *The Literary and Historical Society, 1955–2005* (Dublin: A&A Farmar, 2005), 87–9.

42 Anonymous, '*Irish Times* debating trophy won by UCD', *Irish Times*, 6 May 1963.

43 Anonymous, 'Highest semi-final standard so far', *Irish Times*, 25 January 1964.

44 Anonymous, '*Irish Times* debating trophy winners', *Irish Times*, 2 March 1964.

45 Anonymous, 'UCD debaters through to final', *Irish Times*, 10 April 1964.

46 Anonymous, '*Observer* debate won by UCD', *Irish Times*, 29 June 1964. See also: B. Dowling, 'An exercise in comedy: 1966–8', in F. Callanan (ed.), *The Literary and Historical Society, 1955–2005* (Dublin: A&A Farmar, 2005), 120–31; P. Whyms, 'Gentle speakers conquered: 1979–83', in F. Callanan (ed.), *The Literary and Historical Society, 1955–2005* (Dublin: A&A Farmar, 2005), 236–45.

47 R. Geoghegan, 'John Charles McQuaid and the L&H', in F. Callanan (ed.), *The Literary and Historical Society, 1955–2005* (Dublin: A&A Farmar, 2005), 95–6; see also: A. McTeirnan, 'Momentous occasion for future president', *Irish Times*, 31 January 1992; M. Webb, *Trinity's Psychiatrists: From Serenity of the Soul to Neuroscience* (Dublin: Trinity College, 2011), pp. 120–3.

48 Personal communication: R. Dudley Edwards, interview with BK (14 June 2019).

49   Personal communication: Colm de Barra, email to BK (17 June 2019).

50   Personal communication: R.M. Murray, interview with BK (25 February 2018).

51   A.W. Clare, 'General Costello and NATO', *Irish Times*, 20 February 1962.

52   A.W. Clare, 'A question of numbers', *St Stephen's* (Michaelmas, 1963), 9–11

53   A. Clare, 'Students and intellectual freedom', *Hibernia*, 28, 1 (January 1964), 7–8; see also: Anonymous, 'UCD "ban" on two churchmen', *Irish Times*, 11 January 1964; R. Geoghegan, 'John Charles McQuaid and the L&H', in F. Callanan (ed.), *The Literary and Historical Society, 1955–2005* (Dublin: A&A Farmar, 2005), 95–6.

54   P. Cosgrave, 'The ambiguities of attitude', *St Stephen's* (Trinity, 1962), 18–22; P. Cosgrave, 'The Marxist legacy', *St Stephen's* (Trinity, 1963), 39–45. See also: R. Dudley Edwards, 'Patrick Cosgrave – Tory rebel', in F. Callanan (ed.), *The Literary and Historical Society, 1955–2005* (Dublin: A&A Farmar, 2005), 87–9.

55   Personal communication: J. Clare, email to MH and BK (14 January 2019). See also: J. Clare, 'Family ties', *Sunday Tribune*, 17 September 1995.

56   E.J. Dickson, 'Hometown: Anthony Clare, Dublin', *The Times*, 14 October 1995. See also: J. Diski, 'Who's been sitting in my chair?', *Observer*, 9 August 1998.

57   Personal communication: E. Philbin Bowman, email to BK (1 June 2018).

58   H. Crawley, 'Applause is a hard drug: 1961–6', in F. Callanan (ed.), *The Literary and Historical Society, 1955–2005* (Dublin: A&A Farmar, 2005), 97–114; V. Browne, 'Wasted lives', in F. Callanan (ed.), *The Literary and Historical Society, 1955–2005* (Dublin: A&A Farmar, 2005), 117–19.

59   Personal communication: J. Clare, interview with BK (10 May 2018).

60   G. Sinnott, 'Hip hiatuses and a return to history: 1996–8', in F. Callanan (ed.), *The Literary and Historical Society, 1955–2005* (Dublin: A&A Farmar, 2005), 314–23.

61   H. Kelly, 'Move over McGonagall', in F. Callanan (ed.), *The Literary and Historical Society, 1955–2005* (Dublin: A&A Farmar, 2005), 132–6; W. Earley, 'A natural resting place: 1968–70', in F. Callanan (ed.), *The Literary and Historical Society, 1955–2005* (Dublin: A&A Farmar, 2005), 137–47; P. Leahy, 'A good time for debating: 1990–2', in F. Callanan (ed.), *The Literary and Historical Society, 1955–2005* (Dublin: A&A Farmar, 2005), 279–87; M. MacNicholas, 'Seedy glamour: 1992–6', in F. Callanan (ed.), *The Literary and Historical Society, 1955–2005* (Dublin: A&A Farmar, 2005), 288–304.

62   P. Smyth, 'Drama and Life', in F. Callanan (ed.), *The Literary and Historical Society, 1955–2005* (Dublin: A&A Farmar, 2005), 342–3; M. McDowell, 'Braving the cockpit of controversy', *Irish Times*, 12 March 2005; C. Walsh, 'Loss of a vibrant voice', *Irish Times*, 3 November 2007. See also: P. McGarry, 'Schizophrenia Ireland's "Lucia Day" highlights Joyce family's tragedy to heighten awareness of mental illness', *Irish Times*, 27 July 1998.

63   E. Curran, 'Ripe for expansion: 1998–2002', in F. Callanan (ed.), *The Literary and Historical Society, 1955–2005* (Dublin: A&A Farmar, 2005), 326–37; p. 330.

64   Personal communication: J. Clare, email to MH and BK (14 January 2019).

65   S. Hogan, *History of Irish Steel* (Dublin: Gill and Macmillan Ltd., 1980).

66   A. Wallace, 'Ireland's greatest rugby legislator', *Irish Times*, 2 March 2018.

67   S. Cody, 'Anthony Clare: In the Psychiatrist's Chair', unpublished interview, 1 May 1984; Personal communication: S. Cody, email to BK and MH (6 April 2019).

68   A. Clare, *On Men: Masculinity in Crisis* (London: Chatto & Windus, 2000).

69   K. Holmquist, 'Men in crisis – or is it just me?', *Irish Times*, 27 July 2000.

70   Personal communication: J. Clare, interview with BK (23 June 2018).

2. THE MAKING OF A PSYCHIATRIST (1966–76)

1   C. Richmond, 'Obituary: Anthony Clare', *Guardian*, 31 October 2007.

2   Personal communication: J. Clare, interview with BK (7 June 2018).

3   K. Holmquist, 'Men in crisis – or is it just me?', *Irish Times*, 27 July 2000.

4   Personal communication: R. Clare, interview with BK (7 March 2019).

5   D. Brennan, *Irish Insanity, 1800–2000* (Abingdon, Oxon.: Routledge, 2014), p. 2; B.D. Kelly, 'Mental health services: where does Ireland stand internationally?', *Medical Independent*, 15 March 2018.

6   Commission of Inquiry on Mental Illness, *Report of the Commission of Inquiry on Mental Illness* (Dublin: The Stationery Office, 1967) (hereafter 'Commission'), p.xv; *Irish Times* Reporter, 'Ireland has high mental illness rate', *Irish Times*, 29 March 1967; *Irish Times*, 16 November 1967.

7   A.W. Clare, 'Swift, mental illness and St Patrick's Hospital', *Irish Journal of Psychological Medicine*, 15, 3 (September 1998), 100–4.

8   Kelly, *Hearing Voices: The History of Psychiatry in Ireland*, p. 22.

9   A.W. Clare, 'St. Patrick's Hospital', *American Journal of Psychiatry*, 155, 11 (November 1998), 1599.

10   E. Malcolm, *Swift's Hospital: A History of St Patrick's Hospital, Dublin, 1746–1989* (Dublin: Gill and Macmillan, 1989), p. 259.

11   A.W. Clare and J.G. Cooney, 'Alcoholism and road accidents', *Journal of the Irish Medical Association*, 66, 11 (9 June 1973), 281–6.

12   A. Clare, 'El Vino veritas', *The Listener*, 27 September 1984; A. Clare and M. Bristow, 'Drinking drivers: the needs for research and rehabilitation', *British Medical Journal (Clinical Research Edition)*, 295, 6611 (5 December 1987), 1432–3.

13   S. Perera, 'Currie claims success for anti-drug campaign', *Guardian*, 30 October 1987.

14   Personal communication: J. Clare, interview with BK (7 June 2018).

15   A.W. Clare, 'John Norman Parker Moore (obituary)', *Psychiatric Bulletin*, 20, 12 (1 December 1996), 771–3.

16   Personal communication: I. Browne, interview with BK (7 July 2018).

17   RTÉ website: www.rte.ie/archives/2013/0726/464758-the-dangers-of-scientology (Accessed 16 January 2020).

18   Personal communication: R. Clare, interview with BK (7 March 2019).

19   For more on Maudsley, see: T. Turner, 'Henry Maudsley – psychiatrist, philosopher and entrepreneur', *Psychological Medicine*, 18, 3 (August 1988), 551–74.

20   Clare later wrote about the psychological effects of war: A. Clare, 'Wounded minds that find no peace when the war is over', *Sunday Express*, 17 January 1993.

21   For more on Mapother, see: A. Lewis, 'Edward Mapother and the making of the Maudsley Hospital', *British Journal of Psychiatry*, 115, 529 (December 1969), 1349–66.

22   For more on Lewis, see: M. Shepherd, 'Aubrey Lewis 1900–1975', *American Journal of Psychiatry*, 132, 8 (August 1975), 872.

23   See, for example: A.W. Clare, 'Training of psychiatrists', *Lancet*, 300, 7780 (7 October 1972), 753–6.

24   Physician at the Bethlem Royal and Maudsley Hospitals, London. See: M.S., 'Obituary: Frederick Kräupl Taylor', *Psychiatric Bulletin*, 13, 7 (July 1989), 394–5.

25   F.K. Taylor, 'Prokaletic measures derived from psychoanalytic technique', *British Journal of Psychiatry*, 115, 521 (April 1969), 407–19; J. Neeleman and A.H. Mann, 'Treatment of hysterical aphonia with hypnosis and prokaletic therapy', *British Journal of Psychiatry*, 163, 6 (December 1993), 816–19.

26   Personal communication: A. Mann, interview with BK (2 July 2018).

27   R.M. Murray, 'Obituary: Professor Anthony Clare', *Psychiatric Bulletin*, 32, 3 (1 March 2008), pp. 118–19.

28   Personal communication: R.M. Murray, interview with BK (25 February 2018).

29   Webb, *Trinity's Psychiatrists: From Serenity of the Soul to Neuroscience*, p. 121.

30   T. Bewley, *Madness to Mental Illness: A History of the Royal College of Psychiatrists* (London: RCPsych Publications, 2008), pp. 12, 60.

31   J. Bird, P. Campbell, A. Clare, J. Hamilton, A. Maiden, W. Marsh, A. McDowall, P. O'Farrell, E. Owens, D. Storer, R. Symonds and E. Worrall, 'Association of Psychiatrists in Training', *Lancet*, 298, 7724 (11 September 1971), 597.

32   R.C. Adams and over 300 others including A.W. Clare, 'Examination for the MRCPsych', *Lancet*, 298, 7724 (11 September 1971), 598–9.

33   *Lancet*, 'College capers', *Lancet*, 298, 7724 (11 September 1971), 587–8. See also: Bewley, *Madness to Mental Illness: A History of the Royal College of Psychiatrists*, pp. 67–70.

34   Our Medical Reporter, 'GMC wants details of psychiatry training', *The Times*, 13 November 1971. For Clare's later thoughts on the GMC, see: A. Clare,

'Secrecy in the personal interest', *The Listener*, 5 February 1987.

35 A.W. Clare, 'Training of psychiatrists', *Lancet*, 300, 7780 (7 October 1972), 753–6.

36 P. Bowden and A.W. Clare, 'Redeployment of registrar and senior-registrar posts', *Lancet*, 302, 7833 (13 October 1973), 856–7.

37 For more on Paine (1921–2013), see: G. Russell, 'Obituary: Mr Leslie Paine MA (Oxon), OBE, formerly House Governor of the Bethlem Royal and Maudsley Hospital (1963–1985)', *Psychiatric Bulletin*, 38, 5 (October 2013), 253–4. For more on tennis, see: A. Clare, 'Endpiece', *The Listener*, 14 July 1983; A. Clare, 'Sport's smokescreen', *The Listener*, 6 February 1986; A. Clare, 'Why success means more than winning', *The Listener*, 31 July 1986.

38 Personal communication: R.M. Murray, interview with BK (25 February 2018). Clare remained concerned with trainees' conditions throughout his career; see: A. Ballantyne, 'Psychiatrist says long hours harm junior doctors' health', *Guardian*, 10 April 1989.

39 For more on Rawnsley (1926–92), president of the Royal College of Psychiatrists (1981–4), see: M. Roth, 'Obituary: Kenneth Rawnsley, CBE, formerly Professor of Psychiatry in the Welsh National School of Medicine and President of the Royal College of Psychiatrists', *Psychiatric Bulletin*, 16, 9 (September 1992), 587–9.

40 R.D. Laing, *The Divided Self* (Harmondsworth, Middlesex: Penguin, 1960). See also: A.W. Clare, 'Ronald David Laing 1927–1989: an appreciation', *Psychiatric Bulletin*, 14, 2 (1 February 1990), 87–8.

41 T. Szasz, *The Myth of Mental Illness: Foundations of a Theory of Personal Conduct* (New York: Harper & Row, 1961).

42 A. Clare, 'The price Laing paid', *The Listener*, 6 June 1985.

43 A. Ferriman, '"Threat" of institutional psychiatry described at mental health meeting', *The Times*, 9 December 1977.

44 A. Clare, *Psychiatry in Dissent: Controversial Issues in Thought and Practice* (London: Tavistock Publications Ltd, 1976), pp. 38–74, 325–69. See also: A. Clare, 'Depth psychology', *The Listener*, 15 December 1977.

45 Personal communication: J. Lucey, interview with BK (30 August 2018).

46 A.W. Clare, 'Diazepam, alcohol, and barbiturate abuse', *British Medical Journal*, 4, 5783 (6 November 1971), 340.

47 E. Shorter, *A History of Psychiatry: From the Era of the Asylum to the Age of Prozac* (New York: John Wiley and Sons, Inc., 1997), pp. 318–19.

48 A.W. Clare, 'Training of psychiatrists', *Lancet*, 300, 7780 (7 October 1972), 753–6.

49 *Irish Times*, 3 November 2007.

50 Personal communication: R.M. Murray, interview with BK (25 February 2018).

51 A.W. Clare, 'A Study of Psychiatric Illness in an Immigrant Irish Population' (MPhil (Psychiatry) Thesis, London University, 1972).

52 Kelly, *Hearing Voices: The History of Psychiatry in Ireland*, pp. 206–9.

53 A.W. Clare, 'Alcoholism and schizophrenia in Irishmen in London – a reassessment', *British Journal of Addiction to Alcohol and Other Drugs*, 69, 3 (September 1974), 207–12.

54 P. Maume, 'Clare, Anthony Ward', in J. McGuire and J. Quinn (eds), *Dictionary of Irish Biography From the Earliest Times to 2002* (Dublin and Cambridge: Royal Irish Academy and Cambridge University Press, 2014).

55 M. Brankin, 'The legacy of Anthony Clare', *Irish Times*, 15 November 2007.

56 A.W. Clare and J.G. Cooney, 'Alcoholism and road accidents', *Journal of the Irish Medical Association*, 66, 11 (9 June 1973), 281–6.

57 A.W. Clare, 'Mental illness in the Irish emigrant', *Journal of the Irish Medical Association*, 67, 1 (12 January 1974), 20–4.

58 A. Clare and M. Bristow, 'Drinking drivers: the needs for research and rehabilitation', *British Medical Journal (Clinical Research Edition)*, 295, 6611 (5 December 1987), 1432–3; T. Prentice, 'Doctors back lower drink-drive limit and random testing', *The Times*, 5 December 1987.

59 A.W. Clare, 'The causes of alcoholism', *British Journal of Hospital Medicine*, 21, 4 (April 1979), 403–11.

60 K. O'Sullivan, P. Whillans, M. Daly, B. Carroll, A. Clare and J. Cooney, 'A comparison of alcoholics with and without co-existing affective disorder', *British Journal of Psychiatry*, 143, 2

(August 1983), 133–8; K. O'Sullivan, C. Rynne, J. Miller, S. O'Sullivan, V. Fitzpatrick, M. Hux, J. Cooney and A. Clare, 'A follow-up study on alcoholics with and without co-existing affective disorder', *British Journal of Psychiatry*, 152, 6 (1 June 1988), 813–19.

61 A.W. Clare, 'Developing a policy for a district alcohol service', *Practitioner*, 231, 1425 (8 March 1987), 318–21; R. Gledhill, 'Pope resists moves to soften encyclical', *The Times*, 18 September 1993.

62 A.W. Clare, 'Alcohol education and the medical student', *Alcohol and Alcoholism*, 19, 4 (1 January 1984), 291–6; F. Adshead and A.W. Clare, 'Doctors' double standards on alcohol', *British Medical Journal (Clinical Research Edition)*, 293, 6562 (20–27 December 1986), 1590–1. See also: Anonymous, 'Sobering plight of student doctors', *Guardian*, 24 April 1982.

63 A.W. Clare, 'Immigration: new challenges for psychiatry and mental health services in Ireland', *Irish Journal of Psychological Medicine*, 19, 1 (March 2002), 3.

64 P. MacÉinrí, *Immigration into Ireland* (Cork: Irish Centre For Migration Studies, 2001).

65 A. Lewis, 'Health as a social concept', *British Journal of Sociology*, 4, 2 (June 1953), 109–14.

66 M. Binchy, 'The race that God made mad', *Irish Times*, 7 June 1976.

67 Personal communication: J. Clare, interview with BK (10 May 2018).

68 Personal communication: J. Clare, interview with BK (7 June 2018).

69 Personal communication: R. Clare, interview with BK (7 March 2019).

70 Personal communication: P. Clare, interview with BK (9 February 2019).

71 Personal communication: R. Clare, interview with BK (7 March 2019).

72 Personal communication: R. Dudley Edwards, interview with BK (14 June 2019).

73 Personal communication: R.M. Murray, interview with BK (25 February 2018).

74 Personal communication: J. Clare, interview with BK (10 May 2018).

75 A. Clare, 'Lucky loonies?', *The Listener*, 26 June 1980; A. Clare, 'Lucky loonies?', *The Listener*, 3 July 1980; A. Clare, K. Rawnsley and M. Roth, 'Dr Anatoly Koryagin', *Psychiatric Bulletin*, 9, 4 (1 April 1985), 80; A. Clare, 'A challenge to honour', *The Listener*, 25 April 1985.

76 Personal communication: R.M. Murray, interview with BK (25 February 2018).

77 A.W. Clare, 'A question of numbers', *St Stephen's* (Michaelmas, 1963), 9–11.

78 A.W. Clare, 'Doctors and the pill', *Irish Times*, 7 August 1968.

79 A. Clare, 'The humanist and abortion', *Irish Times*, 25 May 1970.

80 J. Duggan, 'The humanist and abortion', *Irish Times*, 30 May 1970.

81 K. Lorenz, *On Aggression* (London: Methuen, 1966).

82 A.W. Clare, 'Is aggression instinctive? Konrad Lorenz's theories re-assessed', *Studies: An Irish Quarterly Review*, 58, 230 (Summer 1969), 153–65; p. 153.

83 Ibid., pp. 163–4.

84 A. Clare, 'Explorers of inner space', *Irish Times*, 27 June 1970.

85 A. Clare, 'The new neurosis', *Irish Times*, 14 August 1971.

86 A. Clare, 'Psychoanalysis on the defensive?', *Irish Times*, 17 July 1971.

87 R. Bowman, 'Does psychoanalysis work?', *Irish Times*, 25 January 1971.

88 A. Clare, 'Does psychoanalysis work?', *Irish Times*, 20 January 1971.

89 A. Clare, 'Is analysis a Freudian slip?', *The Times*, 8 July 1985; A. Clare, 'Myth or medicine?', *The Times*, 9 July 1985; A. Clare, 'Endpiece', *The Listener*, 21 July 1983; A. Clare, 'Psychoanalysis has been over taken by knowledge and events', *The Listener*, 2 May 1985.

90 A.W. Clare, 'Ireland's smug medicine', *Irish Times*, 7 January 1971.

91 A. Clare, 'How sick is the North?', *Irish Times*, 30 August 1971.

92 J.M. Bell, 'Responsibilities', *Irish Times*, 3 September 1971.

93 T.S. Szasz, *The Manufacture of Madness* (London: Routledge and Kegan Paul, 1972).

94 A. Ferriman, '"Threat" of institutional psychiatry described at mental health meeting', *The Times*, 9 December 1977.

95 A. Clare, 'The new inquisition', *Irish Times*, 16 March 1972.

96 A. Clare, 'What are psychiatrists doing?', *The Spectator*, 12 August 1972.

97 E. Pearce, 'Patrick Cosgrave: English-loving Irish journalist who blasted Edward Heath', *Guardian*, 17 September 2001.

98 A.W. Clare, 'Jensen's reply', *The Spectator*, 18 August 1973.

99 A. Clare, 'Balls up', *The Spectator*, 26 June 1976.

100 A.W. Clare, 'Jung confusions', *The Spectator*, 30 June 1973.

101 A. Clare, 'Herrema siege', *The Spectator*, 15 November 1975.

102 A. Clare, 'The drugging of prisoners', *The Spectator*, 17 December 1977.

103 A.W. Clare, 'Laing returns to the fold', *The Spectator*, 3 February 1973.

104 M. Williams, 'Laing's return?', *The Spectator*, 24 February 1973.

105 A.W. Clare, 'Laing's return', *The Spectator*, 17 March 1973.

106 A.W. Clare, 'Eysenck the controversialist', *The Spectator*, 21 April 1973.

107 A. Clare, 'Eysenck and the Irish', *Irish Times*, 5 August 1971.

108 H.J. Eysenck, 'Controversial Eysenck', *The Spectator*, 5 May 1973.

109 A.W. Clare, 'Controversial Eysenck', *The Spectator*, 19 May 1973.

110 A. Clare, 'Neurotics anonymous', *The Listener*, 16 June 1977; A. Clare, 'Eysenck is a behavioural conquistador with eyes on Freud's territory', *The Listener*, 29 August 1985.

111 E. Pearce, 'Patrick Cosgrave: English-loving Irish journalist who blasted Edward Heath', *Guardian*, 17 September 2001. Courtesy of *Guardian* News & Media Ltd.

112 R. Dudley Edwards, 'Patrick Cosgrave – Tory rebel', in F. Callanan (ed.), *The Literary and Historical Society, 1955–2005* (Dublin: A&A Farmar, 2005), 87–9.

113 P. Cosgrave, *Margaret Thatcher: A Tory and Her Party* (London: Hutchinson, 1978).

114 P. Cosgrave, 'The ambiguities of attitude', *St Stephen's* (Trinity, 1962), 18–22; P. Cosgrave, 'The Marxist legacy', *St Stephen's* (Trinity, 1963), 39–45.

115 A. Clare, 'Langham Diary', *The Listener*, 12 May 1983.

116 J. Crowley, 'Patrick Cosgrave: immigrant chic', *Irish Times*, 28 January 1978.

117 Personal communication: R.M. Murray, interview with BK (25 February 2018).

118 A. Clare, 'Obsessed with being reasonable', *Irish Times*, 5 July 1977.

119 A. Clare, 'A rust bowl', *New Statesman*, 18 December 2000; A. Clare, 'The lust for life', *New Statesman*, 16 April 2001.

120 Our Medical Reporter, 'GMC wants details of psychiatry training', *The Times*, 13 November 1971.

121 J. Cunningham, 'Mental health plans', *Guardian*, 3 March 1973.

122 M. Binchy, 'The race that God made mad', *Irish Times*, 7 June 1976.

123 A.W. Clare, 'The mind of the kidnapper', *Nursing Mirror and Midwives Journal*, 142, 15 (8 April 1976), 47–8.

124 A.W. Clare, 'Psychiatry in dissent', *Nursing Mirror and Midwives Journal*, 143, 15 (7 October 1976), 61–2.

125 A.W. Clare, 'One Flew Over the Cuckoo's Nest (film review)', *Lancet*, 307, 7964 (17 April 1976), 851.

126 Personal communication: R. Clare, interview with BK (7 March 2019).

127 Personal communication: D. Knowles, interview with MH (12 November 2018).

128 P. Nolan, 'Anthony Clare: A man of compassion', *Mental Health Practice*, 11, 5 (February 2008), 11.

3. WRITER: *PSYCHIATRY IN DISSENT* (1976)

1 E. Goffman, *Asylums: Essays on the Social Situation of Mental Patients and Other Inmates* (New York: Anchor Books, Doubleday & Co., 1961).

2 M. Foucault, *Folie et Déraison: Histoire de la Folie à l'Âge Classique* (Paris: Plon, 1961); M. Foucault, *History of Madness* (London and New York: Routledge, 2006).

3 T. Szasz, *The Myth of Mental Illness: Foundations of a Theory of Personal Conduct* (New York: Harper & Row, 1961).

4 K. Kesey, *One Flew Over the Cuckoo's Nest* (New York: Viking Press, 1962). See also: Shorter, *A History of Psychiatry: From the Era of the Asylum to the Age of Prozac*, pp. 272–7.

5 A.W. Clare, 'One Flew Over the Cuckoo's Nest (film review)', *Lancet*, 307, 7964 (17 April 1976), 851.

6 R.D. Laing, *The Divided Self* (Harmondsworth, Middlesex: Penguin, 1960). For a discussion of Laing with reference to Clare, see: R. Boston, 'In the late 1960s confusion of the psychic, the psychotic and the psychedelic, Dr Laing's homage to catatonia went down beautifully', *Guardian*, 3 August 1976. See also: A.W. Clare, 'Ronald David Laing 1927–1989: an appreciation', *Psychiatric Bulletin*, 14, 2 (1 February 1990), 87–8.

7 Personal communication: R.M. Murray, interview with BK (25 February 2018).

8 D. Stafford-Clark, *Psychiatry Today* (Harmondsworth, Middlesex: Penguin, 1952).

9 G. Miller, 'David Stafford-Clark (1916–1999): seeing through a celebrity psychiatrist', *Wellcome Open Research*, 2 (2017), 30.

10 A. Clare, *Psychiatry in Dissent: Controversial Issues in Thought and Practice* (London: Tavistock Publications Ltd, 1976).

11 Personal communication: A. Mann, interview with BK (2 July 2018).

12 Kelly, *Hearing Voices: The History of Psychiatry in Ireland*, pp. 229–32.

13 B.D. Kelly and L. Feeney, 'Psychiatry: no longer in dissent?', *Psychiatric Bulletin*, 30, 9 (1 September 2006), 344–5.

14 For some of Clare's later thoughts on this theme, see: A. Clare, 'Brain scan', *The Listener*, 15 September 1988; A.W. Clare, 'Psychiatry's future', *Journal of Mental Health*, 8, 2 (1999), pp. 109–11.

15 Personal communication: R. Clare, interview with BK (7 March 2019). See also: C. Stott, 'Relative values: shrink resistant', *Sunday Times*, 12 April 1992.

16 P. Tyrer, 'From the Editor's Desk', *British Journal of Psychiatry*, 192, 1 (1 January 2008), 82.

17 Szasz, *The Myth of Mental Illness: Foundations of a Theory of Personal Conduct*; B.D. Kelly, P. Bracken, H. Cavendish, N. Crumlish, S. MacSuibhne, T. Szasz and T. Thornton, 'The Myth of Mental Illness 50 years after publication: what does it mean today?', *Irish Journal of Psychological Medicine*, 27, 1 (March 2010), 35–43.

18 Some of this section is adapted from: B.D. Kelly and L. Feeney, 'Psychiatry: no longer in dissent?', *Psychiatric Bulletin*, 30, 9 (1 September 2006), 344–5. Reprinted with permission (Cambridge University Press).

19 Clare, *Psychiatry in Dissent*, p. 20.

20 S.M. White, 'Preventive detention must be resisted by the medical profession', *Journal of Medical Ethics*, 28, 2 (April 2002), 95–8.

21 World Health Organisation, *ICD-10 Classification of Mental and Behavioural Disorders* (Geneva: World Health Organisation, 1992), pp. 1–3; American Psychiatric Association, *Diagnostic and Statistical Manual of Mental Disorders (Fourth Edition, Text Revision)* (Washington DC: American Psychiatric Association, 2000); American Psychiatric Association, *Diagnostic and Statistical Manual of Mental Disorders (Fifth Edition)* (Washington DC: American

Psychiatric Association, 2013), p. 19.

22 Clare, *Psychiatry in Dissent*, p. 156.

23 S. Bloch and P. Reddaway, *Soviet Psychiatric Abuse: The Shadow Over World Psychiatry* (London: Victor Gollancz Ltd, 1984); see also: A. Clare, 'Lucky loonies?', *The Listener*, 26 June 1980; A. Clare, 'Lucky loonies?', *The Listener*, 3 July 1980; A. Clare, K. Rawnsley and M. Roth, 'Dr Anatoly Koryagin', *Psychiatric Bulletin*, 9, 4 (1 April 1985), 80; A. Clare, 'A challenge to honour', *The Listener*, 25 April 1985.

24 R. Munro, 'Judicial psychiatry in China and its political abuses', *Columbia Journal of Asian Law*, 14, 1 (Spring 2000), 1–125.

25 Clare, *Psychiatry in Dissent*, p. 32.

26 H. Verdoux and J. van Os, 'Psychotic symptoms in non-clinical populations and the continuum of psychosis', *Schizophrenia Research*, 54, 1–2 (1 March 2002), 59–65.

27 Clare, *Psychiatry in Dissent*, p. 33.

28 N.C. Andreasen, *Brave New Brain: Conquering Mental Illness in the Era of the Genome* (Oxford: Oxford University Press, 2001), pp. 26–9.

29 P. Thomas and P. Bracken, 'Critical psychiatry in practice', *Advances in Psychiatric Treatment*, 10, 5 (1 August 2004), 361–70.

30 D. Healy and D. Cattell, 'Interface between authorship, industry and science in the domain of therapeutics', *British Journal of Psychiatry*, 183, 1 (1 July 2003), 22–7.

31 D.K. Hsieh and S.A. Kirk, 'The effect of social context on psychiatrists' judgements of adolescent antisocial behaviour', *Journal of Child Psychology and Psychiatry*, 44, 6 (September 2003), 877–87.

32 D.L. Sackett, W.M.C. Rosenberg, J.A. Gray, R.B. Haynes and W.S. Richardson, 'Evidence based medicine: what it is and what it isn't', *BMJ*, 312, 7023 (13 January 1996), 71–2.

33 Clare, *Psychiatry in Dissent*, pp. 214–15.

34 Ibid., p. 306.

35 A. Neustatter, 'Mental disorder', *Guardian*, 5 May 1976. Courtesy of Guardian News & Media Ltd.

36 W.H. Trethowan, 'Book review: *Psychiatry in Dissent*', *British Medical Journal*, 2, 6041 (16 October 1976), 948.

37 H. Baruk, 'Book review: *Psychiatry in Dissent: Controversial Issues in Thought and Practice*', *International Journal of*

Social Psychiatry, 25, 3 (1 September 1979), 227.

38 J. Berger, 'Book review: *Psychiatry in Dissent: Controversial Issues in Thought and Practice*', *Canadian Journal of Psychiatry*, 24, 1 (1 February 1979), 95–7.

39 P. Sedgwick, 'Shrinking world', *Guardian*, 27 May 1976. Courtesy of Guardian News & Media Ltd.

40 Clare, *Psychiatry in Dissent*, pp. 24–5.

41 P. Sedgwick, *PsychoPolitics* (London: Pluto Press, 1982).

42 M. Binchy, 'The race that God made mad', *Irish Times*, 7 June 1976.

43 See, for example: R. Boston, 'In the late 1960s confusion of the psychic, the psychotic and the psychedelic, Dr Laing's homage to catatonia went down beautifully', *Guardian*, 3 August 1976; J. Candy, 'Shock wave', *Guardian*, 16 May 1978.

44 A.W. Clare, 'Psychiatry in dissent', *Nursing Mirror and Midwives Journal*, 143, 15 (7 October 1976), 61–2.

45 A. Clare, *Psychiatry in Dissent: Controversial Issues in Thought and Practice (Second Edition)* (London and New York: Routledge, 1980).

46 J.S. Norell, 'Book review: *Psychiatry in Dissent: Controversial Issues in Thought and Practice (Second Edition)*', *Journal of the Royal College of General Practitioners*, 30, 220 (November 1980), 702.

47 J. Holmes, 'Ten books', *British Journal of Psychiatry*, 179, 5 (1 November 2001), pp. 468–71.

48 A. Beveridge, 'Ten books', *British Journal of Psychiatry*, 191, 6 (1 November 2007), 567–70.

49 D. Cunningham Owens, 'Ten books', *British Journal of Psychiatry*, 199, 2 (1 August 2011), 160–3.

50 T. Turner, 'Ten books', *British Journal of Psychiatry*, 209, 2 (1 August 2016), 175–7.

51 S. Wessely, 'Ten books', *British Journal of Psychiatry*, 181, 1 (1 July 2002), 81–4. For a good-natured exchange of letters between Wessely, Clare and colleagues, see: P.D. White, W.D.A. Bruce-Jones, J.M. Thomas, J. Amess and A.W. Clare, 'Viruses, neurosis and fatigue', *Journal of Psychosomatic Research*, 39, 3 (April 1995), 379.

52 Personal communication: S. Wessely, interview with BK (2 October 2017). See also: C. Kelleher, 'Literary, but not hysterical? Trying to come of age in Dublin's 1970s', in F. Callanan (ed.), *The Literary and Historical Society, 1955–2005* (Dublin: A&A Farmar, 2005), 220–3.

53 Personal communication: T. Fahy, email to BK (26 February 2018).

54 S. Cody, 'Anthony Clare: In the Psychiatrist's Chair', unpublished interview, 1 May 1984; Personal communication: S. Cody, email to BK and MH (6 April 2019).

55 B.D. Kelly and L. Feeney, 'Psychiatry: no longer in dissent?', *Psychiatric Bulletin*, 30, 9 (1 September 2006), 344–5; D.B. Double, 'Twenty years of the Critical Psychiatry Network', *British Journal of Psychiatry*, 214, 2 (1 February 2019), 61–2.

56 Anonymous, 'AGM Minutes – 2007 Thirty-Sixth Annual Meeting [of the Royal College of Psychiatrists]', *Psychiatric Bulletin*, 31, 12 (1 December 2007), 470–9.

57 D. Cunningham Owens, 'Ten books', *British Journal of Psychiatry*, 199, 2 (1 August 2011), 160–3.

58 Personal communication: A.W. Clare, correspondence to BK (7 September 2005).

59 B.D. Kelly and L. Feeney, 'Psychiatry: no longer in dissent?', *Psychiatric Bulletin*, 30, 9 (1 September 2006), 344–5.

60 American Psychiatric Association, *Diagnostic and Statistical Manual of Mental Disorders (Fourth Edition, Text Revision)* (Washington DC: American Psychiatric Association, 2000).

61 World Health Organisation, *ICD-10 Classification of Mental and Behavioural Disorders* (Geneva: World Health Organisation, 1992).

62 Personal communication: A.W. Clare, correspondence to BK (1 September 2006). For more on stigma, see: A. Clare, 'Scepticism is the first refuge of the wise', *The Listener*, 26 April 1984.

63 D. Stafford-Clark, *Psychiatry Today* (Harmondsworth, Middlesex: Penguin, 1952).

64 T. Burns, *Our Necessary Shadow: The Nature and Meaning of Psychiatry* (London: Allen Lane/Penguin Group, 2013).

65 Personal communication: T. Burns, email to BK (26 September 2018).

4. PSYCHIATRIST, SCIENTIST, PROFESSOR (1976–89)

1 Personal communication: R. Clare, interview with BK (7 March 2019).

2 Personal communication: P. Clare, interview with BK (9 February 2019).

3 Personal communication: R. Clare, interview with BK (7 March 2019).

4 G. Russell, 'Michael Shepherd (obituary)', *Psychiatric Bulletin*, 20, 10 (October 1996), 632–7.

5 D.P. Goldberg and B. Blackwell, 'Psychiatric illness in general practice: a detailed study using a new method of case identification', *British Medical Journal*, 1, 5707 (23 May 1970), 439–43.

6 Personal communication: R.M. Murray, interview with BK (25 February 2018).

7 Personal communication: A. Mann, interview with BK (2 July 2018).

8 Personal communication: A.W. Clare, correspondence (4 January 1978).

9 Falloon was a psychiatrist and pioneer of greater family involvement in mental health care: I.R. Falloon, 'Family interventions for mental disorders: efficacy and effectiveness', *World Psychiatry*, 2, 1 (February 2003), 20–8; M. Johnston, 'Pioneer psychiatrist brought families in', *New Zealand Herald*, 21 July 2006.

10 Personal communication: R.M. Murray, interview with BK (25 February 2018).

11 For more on Hill, see: R.H.C., 'Obituary: Sir (John) Denis Hill, formerly Professor of Psychiatry, Institute of Psychiatry, London SE5', *Bulletin of the Royal College of Psychiatrists*, 6, 11 (November 1982), 206–7.

12 Personal communication: A. Mann, interview with BK (2 July 2018).

13 A.W. Clare and V.E. Cairns, 'Design, development and use of a standardised interview to assess social maladjustment and dysfunction in community studies', *Psychological Medicine*, 8, 4 (November 1978), 589–604.

14 A.W. Clare and V.E. Cairns, 'A standardised interview to assess social maladjustment and dysfunction', in P. Williams and A. Clare (eds), *Psychosocial Disorders in General Practice* (London and New York: Academic Press and Grune and Stratton, 1979), 29–43.

15 P. Williams and A. Clare (eds), *Psychosocial Disorders in General Practice* (London and New York: Academic Press and Grune and Stratton, 1979).

16 P. Williams and A.W. Clare, 'Preface', in P. Williams and A. Clare (eds), *Psychosocial Disorders in General Practice* (London and New York: Academic Press and Grune and Stratton, 1979), xi–xii.

17 M. Shepherd, 'Foreword', in P. Williams and A. Clare (eds), *Psychosocial Disorders in General Practice* (London and New York: Academic Press and Grune and Stratton, 1979), vii–viii.

18 D. Morrell, 'Foreword', in P. Williams and A. Clare (eds), *Psychosocial Disorders in General Practice* (London and New York: Academic Press and Grune and Stratton, 1979), ix.

19 P. Williams and A.W. Clare, 'Introduction', in P. Williams and A. Clare (eds), *Psychosocial Disorders in General Practice* (London and New York: Academic Press and Grune and Stratton, 1979), 3–7.

20 A.W. Clare and P. Williams, 'Future trends in research into primary care psychiatry: a personal view', in P. Williams and A. Clare (eds), *Psychosocial Disorders in General Practice* (London and New York: Academic Press and Grune and Stratton, 1979), 325–32.

21 A.W. Clare, 'Community mental health centres', *Journal of the Royal Society of Medicine*, 73, 1 (January 1980), 75–6.

22 P. Williams, A. Tarnopolsky and A.W. Clare, 'Recent advances in the epidemiological study of minor psychiatric disorder', *Journal of the Royal Society of Medicine*, 73, 9 (September 1980), 679–80.

23 M. Shepherd, B. Cooper, A.C. Brown and G. Kalton (eds), *Psychiatric Illness in General Practice (Second Edition)* (Oxford: Oxford University Press, 1981).

24 A. Lewis, 'Foreword', in M. Shepherd, B. Cooper, A.C. Brown and G. Kalton (eds), *Psychiatric Illness in General Practice (Second Edition)* (Oxford: Oxford University Press, 1981), v–vi.

25 G. Russell, 'Michael Shepherd (obituary)', *Psychiatric Bulletin*, 20, 10 (October 1996), 632–7.

26 Personal communication: R.M. Murray, interview with BK (25 February 2018).

27 M. Shepherd, B. Cooper, A.C. Brown and G.W. Kalton (eds), *Psychiatric Illness in General Practice* (Oxford: Oxford University Press, 1966).

28 M. Shepherd and A. Clare, 'Addendum: developments since 1966', in M. Shepherd, B. Cooper, A.C. Brown and G. Kalton, *Psychiatric Illness in General Practice*

(Second Edition) (Oxford: Oxford University Press, 1981), 208–27.

29　A.W. Clare and M. Lader (eds), *Psychiatry and General Practice* (London: Academic Press, 1982).

30　A.W. Clare and M. Lader, 'Preface', in A.W. Clare and M. Lader (eds), *Psychiatry and General Practice* (London: Academic Press, 1982), xi–xiv.

31　G. Young, 'Foreword', in A.W. Clare and M. Lader (eds), *Psychiatry and General Practice* (London: Academic Press, 1982), vii–x.

32　A.W. Clare, 'Problems of psychiatric classification in general practice', in A.W. Clare and M. Lader (eds), *Psychiatry and General Practice* (London: Academic Press, 1982), 15–25.

33　A.W. Clare and K. Sabbagh, 'Appendix: general practice consultation video exercise', in A.W. Clare and M. Lader (eds), *Psychiatry and General Practice* (London: Academic Press, 1982), 26–32.

34　D. Pereira Gray, 'Psychiatry and general practice (book review)', *Psychological Medicine*, 14, 1 (February 1984), 233–6.

35　M.E. Briscoe and A.W. Clare, 'The health visitor and prevention', *British Medical Journal (Clinical Research Edition)*, 285, 6343 (11 September 1982), 740. This letter was written in response to: R.P. Snaith, 'The health visitor and prevention', *British Medical Journal (Clinical Research Edition)*, 285, 6340 (14 August 1982), 512; that, in turn, was in response to: S. Goodwin, 'The health visitor and prevention', *British Medical Journal (Clinical Research Edition)*, 285, 6336 (17 July 1982), 182–3.

36　R.H. Corney, A.W. Clare and J. Fry, 'The development of a self-report questionnaire to identify social problems: a pilot study', *Psychological Medicine*, 12, 4 (November 1982), 903–9.

37　A.W. Clare, 'Psycho-social morbidity in general practice', *Practitioner*, 227, 1375 (January 1983), 35–44.

38　A.W. Clare, R.H. Corney and V.E. Cairns, 'Social adjustment: the design and use of an instrument for social work and social work research', *British Journal of Social Work*, 14, 1 (1 January 1984), 323–36. See also: R.H. Corney and A.W. Clare, 'The construction, development and testing of a self-report questionnaire to identify social problems', *Psychological Medicine*, 15, 3 (August 1985), 637–49.

39　R.H. Corney and A.W. Clare, 'The effectiveness of attached social workers in the management of depressed women in general practice', *British Journal of Social Work*, 13, 1 (1 January 1983), 57–74.

40　A.W. Clare, 'Psychiatry in general practice', *Journal of the Royal College of General Practitioners*, 33, 249 (April 1983), 195–8.

41　C.V. Blacker and A.W. Clare, 'Depression in general practice', *British Journal of Psychiatry*, 148, 3 (1 March 1986), 333–5; C.V. Blacker and A.W. Clare, 'Depressive disorder in primary care', *British Journal of Psychiatry*, 150, 6 (1 June 1987), 737–51; C.V. Blacker and A.W. Clare, 'The prevalence and treatment of depression in general practice', *Psychopharmacology*, 95, 1 (suppl.) (March 1988), S14–17.

42　R.H. Corney, A. Cooper and A.W. Clare, 'Seeking help for marital problems: the role of the general practitioner', *Journal of the Royal College of General Practitioners*, 34, 265 (August 1984), 431–3.

43　The *International Statistical Classification of Diseases and Related Health Problems* (ICD) is the World Health Organization's international standard diagnostic tool for epidemiology, health management and clinical purposes. The ninth edition of their *International Classification of Mental and Behavioural Disorders* (ICD-9) was published in 1978: World Health Organization, *The ICD-9 Classification of Mental and Behavioral Disorders: Clinical Descriptions and Diagnostic Guidelines* (Geneva: World Health Organization, 1978).

44　Personal communication: R.M. Murray, interview with BK (25 February 2018).

45　A.W. Clare, 'Psychiatric and Social Aspects of Premenstrual Complaint' (MD Thesis, University College Dublin, 1980).

46　R.T. Frank, 'The hormonal causes of premenstrual tension', *Archives of Neurology and Psychiatry*, 26, 5 (November 1931), 1053–7.

47　R. Greene and K. Dalton, 'The premenstrual syndrome', *British Medical Journal*, 1, 4818 (9 May 1953), 1007–14.

48　A. Clare, 'A beneficial treatment hijacked by the affluent', *The Times*, 21 February 1994; L. Berrington, 'Weldon fails to lift curse of therapy', *The Times*, 24 February 1994.

49　D. Goldberg, *The Detection of Psychiatric Illness by Questionnaire (Maudsley*

Monograph No. 21) (London: Oxford University Press, 1972).

50 R.H. Moos, 'The development of a menstrual distress questionnaire', *Psychosomatic Medicine*, 30, 6 (November–December 1968), 853–67; R.H. Moos, 'Assessment of psychological concomitants of oral contraceptives', in H.A. Salhanick, D.M. Kipnis and R.L. Vande Wiele (eds), *Metabolic Effects of Gonadal Hormones and Contraceptive Steroids* (New York: Plenum, 1969), 676–705; R.H. Moos, 'Typology of menstrual cycle symptoms', *American Journal of Obstetrics and Gynecology*, 103, 3 (1 February 1969), 390–402.

51 A.W. Clare, 'Psychological profiles of women complaining of premenstrual symptoms', *Current Medical Research and Opinion*, 4, suppl. 4 (1977), 23–8.

52 D.E. Friedman, A.W. Clare, L.H. Rees and A. Grossman, 'Should impotent males who have no clinical evidence of hypogonadism have routine endocrine screening?', *Lancet*, 327, 8488 (3 May 1986), 1041.

53 A. Clare, *On Men: Masculinity in Crisis* (London: Chatto & Windus, 2000).

54 Personal communication: J. Clare, interview with BK (7 June 2018).

55 K. Holmquist, 'Men in crisis – or is it just me?', *Irish Times*, 27 July 2000.

56 A.W. Clare, 'Psychological profiles of women complaining of premenstrual symptoms', *Current Medical Research and Opinion*, 4, suppl. 4 (1977), 23–8.

57 A.W. Clare, 'The treatment of premenstrual symptoms', *British Journal of Psychiatry*, 135, 6 (December 1979), 576–9.

58 A.W. Clare, 'Progesterone, fluid, and electrolytes in premenstrual syndrome', *British Medical Journal*, 281, 6234 (20 September 1980), 810–11. This letter was written in response to: K. Dalton, 'Progesterone, fluid, and electrolytes in premenstrual syndrome', *British Medical Journal*, 281, 6232 (5 July 1980), 61. Dalton responded to Clare on 11 October 1980: K. Dalton, 'Progesterone, fluid, and electrolytes in premenstrual syndrome', *British Medical Journal*, 281, 6246 (11 October 1980), 1008–9.

59 A.W. Clare, 'Premenstrual syndrome', *British Journal of Psychiatry*, 138, 1 (1 January 1981), 82–3. This letter was written in response to: K. Dalton, 'Premenstrual syndrome', *British Journal of Psychiatry*, 137, 2 (1 August 1980), 199; that, in turn, was in response to: G.A. Sampson, 'Premenstrual syndrome: a double-blind controlled trial of progesterone and placebo', *British Journal of Psychiatry*, 135, 3 (1 September 1979), 209–15.

60 A.W. Clare, 'Psychiatric and social aspects of premenstrual complaint', *Psychological Medicine Monograph Supplement*, 4 (1983), 1–58.

61 R.W. Taylor, 'Book review: Psychiatric and social aspects of premenstrual complaint', *Psychological Medicine*, 14, 3 (August 1984), 706–7.

62 A.W. Clare, 'Premenstrual tension: psychological aspects', *Irish Journal of Medical Science*, 152 (suppl. 2) (June 1983), 33–43.

63 A.W. Clare, 'The relationship between psychopathology and the menstrual cycle', *Women and Health*, 8, 2–3 (Summer–Fall 1983), 125–36.

64 A.W. Clare, 'Premenstrual syndrome: single or multiple causes?', *Canadian Journal of Psychiatry*, 30, 7 (November 1985), 474–82.

65 A.W. Clare, 'Hormones, behaviour and the menstrual cycle', *Journal of Psychosomatic Research*, 29, 3 (1985), 225–33.

66 A.W. Clare, 'Behavior and the menstrual cycle (sexual behavior series, vol. 1) (book review)', *Journal of Psychosomatic Research*, 28, 4 (1984), 349.

67 R.H. Corney and A.W. Clare, 'The treatment of premenstrual syndrome', *Practitioner*, 233, 1463 (22 February 1989), 233–6.

68 A.W. Clare, 'Premenstrual problems', *The Times*, 26 November 1981.

69 R. Jenkins and A.W. Clare, 'Women and mental illness', *British Medical Journal (Clinical Research Edition)*, 291, 6508 (30 November 1985), 1521–2.

70 Personal communication: R. Jenkins, email to BK (2 August 2018).

71 R. Jenkins and A.W. Clare, 'Women and mental illness', *British Medical Journal (Clinical Research Edition)*, 291, 6508 (30 November 1985), 1521–2. See also: N. Timmins, 'Depression in women "caused by poor life"', *The Times*, 29 November 1985.

72 D. Purcell, 'Clare headed', *Sunday Tribune*, 11 January 1987. See also: A. Clare, 'Langham Diary', *The Listener*, 16 February 1984.

73 Personal communication: J. Clare, interview with BK (10 May 2018).

74 Personal communication: R. Clare, interview with BK (7 March 2019).

75 Personal communication: R.M. Murray, interview with BK (25 February 2018).

76 Personal communication: A. Mann, interview with BK (2 July 2018).

77 Personal communication: R. Clare, interview with BK (7 March 2019). See also: V. Kewley and A. Clare, 'My hols', *Sunday Times*, 5 October 1997.

78 A.W. Clare, '"The other half of medicine" and St Bartholomew's Hospital', *British Journal of Psychiatry*, 146, 2 (1 February 1985), 120–6.

79 Personal communication: R.M. Murray, interview with BK (25 February 2018).

80 Medical College of Saint Bartholomew's Hospital in the City of London, *Annual Report 1986* (London: University of London, 1986).

81 Personal communication: T. Dinan, email to BK (3 July 2018).

82 Anonymous, 'The powers that will be', *Sunday Times*, 22 November 1987.

83 D. Purcell, 'Clare headed', *Sunday Tribune*, 11 January 1987.

84 A.W. Clare, 'Handbook for inceptors and trainees in psychiatry (book review)', *Psychiatric Bulletin*, 1, 2 (1 August 1977), 15.

85 B.K. Toone, R. Murray, A. Clare, F. Creed and A. Smith, 'Psychiatrists' models of mental illness and their personal backgrounds', *Psychological Medicine*, 9, 1 (February 1979), 165–78.

86 Personal communication: Damian Mohan, interview with MH (8 November 2018).

87 D. Purcell, 'Clare headed', *Sunday Tribune*, 11 January 1987. For more of Clare's thoughts on AIDS, see: A. Clare, 'AIDS and medical hubris', *The Listener*, 1 January 1987; A. Clare, 'The Royal Touch', *The Listener*, 23 April 1987.

88 For more of Clare's thoughts on the NHS, see: A. Clare, 'Cinderella story', *The Listener*, 30 August 1984; A. Clare, 'Tomorrow's golden eggs', *The Listener*, 23 May 1985; A. Clare, 'Safe in a grip of iron', *The Listener*, 9 July 1987.

89 Personal communication: R. Clare, interview with BK (7 March 2019).

90 Anonymous, 'A loner "living in fantasy world of violence"', *The Times*, 20 August 1987.

91 G.M. Besser, A.W. Clare, C.J. Dickinson, N. Joels, O.J. Lewis, D.F.J. Mason, G.M. Rees, M.R. Salkind, E.D.R. Stone and R.F.M. Wood, 'Future of Bart's preclinical school', *Lancet*, 327, 8483 (29 March 1986), 741. See also: A. Clare, 'Peer pressure', *The Listener*, 29 May 1986.

92 A. Clare, 'Why closing Bart's is an act of madness', *Evening Standard*, 17 December 1992.

93 For a discussion of a controversial mural painted on the wall of the nurses' swimming pool in Bart's, see: A. Clare, 'The writing on the wall', *The Listener*, 20 June 1985.

94 World Health Organisation, *ICD-10 Classification of Mental and Behavioural Disorders* (Geneva: World Health Organisation, 1992), pp. 312, 322.

95 Clare, *Psychiatry in Dissent: Controversial Issues in Thought and Practice*, pp. 75–115.

96 A. Clare, W. Gulbinat and N. Sartorius, 'A triaxial classification of health problems presenting in primary health care: a World Health Organization multi-centre study', *Social Psychiatry and Psychiatric Epidemiology*, 27, 3 (May 1992), 108–16.

97 P. Hildrew, 'Old hands on new body', *Guardian*, 28 February 1987.

98 A. Clare, 'Obsessed with being reasonable', *Irish Times*, 5 July 1977.

99 D. Purcell, 'Clare headed', *Sunday Tribune*, 11 January 1987.

100 *Irish Times*, 3 November 2007.

101 A.W. Clare, 'Psychiatry: beyond analysis (book review)', *Nature*, 314, 6013 (25 April 1985), 696–7; A.W. Clare, 'Myth, magic and the common solution (book review)', *Nature*, 316, 6029 (15 August 1985), 584; A.W. Clare, 'Where lies the science? (book review)', *Nature*, 318, 6042 (14 November 1985), 112–13; A.W. Clare, 'Going into a trance (book review)', *Nature*, 324, 6098 (18 December 1986), 624.

102 See, for example: A. Clare, 'Is analysis a Freudian slip?', *The Times*, 8 July 1985; A. Clare, 'Myth or medicine?', *The Times*, 9 July 1985.

103 See, for example: A. Clare, 'Come to think of it, I must be mad to be a psychiatrist', *Daily Mail*, 17 September 1991.

104 See, for example: A. Clare, 'Let's talk, and keep peace hopes alive', *Sunday Times*, 1 August 1993; A. Clare, 'The prisoner', *Sunday Times*, 3 October 1993; A. Clare, 'Pick of the year', *Sunday Times*, 19 November 1995.

105 See, for example: A. Clare, 'Is Nixon nuts?', *Sunday Telegraph*, 31 July 1977.

106 See, for example: A. Clare, 'Wounded minds that find no peace when the war is over', *Sunday Express*, 17 January 1993; A. Clare, 'Relative values that Albert Einstein forgot', *Sunday Express*, 5 September 1993.

107 See, for example: A. Clare, 'Standard works', *New Society*, 21 April 1977; A. Clare, 'Freud for fun', *New Society*, 6 April 1978.

108 See, for example: A. Clare, 'The drugging of prisoners', *The Spectator*, 17 December 1977. His contributions were frequently controversial; see, for example: M. Williams, 'Laing's return?', *The Spectator*, 24 February 1973.

109 A. Clare, 'Rage for happiness', *The Listener*, 21 June 1984.

110 See, for example: A. Clare, '"Let's talk about me" – the other person's need for therapy', *The Listener*, 5 October 1978; A. Clare, 'The time for grown-up talk – and the time for screaming', *The Listener*, 19 October 1978; A. Clare, 'Psychotherapy and the search for meaning', *The Listener*, 9 November 1978.

111 A. Clare, 'The time for grown-up talk – and the time for screaming', *The Listener*, 19 October 1978.

112 A. Clare, 'Autistic brilliance', *The Listener*, 23 February 1978.

113 A. Clare, 'Neurotics anonymous', *The Listener*, 16 June 1977.

114 A. Clare, 'Sigmund's stories', *The Listener*, 27 September 1979.

115 A. Clare, 'Standard works', *New Society*, 21 April 1977.

116 A. Clare, 'Facing up to cancer', *The Listener*, 29 November 1979; A. Clare, 'Help at the end of the phone', *The Listener*, 7 November 1985.

117 A. Clare, 'Flagellomania', *The Listener*, 20 July 1978.

118 A. Clare, 'Massification and personhood', *The Listener*, 3 May 1979.

119 A. Clare, 'The guilty sick', *The Listener*, 22 February 1979; S. Sontag, *Illness as Metaphor* (London: Allen Lane, 1979).

120 A. Clare, 'Menopause for thought on sexual politics ...', *Daily Mail*, 12 November 1991.

121 A. Clare, 'No sense of proportion', *The Listener*, 3 April 1986; A. Clare, 'How to put spice into politics', *The Listener*, 21 May 1987.

122 A. Clare, 'Answers for everything', *The Listener*, 31 January 1985.

123 A. Clare, 'Langham Diary', *The Listener*, 4 November 1982; A. Clare, 'Margaret Thatcher: a psychiatrist's view', *The Listener*, 9 June 1983; A. Clare, 'Endpiece', *The Listener*, 4 August 1983; A. Clare, 'Endpiece', *The Listener*, 11 August 1983; A. Clare, 'Face to face with a TV megastar', *The Listener*, 15 August 1985; A. Clare, 'The seductive lady problem', *The Listener*, 5 December 1985; A. Clare, 'Safe in a grip of iron', *The Listener*, 9 July 1987; A. Clare, 'The despotism of desperate times', *The Listener*, 3 March 1988.

124 A. Clare, 'Langham Diary', *The Listener*, 12 May 1983; A. Clare, 'A moderate's voice', *The Listener*, 25 October 1984.

125 A.W. Clare, 'Premenstrual problems', *The Times*, 26 November 1981.

126 A.W. Clare, 'Implications in N Ireland of hanging', *The Times*, 6 July 1983.

127 A. Clare and L. Gostin, 'More than a second opinion needed about Broadmoor', *Guardian*, 2 February 1980.

128 L. Gostin and A. Clare, 'How health charges will put extra strain on mental patients', *Guardian*, 2 March 1982; A.W. Clare, 'Letter to the editor', *Guardian*, 24 April 1982. See also: A. Clare, 'Langham Diary', *The Listener*, 4 November 1982; A. Clare, 'A suitable case for treatment?', *The Listener*, 24 May 1984.

129 A. King, 'Agony in the office', *The Times*, 7 September 1988.

130 S. Tirbutt, 'Bedtime is something our brains have dreamed up', *Guardian*, 28 January 1983; for an exploration of some of the perils of commenting in the media, see: A. Clare, 'Jumping the gun', *The Listener*, 17 September 1987.

131 Anonymous, 'Schizophrenia video launch', *The Times*, 8 September 1987.

132 A.W. Clare, 'Sex and mood', *Health and Hygiene: Journal of the Royal Institute of Public Health and Hygiene*, 6 (1985), 43–60.

133 A. Clare, *Power and the Public Man (Lecture)* (London: Institute of Contemporary Arts, 1985).

134 Personal communication: J. Clare, interview with BK (7 June 2018).

135 A. Clare, 'Endpiece', *The Listener*, 28 July 1983.

136 Anonymous, 'Dinners', *The Times*, 20 September 1986.

137 Anonymous, 'Dinners', *The Times*, 18 September 1987.

138 Personal communication: R.M. Murray, interview with BK (25 February 2018).

139 D. Purcell, 'Clare headed', *Sunday Tribune*, 11 January 1987.

140 B. Levin, 'Society's safety catch', *The Times*, 7 September 1987; B. Levin, 'You analyse; I'd rather just listen', *The Times*, 3 April 1997. For Clare on Levin, see: A. Clare, 'Eskimo Bernard', *The Listener*, 6 March 1986.

141 Personal communication: J. Clare, interview with BK (7 June 2018).

142 A. Clare, 'Is analysis a Freudian slip?', *The Times*, 8 July 1985; A. Clare, 'Myth or medicine?', *The Times*, 9 July 1985. See also: A. Clare, 'Sigmund's stories', *The Listener*, 27 September 1979; A. Clare, 'Fears after Freud', *The Listener*, 29 April 1982.

143 C. Yorke, 'Analytical slips on Freudian analysis', *The Times*, 13 July 1985.

144 L.D. Phillips, 'Myth or medicine?', *The Times*, 15 July 1985.

145 D. Friedman, 'Myth or medicine?', *The Times*, 15 July 1985.

146 A.W. Clare, 'The causes of alcoholism', *British Journal of Hospital Medicine*, 21, 4 (April 1979), 403–11. In relation to cannabis, see: A. Clare, 'Righteous indignation', *The Listener*, 28 February 1985.

147 K. O'Sullivan, P. Whillans, M. Daly, B. Carroll, A. Clare and J. Cooney, 'A comparison of alcoholics with and without co-existing affective disorder', *British Journal of Psychiatry*, 143, 2 (August 1983), 133–8; K. O'Sullivan, C. Rynne, J. Miller, S. O'Sullivan, V. Fitzpatrick, M. Hux, J. Cooney and A. Clare, 'A follow-up study on alcoholics with and without co-existing affective disorder', *British Journal of Psychiatry*, 152, 6 (1 June 1988), 813–19.

148 A.W. Clare, 'Developing a policy for a district alcohol service', *Practitioner*, 231, 1425 (8 March 1987), 318–21; R. Gledhill, 'Pope resists moves to soften encyclical', *The Times*, 18 September 1993.

149 A.W. Clare, 'Alcohol education and the medical student', *Alcohol and Alcoholism*, 19, 4 (1 January 1984), 291–6; F. Adshead and A.W. Clare, 'Doctors' double standards on alcohol', *British Medical Journal (Clinical Research Edition)*, 293, 6562 (20–27 December 1986), 1590–1.

150 J.C. Cutting, A.W. Clare and A.H. Mann, 'Cycloid psychosis: an investigation of the diagnostic concept', *Psychological Medicine*, 8, 4 (November 1978), 637–48.

151 J. Murray, P. Williams and A. Clare, 'Health and social characteristics of long-term psychotropic drug-takers', *Social Science and Medicine*, 16, 18 (1982), 1595–8; P. Williams, J. Murray and A. Clare, 'A longitudinal study of psychotropic drug prescription', *Psychological Medicine*, 12, 1 (February 1982), 201–6. See also: A. Clare, 'What is an acceptable risk?', *The Listener*, 3 January 1985.

152 A.W. Clare, 'The dying don't need analytic psychotherapy', *Journal of Medical Ethics*, 8, 4 (December 1982), 213. This letter was written in response to: L. Goldie, 'The ethics of telling the patient', *Journal of Medical Ethics*, 8, 3 (September 1982), 128–33.

153 A.W. Clare, 'Therapeutic and ethical aspects of electro-convulsive therapy: a British perspective', *International Journal of Law and Psychiatry*, 1, 3 (1978), 237–45.

154 Clare, *Psychiatry in Dissent: Controversial Issues in Thought and Practice*, pp. 223–67.

155 A. Clare and L. Gostin, 'More than a second opinion needed about Broadmoor', *Guardian*, 2 February 1980.

156 P. Bebbington, J.L.T. Birley, A.W. Clare, J. Cutting, R. Kumar, A. Mann, P. Mullen, P. Williams and D.H. Bennett, 'Unmodified ECT', *Lancet*, 315, 8168 (Pt 1) (15 March 1980), 599. This letter was written in response to: D.A. Pond, 'ECT at Broadmoor', *Lancet*, 315, 8165 (23 February 1980), 430; that, in turn, was in response to: Lancet, 'ECT at Broadmoor', *Lancet*, 315, 8164 (16 February 1980), 348–9 (which, in turn, cited the letter Clare had co-written to the *Guardian* two weeks earlier; see above).

157 R. Deitch, 'Commentary from Westminster', *Lancet*, 315, 8165 (23 February 1980), 433–4; J. Crammer, 'Unmodified ECT', *Lancet*, 315, 8166 (1 March 1980), 486; P.G. McGrath, 'ECT at Broadmoor', *Lancet*, 315, 8167 (8 March 1980), 550; R. Deitch, 'Commentary from Westminster', *Lancet*, 315, 8169 (22 March 1980), 663–4.

158 A.W. Clare, 'Clinical responsibility: II. Where does the patient stand? When did you last see your psychiatrist?',

British Medical Journal, 2, 6103 (24–31 December 1977), 1637–42.

159 T. Szasz, 'The case against compulsory psychiatric interventions', *Lancet*, 311, 8072 (13 May 1978), 1035–6.

160 A.W. Clare, 'In defence of compulsory psychiatric intervention', *Lancet*, 311, 8075 (3 June 1978), 1197–8. Clare was by no means alone in criticising Szasz's contribution: F.A. Jenner, 'Compulsory psychiatry', *Lancet*, 311, 8074 (27 May 1978), 1150; A. White, 'Compulsory psychiatry', *Lancet*, 311, 8074 (27 May 1978), 1150; D.G. Wilkinson, 'Compulsory psychiatry', *Lancet*, 311, 8074 (27 May 1978), 1150.

161 Clare, *Psychiatry in Dissent: Controversial Issues in Thought and Practice*, pp. 325–69.

162 A.W. Clare, 'Treatment or torture', *Midwife, Health Visitor and Community Nurse*, 14, 7 (July 1978), 205–6.

163 A.W. Clare, 'Consent to treatment', *Journal of the Royal Society of Medicine*, 74, 11 (November 1981), 787–9.

164 A.W. Clare, 'Ethical issues in psychiatry', *Practitioner*, 223, 1333 (July 1979), 89–96. See also: Clare, *Psychiatry in Dissent: Controversial Issues in Thought and Practice*, pp. 268–324; A. Clare, 'Secrecy in the personal interest', *The Listener*, 5 February 1987.

165 A.W. Clare, 'Doctors and the death penalty: an international issue', *British Medical Journal (Clinical Research Edition)*, 294, 6581 (9 May 1987), 1180–1; see also: A. Clare, 'Endpiece', *The Listener*, 30 June 1983.

166 A.W. Clare, 'The clinical process in psychiatry (book review)', *Journal of Neurology, Neurosurgery and Psychiatry*, 50, 8 (August 1987), 1089–90.

167 A.W. Clare, 'Fringe medicine and beyond', *Journal of the Irish Medical Association*, 72, 12 (suppl) (1979), 30–4.

168 C.J. Haughey, 'Opening address', *Journal of the Irish Medical Association*, 72, 12 (suppl) (1979), 7–8.

169 A.W. Clare, 'Letter to the editor', *Guardian*, 24 April 1982. Courtesy of Guardian News & Media Ltd. This letter was written in response to a *Guardian* editorial: *Guardian*, 'Battles beyond the mind', *Guardian*, 22 April 1982; see also: R. Sang, 'Letter to the editor', *Guardian*, 24 April 1982; A. Veitch, 'MIND adviser quits over law change', *Guardian*, 24 April 1982.

170 J. Picardie and D. Wade, 'Closure call over women's jail wing', *Sunday Times*, 28 July 1985.

171 T. Prentice, 'Daily spending on mentally ill "only cost of a cup of tea"', *The Times*, 31 August 1991.

172 M. Wallace, R. Bluglass, F. Caldicott, A. Clare, M. Lader, C. Thompson, A. Tylee and M. Weller, 'Mental health propaganda', *Independent*, 13 June 1995.

173 Personal communication: R.M. Murray, interview with BK (25 February 2018).

5. BROADCASTER: *IN THE PSYCHIATRIST'S CHAIR* (1982–2001)

1 A.W. Clare with S. Thompson, *Let's Talk About Me: A Critical Examination of the New Psychotherapies* (London: BBC, 1981).

2 D. Wade, 'Minds matter', *The Times*, 21 November 1988.

3 Clare, *In the Psychiatrist's Chair* (1992), p. 218; M. Hickling, 'Clare thoughts', *Yorkshire Post*, 22 October 1982; L. Taylor, 'Are you sitting uncomfortably? Then I'll begin ...', *Mail on Sunday*, 5 June 1983; M. M. Davies, 'Reasons why', *Radio Times*, 23 June 1983; P. Bailey, 'The gentle persuader', *Sunday Times*, 24 July 1983; I. Rowan, 'Dr Clare gets a grilling', *Sunday Telegraph*, 14 August 1983.

4 D. Hackett, 'A model of self-possession', *The Times*, 26 July 1983; N. Banks-Smith, 'Macho', *Guardian*, 2 August 1983; P. Ackroyd, 'Modest virtues', *The Times*, 2 August 1983; M. Hoyle, 'Curious character', *The Times*, 9 August 1983; G. Wilkinson, 'Medicine and the media', *British Medical Journal*, 287, 6393 (3 September 1983), 683; A. Clare, 'The seductive lady problem', *The Listener*, 5 December 1985.

5 A. Clare, *Lovelaw: Love, Sex and Marriage Around the World* (London: BBC Publications, 1986). See also: P. Toynbee, 'The unequal partnership', *Guardian*, 22 September 1986; M. Wainwright, 'Touch of Venus beyond our Ken', *Guardian*, 26 September 1986; B. Nicholson, 'Revealing languages of love', *The Times*, 27 September 1986; A. Hislop, 'If at first you don't succeed', *The Times*, 20 October 1986; H. Hebert, 'The end of the affair', *Guardian*, 10 November 1986; N. Shakespeare, 'Naughty but nicely done', *The Times*, 10 November 1986.

6 S. Cody, 'Anthony Clare', *Guardian*, 31 October 2007.

7 M. Riddell, 'A grumpy psychiatrist in the chair', *The Times*, 5 August 1996.

8 A. Clare, 'How to be professional moms and dads', *The Listener*, 24 November 1983; D. Berry, 'All in the mind', *Guardian*, 6 August 1986; J. Erlichman, '"IQ" vitamin claims prompt inquiry', *Guardian*, 15 June 1988.

9 M. Proops, 'What's your problem with agony aunts like me?', *Daily Mirror*, 24 April 1995; R. Johnson, 'Somehow it's less frightening in full colour', *The Times*, 29 April 1995.

10 See, for example: A. Clare, 'The phone-in physician', *The Listener*, 28 March 1985; A. Clare, 'Looking after number one', *The Listener*, 6 August 1987.

11 BBC Radio 4 Extra website: www.bbc.co.uk/programmes/b039dks7 (Accessed 3 December 2019).

12 A. Clare, *In the Psychiatrist's Chair* (London: Chatto & Windus/The Hogarth Press, 1984); A. Clare, *In the Psychiatrist's Chair* (London: William Heinemann Ltd, 1992); A. Clare, *In the Psychiatrist's Chair II* (London: Mandarin/William Heinemann Ltd, 1995); A. Clare, *In the Psychiatrist's Chair III* (London: Chatto & Windus/Random House, 1998).

13 Anonymous, 'Michael Ember, BBC Radio "talks" producer – obituary', *The Telegraph*, 11 April 2017.

14 V. Arnold-Forster, 'All huff and puff', *Guardian*, 17 June 1983.

15 Clare, *In the Psychiatrist's Chair* (1984), p.ix. See also: P. Dunn, 'Putting Dr Clare in the chair', *Sunday Times*, 12 September 1982.

16 Clare and Thompson, *Let's Talk About Me: A Critical Examination of the New Psychotherapies*.

17 A. Clare, 'The recurrent message is that none of us is free from flaw', *The Listener*, 5 August 1982; for Clare's visit to Freeman in the US in September 1988, see: Clare, *In the Psychiatrist's Chair* (1992), p. 217; *Face to Face* was revived from 1989 to 1998, with Jeremy Isaacs interviewing.

18 Clare, *In the Psychiatrist's Chair* (1984), p.x.

19 Ibid., p.xi.

20 R. Ottaway, 'Highlights this week', *Radio Times*, 31 July – 6 August 1982.

21 Clare, *In the Psychiatrist's Chair* (1984), p.xiv.

22 Ibid., p. 6. In relation to the opening question, see: J.G. Ballard, 'Has the interview become a media game?', *Daily Telegraph*, 3 October 1992.

23 Clare, *In the Psychiatrist's Chair* (1984), p. 16.

24 Ibid., p. 17.

25 D. Hendy, *Life On Air: A History of Radio Four* (Oxford: Oxford University Press, 2007), p. 236.

26 Clare, *In the Psychiatrist's Chair III*, p. 413.

27 A. Clare, 'At Her Majesty's pleasure ...', *The Listener*, 18 July 1985.

28 S. Milligan and A. Clare, *Depression and How to Survive It* (London: Ebury Press/Random House Group, 1993).

29 D. Wade, 'The public face of privacy', *The Times*, 14 August 1982.

30 A. Clare, 'The recurrent message is that none of us is free from flaw', *The Listener*, 5 August 1982.

31 Anonymous, 'How to couch the best questions', *Guardian*, 14 August 1982. Courtesy of Guardian News & Media Ltd.

32 L. Taylor, 'Curiouser and curiouser', *The Times*, 13 April 1984. See also: A. Levin, 'Swapping chairs with Clare', *You Magazine*, 27 September 1992; A. Picard, 'Shrink wrapped in an enigma', *Sunday Telegraph*, 5 September 1999.

33 A.T. Ellis, 'Speaking their minds', *The Times*, 14 October 1995.

34 S. Cody, 'Anthony Clare: In the Psychiatrist's Chair', unpublished interview, 1 May 1984.

35 S. Cody, 'Anthony Clare: In the Psychiatrist's Chair', unpublished interview, 1 May 1984; Personal communication: S. Cody, email to BK and MH (6 April 2019).

36 S. Cody, 'Anthony Clare: In the Psychiatrist's Chair', unpublished interview, 1 May 1984.

37 Personal communication: S. Cody, email to MH and BK (7 April 2019).

38 A. W. Clare, correspondence to S. Cody, 22 June 1984.

39 S. Cody, 'Anthony Clare: In the Psychiatrist's Chair', unpublished interview, 1 May 1984; Personal communication: S. Cody, email to BK and MH (6 April 2019).

40 G. Bradberry, 'In the chair and off guard', *The Times*, 20 August 1996.

41 Personal communication: V. Ashkenazy, interview with BK (15 May 2018).

42 Personal communication: B. Kent, email to BK (7 May 2018).

43 V. Arnold-Forster, 'Crime on the couch', *Guardian*, 5 July 1985. Courtesy of Guardian News & Media Ltd.

44 G. Bradberry, 'In the chair and off guard', *The Times*, 20 August 1996.

45 Clare, *In the Psychiatrist's Chair III*, p. 296.

46 Personal communication: W. Savage, email to BK (30 September 2018).

47 V. Arnold-Forster, 'Electric chair', *Guardian*, 30 August 1986. Courtesy of Guardian News & Media Ltd.

48 Clare, *In the Psychiatrist's Chair* (1992), p. 1. See also: P. Cheston, 'Flirting, arrogance and me by Edwina', *Evening Standard*, 17 August 1988; S. Cook, 'An arguably interesting session on the couch with Edwina Currie', *Guardian*, 18 August 1988.

49 Personal communication: E. Currie, email to BK (11 May 2018).

50 Personal communication: N. Lawson, email to BK (9 May 2018).

51 Clare, *In the Psychiatrist's Chair III*, p. 412.

52 Ibid., pp. 428–9.

53 Ibid., p. 435.

54 Ibid., p. 452.

55 Personal communication: A. Widdecombe, interview with BK (10 May 2018).

56 Clare, *In the Psychiatrist's Chair III*, p. 413; see also: A. Clare, 'Sex and the confused parent', *The Listener*, 2 October 1986; A. Clare, 'Sex education: who'll tell the children?', *Time Out*, 29 October 1986.

57 Clare, *In the Psychiatrist's Chair* (1984).

58 E. Philbin Bowman, 'Clare's chair', *Irish Times*, 2 June 1984.

59 Personal communication: E. Philbin Bowman, email to BK (1 June 2018).

60 H. Kinlay, 'Sessions with the shrink', *Irish Times*, 21 August 1984.

61 Clare, *In the Psychiatrist's Chair* (1984), pp.ix–x.

62 R. Twisk, 'Doctor, what's wrong here?', *Observer*, 5 August 1990.

63 V. Arnold-Forster, 'Sounds of battle', *Guardian*, 7 August 1982. Courtesy of Guardian News & Media Ltd. See also: A. Clare, 'Truth and treachery', *The Listener*, 19 April 1984.

64 B. Sibley, 'Compelling illusion', *The Times*, 2 July 1983. See also: R. Hanks, 'In the psychiatrist's easy chair', *The Independent*, 3 August 1992; R. McKie, 'The chair man', *Observer*, 13 May 2001.

65 J. Hepburn, 'Heard the one about radio's new comics?', *The Times*, 21 August 1993.

66 G. Bradberry, 'In the chair and off guard', *The Times*, 20 August 1996.

67 L. Taylor, 'New tunes from Joanna', *The Times*, 16 July 1994. See also: R. Syal, 'Absolutely furious: Lumley's sister demands apology for sanity slur', *Sunday Times*, 9 July 1995.

68 Clare, *In the Psychiatrist's Chair II*, p. 209.

69 Personal communication: J. Lumley, email to BK (21 May 2018). See also: J. Taylor, 'Putting Anthony Clare in a psychiatrist's chair', *Daily Express*, 29 September 1995.

70 J. Rook, 'A shrink who cuts everyone down to size', *Daily Express*, 7 August 1991; P. Foster, 'High-profile victims mourn their quiet but unyielding interrogator', *The Times*, 31 October 2007.

71 Clare, *In the Psychiatrist's Chair* (1992), p. 219.

72 Ibid., p. 218.

73 Personal communication: E. Rantzen, interview with BK (18 May 2018).

74 Hendy, *Life On Air: A History of Radio Four*, p. 237.

75 Clare, *In the Psychiatrist's Chair* (1992), p. 220.

76 City Diary, 'Unshrinking', *The Times*, 26 September 1998.

77 Clare, *In the Psychiatrist's Chair II*, p. 344.

78 Ibid., pp. 348–9.

79 Personal communication: E. Rantzen, interview with BK (18 May 2018).

80 Clare, *In the Psychiatrist's Chair II*, p. 352.

81 P. Donovan, 'Parkinson's sadness over daughter he has never seen', *Sunday Times*, 25 July 1993.

82 Personal communication: J. Clare, interview with BK (10 May 2018).

83 Tattler, 'Out to lunch', *Sunday Express*, 19 July 1992.

84 Clare, *In the Psychiatrist's Chair* (1992), p. 241.

85 Ibid., p. 250.

86 Ibid., p. 254.

87 Ibid., p. 258.

88 Ibid., p. 257.

89 Ibid., pp. 258–9; see also: J. Wheatley, 'The face: A lonely road', *The Times*, 13 January 2006.

90 Clare, *In the Psychiatrist's Chair* (1992), p. 259.

91 Ibid., p. 269.

92 Ibid., p. 241.

93 Ibid., p. 243.

94 Ibid., p. 245.

95 D. Gray and P. Watt, *Giving Victims a Voice: Joint Report into Sexual Allegations Made Against Jimmy Savile* (London: National Society for the Prevention of Cruelty to Children and the Metropolitan Police, 2013), p. 24.

96 Ibid., p. 6.

97 Clare, *In the Psychiatrist's Chair* (1992), p. 269.

98 Ibid., p. 251.

99 Ibid., p. 252.

100 Ibid., p. 277.

101 Anonymous, 'Michael Ember, BBC Radio "talks" producer – obituary', *The Telegraph*, 11 April 2017.

102 Personal communication: E. Rantzen, interview with BK (18 May 2018).

103 Personal communication: A. Widdecombe, interview with BK (10 May 2018).

104 Personal communication: N. Horlick, email to BK (8 May 2018). See also: City Diary, 'Unshrinking', *The Times*, 26 September 1998.

105 Personal communication: G. Slovo, email to BK (15 May 2018).

106 V. Grove, 'Wedding bells ring again for Bayley at 74', *The Times*, 12 January 2000.

107 D. Young, 'Writer's mother libelled by BBC', *The Times*, 4 October 1990; J. Coles, 'BBC pays for Whitehouse slur on Potter's mother', *Guardian*, 4 October 1990.

108 N. Lawson, 'Great shrink show', *The Spectator*, 29 April 1995.

109 M. Binchy, 'If you're Irish … come into the media', *Irish Times*, 31 March 1984.

110 G. Bradberry, 'In the chair and off guard', *The Times*, 20 August 1996.

111 Personal communication: S. Greenfield, interview with BK (1 June 2018).

112 K. Bunce, 'Life, death, footie – and Phil Collins', *The Observer*, 22 October 2000. Courtesy of Guardian News & Media Ltd.

113 T. Wilson, 'Shall we swap livers?', *The Guardian*, 21 October 2000. Courtesy of Guardian News & Media Ltd.

114 G. Bradberry, 'In the chair and off guard', *The Times*, 20 August 1996; A. Treneman, 'Ran's hand is twice its normal size. It is the hand of a witch', *The Times*, 14 March 2000.

115 Personal communication: E. Rantzen, interview with BK (18 May 2018).

116 Ibid; see also: Hendy, *Life On Air: A History of Radio Four*, p. 237.

117 S. Faulks, 'It's my chair and I'll ask what I like', *The Independent*, 19 September 1992; W. Hartston, 'The armchair confessions of an agony uncle', *The Independent*, 19 October 1992; A.T. Ellis, 'Speaking their minds', *The Times*, 14 October 1995; J. Barnes, 'Shrink wrapped', *Sunday Times*, 19 July 1998; R. Campbell-Johnston, 'A life as ordinary', *The Times*, 8 August 1998.

118 Clare, *In the Psychiatrist's Chair* (1992).

119 M. Gaffney, 'The view from the chair', *Irish Times*, 26 September 1992.

120 Clare, *In the Psychiatrist's Chair III*.

121 R. Campbell-Johnston, 'A life as ordinary', *The Times*, 8 August 1998.

122 Personal communication: D. Knowles, interview with MH (12 November 2018).

123 A. Ferriman, 'Aspirin "could prevent strokes"', *Observer*, 3 July 1988; A. Ballantyne, 'Psychiatrist says long hours harm junior doctors' health', *Guardian*, 10 April 1989.

124 F. Gibb, 'Society takes the Mickey', *The Times*, 26 October 1999.

125 N. Wood, 'Parkinson dispute revived', *The Times*, 23 August 1986; T. Rayment and K. Symon, 'Adams tells of his Protestant loves', *Sunday Times*, 6 August 1995; Anonymous, 'Christie: UK lacks respect', *Sunday Times*, 3 September 1995.

126 www.hayfestival.com/p-5500-gitta-sereny-talks-to-anthony-clare.aspx?skinid=16 (Accessed 4 December 2019); https://podcasts.apple.com/gb/podcast/hay-festival/id600478477?i=1000136108008 (Accessed 4 December 2019). See also: E. Hardcastle, 'Authoress Gitta Sereny …', *Daily Mail*, 2 June 1998.

127 Clare, *In the Psychiatrist's Chair II*, pp. 169–208.

128 Personal communication: B. Knight, correspondence to BK (20 May 2018).

129 C. Midgley, 'Questionmaster in the hot seat', *The Times*, 21 May 1997.

130 A. Billen, 'Face to face with an ice maiden', *The Times*, 4 April 2007.

131 R. McKie, 'The chair man', *Observer*, 13 May 2001. Courtesy of Guardian News & Media Ltd.

132 S. Cody, 'Anthony Clare: In the Psychiatrist's Chair', unpublished interview, 1 May 1984; Personal communication: S. Cody, email to BK and MH (6 April 2019).

133 G. Miller, 'David Stafford-Clark (1916–1999): seeing through a celebrity

psychiatrist', *Wellcome Open Research*, 2 (2017), 30.

134 Personal communication: U. Geller, email to BK (8 May 2018).

135 Personal communication: E. Rantzen, interview with BK (18 May 2018). See also: V. Grove, 'Behind the psychiatrist's mask', *Sunday Times*, 14 August 1988.

136 Hendy, *Life On Air: A History of Radio Four*, p. 238.

137 Personal communication: S. Greenfield, interview with BK (1 June 2018).

138 Hendy, *Life On Air: A History of Radio Four*, p. 238.

139 Personal communication: J. Clare, interview with BK (10 May 2018). Clare himself said the same; see: R. Simpson, 'On a Clare day you can see for ever', *Daily Express*, 28 July 1992.

6. RETURN TO IRELAND (1989)

1 Personal communication: P. Clare, interview with BK (9 February 2019).

2 Personal communication: R. Clare, interview with BK (7 March 2019). See also: P. Kennedy, 'In the chair with Doctor Clare', *Daily Express*, 29 August 1988. For Clare's thoughts on Christmas, see: A. Clare, 'Dickens has much to answer for', *The Listener*, 23 December 1982.

3 Personal communication: P. Clare, interview with BK (9 February 2019).

4 J. Adams, 'He tried to shrink away but we got him to expand on love', *Today*, 18 August 1990.

5 A.W. Clare, *St Patrick's Hospital: A Discussion Document Concerning its Current Status and Future Plans in the Light of Trends in Contemporary Psychiatric Theory and Practice* (Dublin: St Patrick's Hospital, 1989), p. 13.

6 J. Lucey, 'Dr Anthony Clare remembered', *Irish Medical Times*, 16 November 2007. See also: Personal communication: A.W. Clare, correspondence (20 March 2000).

7 Personal communication: J. Lucey, interview with BK (30 August 2018).

8 Webb, *Trinity's Psychiatrists: From Serenity of the Soul to Neuroscience*, p. 123.

9 Personal communication: F. O'Donoghue, interview with BK (24 January 2019).

10 P. Burt, 'The man who meets the minds of the famous', *Evening Standard*, 25 July 1991.

11 Personal communication: A.W. Clare, correspondence (12 August 1990).

12 S. Cody, 'Anthony Clare', *Guardian*, 31 October 2007.

13 Personal communication: S. Cody, email to MH and BK (7 April 2019). For more on *Motives*, see: P. Ackroyd, 'Modest virtues', *The Times*, 2 August 1983; G. Wilkinson, 'Medicine and the media', *British Medical Journal*, 287, 6393 (3 September 1983), 683; A. Clare, 'The seductive lady problem', *The Listener*, 5 December 1985.

14 S. Cody, correspondence to A. Clare, 25 April 1986; 24 June 1986.

15 B. Knott, 'Julie's returns', *Financial Times*, 19 October 2019.

16 Personal communication: S. Cody, email to MH and BK (7 April 2019).

17 Ibid.

18 S. Cody, 'Anthony Clare', *Guardian*, 31 October 2007.

19 Personal communications: A.W. Clare, correspondence (22 May 1989 and 28 March 1990). Clare later saw patients at 45 Fitzwilliam Square in Dublin.

20 M. Maher, 'Clare comes a long way from there to here', *Irish Times*, 12 December 1988.

21 Anonymous, 'Emotional problems', *Evening Standard*, 3 March 1988.

22 Personal communication: R.M. Murray, interview with BK (25 February 2018).

23 Personal communication: J. Moriarty, email to BK (14 August 2018).

24 R. Young, 'Baby's kidnapper was convinced she gave birth to twins', *The Times*, 14 September 1993.

25 D. O'Donoghue, 'Shrink rap', *RTÉ Guide*, 1 May 1999.

26 A. Clare, 'My hero: Anthony Clare on John Hume', *Independent*, 7 January 1989.

27 See, for example: A. Clare, 'Television and the death of literacy', *Irish Times*, 29 June 1998.

28 Personal communication: A.W. Clare, correspondence (30 March 1993).

29 Personal communication: A.W. Clare, correspondence to G. Hussey (13 June 1990).

30 G. Hussey, *At the Cutting Edge: Cabinet Diaries 1982–1987* (Dublin: Gill and Macmillan Ltd., 1990).

31 Maume, *Dictionary of Irish Biography From the Earliest Times to 2002*.

32 Personal communication: J. Clare, interview with BK (23 June 2018).

33 Personal communication: D. Knowles, interview with MH (12 November 2018).

34 Maume, *Dictionary of Irish Biography From the Earliest Times to 2002.*

35 Personal communication: R. Clare, interview with BK (7 March 2019).

36 Personal communication: R.M. Murray, interview with BK (25 February 2018).

37 Personal communication: J. Clare, interview with BK (7 June 2018).

38 Personal communication: A. Mann, interview with BK (2 July 2018).

39 S. Milligan and A. Clare, *Depression and How to Survive It* (London: Arrow Books, 1994); H. Griffey, 'Falling from a great Hite', *Guardian*, 23 September 1996.

40 Personal communication: J. Clare, interview with BK (10 May 2018).

41 A. Clare, *On Men: Masculinity in Crisis* (London: Chatto & Windus, 2000).

42 A. Clare, 'Foreword', in E. Lee, *Mental Health Care: A Workbook for Care Workers* (London: Palgrave Macmillan, 1997), v.

43 A. Clare, 'Foreword', in N. Kfir and M. Slevin, *Challenging Cancer: From Chaos to Control* (London and New York: Tavistock/Routledge, 1991), xi. See also: A. Clare, 'The guilty sick', *The Listener*, 22 February 1979; A. Clare, 'Facing up to cancer', *The Listener*, 29 November 1979.

44 A.W. Clare, 'Foreword to the first edition', in M. Slevin and N. Kfir, *Challenging Cancer: Fighting Back, Taking Control, Finding Options (Second Edition)* (London: Class Publishing, 2002), xiii.

45 C. Rayner, 'Foreword to this edition', in M. Slevin and N. Kfir, *Challenging Cancer: Fighting Back, Taking Control, Finding Options (Second Edition)* (London: Class Publishing, 2002), xi–xii.

46 A.W. Clare, 'Foreword', in R.S. Kirby, C.C. Carson, M.G. Kirby and R.N. Farah (eds), *Men's Health (Second Edition)* (London: Taylor & Francis, 2004), xiii.

47 C. Keane, 'Introduction', in C. Keane (ed.), *Mental Health in Ireland* (Dublin: Gill and Macmillan and Radio Telefís Éireann, 1991), 1–3.

48 A. Clare, 'The mad Irish?', in C. Keane (ed.), *Mental Health in Ireland* (Dublin: Gill and Macmillan and Radio Telefís Éireann, 1991), 4–17.

49 See also Clare's contribution to *Nervous Breakdown*, a book accompanying the RTÉ Radio One series of the same title in 1994: A. Clare, 'Nervous breakdown', in C. Keane (ed.), *Nervous Breakdown* (Cork and Dublin: Mercier Press and Radio Telefís Éireann, 1994), 17–26.

50 A.W. Clare, 'Mental health and the media', *Journal of Mental Health*, 1, 1 (1992), 1–2.

51 A. Clare, 'The 1992 Jansson Memorial Lecture: communication in medicine', *European Journal of Disorders of Communication*, 28, 1 (1993), 1–12. See also: A. Clare, 'The relationship', *Daily Telegraph*, 13 June 1989; A. Clare, 'Stressed doctors and angry patients can make each other feel better', *Daily Mail*, 15 October 1991.

52 A.W. Clare, *Violence, Mental Illness and Society: The Stevens Lectures for the Laity 1994*. London: The Royal Society of Medicine, 1994. See also: A.W. Clare, 'Foreword' in P.J. Taylor (ed.), *Violence in Society* (London: Royal College of Physicians of London, 1993), iii–iv. For background to some of Clare's thoughts about violence, see: A. Clare, 'Sense and desensitisation', *The Listener*, 9 January 1986; A. Clare, 'Keeping violence in the family', *The Listener*, 6 November 1986; A. Clare, 'Living death', *The Listener*, 31 March 1988; A. Clare, 'Searching for the truth will never be an easy task', *Daily Mail*, 29 October 1991.

53 A.W. Clare, *Violence, Mental Illness and Society: The Stevens Lectures for the Laity 1994*. London: The Royal Society of Medicine, 1994; p. 5; quotations are reproduced by kind permission of the Royal Society of Medicine.

54 Ibid., p. 17.

55 Ibid., p. 23.

56 Ibid., pp. 27–8.

57 Ibid., p. 28.

58 A.W. Clare, 'Meeting of minds: the import of family and society', in B. Cartledge (ed.), *Mind, Brain and the Environment: The Linacre Lectures 1995–6* (Oxford: Oxford University Press, 1998), 144–57.

59 Clare, *Psychiatry in Dissent*, pp. 68–70; see also: A.W. Clare, 'Psychiatry's future', *Journal of Mental Health*, 8, 2 (1999), pp. 109–11.

60 J.V. Lucey, V. O'Keane, K. O'Flynn, A.W. Clare and T.G. Dinan, 'Gender and age differences in the growth hormone response to pyridostigmine', *International Clinical Psychopharmacology*, 6, 2 (Summer 1991), 105–9; J.V. Lucey, G. Butcher, A.W. Clare and T.G. Dinan, 'Elevated growth hormone responses to pyridostigmine in obsessive-compulsive disorder: evidence of cholinergic supersensitivity', *American Journal of*

Psychiatry, 150, 6 (June 1993), 961–2; J.V. Lucey, G. Butcher, K. O'Flynn, A.W. Clare and G. Dinan, 'The growth hormone response to baclofen in obsessive compulsive disorder: does the GABA-B receptor mediate obsessive anxiety?', *Pharmacopsychiatry*, 27, 1 (January 1994), 23–6.

61 R.H. Corney, R. Stanton, R. Newell and A.W. Clare, 'Comparison of progesterone, placebo and behavioural psychotherapy in the treatment of premenstrual syndrome', *Journal of Psychosomatic Obstetrics and Gynecology*, 11, 3 (1990), 211–20.

62 J.V. Lucey, G. Butcher, A.W. Clare and T.G. Dinan, 'Buspirone induced prolactin responses in obsessive-compulsive disorder (OCD): is OCD a 5-HT2 receptor disorder?', *International Clinical Psychopharmacology*, 7, 1 (Spring 1992), 45–9.

63 E. Ur, T.G. Dinan, V. O'Keane, A.W. Clare, L. McLoughlin, L.H. Rees, T.H. Turner, A. Grossman and G.M. Besser, 'Effect of metyrapone on the pituitary-adrenal axis in depression: relation to dexamethasone suppressor status', *Neuroendocrinology*, 56, 4 (October 1992), 533–8; J.V. Lucey, V. O'Keane, G. Butcher, A.W. Clare and T.G. Dinan, 'Cortisol and prolactin responses to d-fenfluramine in non-depressed patients with obsessive-compulsive disorder: a comparison with depressed and healthy controls', *British Journal of Psychiatry*, 161, 4 (1 October 1992), 517–21; J.V. Lucey, J.V., G. Butcher, A.W. Clare and T.G. Dinan, 'The anterior pituitary responds normally to protirelin in obsessive-compulsive disorder: evidence to support a neuroendocrine serotonergic deficit', *Acta Psychiatrica Scandinavica*, 87, 6 (June 1993), 384–8.

64 M. O'Hanlon, S. Barry, A.W. Clare and T.G. Dinan, 'Serum thyrotropin responses to thyrotropin-releasing hormone in alcohol-dependent patients with and without depression', *Journal of Affective Disorders*, 21, 2 (February 1991), 109–15.

65 R.H. Corney, R. Stanton, R. Newell, A. Clare and P. Fairclough, 'Behavioural psychotherapy in the treatment of irritable bowel syndrome', *Journal of Psychosomatic Research*, 35, 4–5 (1991), 461–9.

66 W.D.A. Bruce-Jones, P.D. White, J.M. Thomas and A.W. Clare, 'The effect of social adversity on the fatigue syndrome, psychiatric disorders and physical recovery, following glandular fever', *Psychological Medicine*, 24, 3 (August 1994), 651–9; P.D. White, P.D., J.M. Thomas, J. Amess, S.A. Grover, H.O. Kangro and A.W. Clare, 'The existence of a fatigue syndrome after glandular fever', *Psychological Medicine*, 25, 5 (September 1995), 907–16; P.D. White, S.A. Grover, H.O. Kangro, J.M. Thomas, J. Amess and A.W. Clare, 'The validity and reliability of the fatigue syndrome that follows glandular fever', *Psychological Medicine*, 25, 2 (September 1995), 917–24; P.D. White, J.M. Thomas, J. Amess, D.H. Crawford, S.A. Grover, H.O Kangro and A.W. Clare, 'Incidence, risk and prognosis of acute and chronic fatigue syndromes and psychiatric disorders after glandular fever', *British Journal of Psychiatry*, 173, 6 (December 1998), 475–81; P.D. White, J.M. Thomas, H.O. Kangro, W.D. Bruce-Jones, J. Amess, D.H. Crawford, S.A. Grover and A.W. Clare, 'Predictions and associations of fatigue syndromes and mood disorders that occur after infectious mononucleosis', *Lancet*, 358, 9297 (8 December 2001), 1946–54.

67 M.C. Sharpe, L.C. Archard, J.E. Banatvala, L.K. Borysiewicz, A.W. Clare, A. David, R.H.T. Edwards, K.E.H. Hawton, H.P. Lambert, R.J.M. Lane, E.M. McDonald, J.F. Mowbray, D.J. Pearson, T.E.A. Peto, V.R. Preedy, A.P. Smith, D.G. Smith, D.J. Taylor, D.A.J. Tyrrell, S. Wessely, P.D. White, P.O. Behan, F. Clifford Rose, T.J. Peters, P.G. Wallace, D.A. Warrell and D.J.M Wright, 'A report: chronic fatigue syndrome: guidelines for research', *Journal of the Royal Society of Medicine*, 84, 2 (February 1991), 118–21. See also: A. Clare, 'Taking "real" illness to the psychiatrist', *Daily Mail*, 1 October 1991.

68 Maume, *Dictionary of Irish Biography From the Earliest Times to 2002*.

69 Personal communication: A.W. Clare, correspondence (22 November 1993).

70 F. Lynch and A. Clare, 'Chronic fatigue syndrome', *Modern Medicine of Ireland*, 29, 5 (May 1999), 22–4.

71 E. Goudsmit, 'Chronic fatigue syndrome', *Modern Medicine of Ireland*, 29, 7/8 (July/August 1999), 67–9.

72 C.K. Farren, A.W. Clare and T.G. Dinan, 'Basal serum cortisol and dexamethasone-induced growth hormone release in the

alcohol dependence syndrome', *Human Psychopharmacology*, 10, 3 (May/June 1995), 207–13; C.K. Farren, A.W. Clare, D. Ziedonis, F.A. Hammeedi and T.G. Dinan, 'Evidence for reduced dopamine D2 receptor sensitivity in postwithdrawal alcoholics', *Alcoholism, Clinical and Experimental Research*, 19, 6 (December 1995), 1520–4; C.K. Farren, D. Ziedonis, A.W. Clare, F.A. Hammeedi and T.G. Dinan, 'D-fenfluramine-induced prolactin responses in postwithdrawal alcoholics and controls', *Alcoholism, Clinical and Experimental Research*, 19, 6 (December 1995), 1578–82; C.K. Farren, A.W. Clare, K.F. Tipton and T.G Dinan, 'Platelet MAO activity in subtypes of alcoholics and controls in a homogenous population', *Journal of Psychiatric Research*, 32, 1 (January–February 1998), 49–54. See also: A. Clare, 'Just another one for the road', *Daily Mail*, 8 October 1991.

73   R.A. Ball and A.W. Clare, 'Symptoms and social adjustment in Jewish depressives', *British Journal of Psychiatry*, 156, 3 (1 March 1990), 379–83; S.A. Montgomery, J. Henry, G. McDonald, T. Dinan, M. Lader, I. Hindmarch, A. Clare and D. Nutt, 'Selective serotonin reuptake inhibitors: meta-analysis of discontinuation rates', *International Clinical Psychopharmacology*, 9, 1 (Spring 1994), 47–53.

74   H. O'Connell and A. Clare, 'Nearly lethal suicide attempt: implications for research and prevention', *Irish Journal of Psychological Medicine*, 21, 4 (December 2004), 131–3.

75   C. Smyth, M. MacLachlan and A. Clare, *Cultivating Suicide? Destruction of Self in a Changing Ireland* (Dublin: The Liffey Press, 2003).

76   Personal communication: M. MacLachlan, email to BK (16 August 2018).

77   G.R. Swanwick and A.W. Clare, 'Suicide in Ireland 1945–1992: social correlates', *Irish Medical Journal*, 90, 3 (April–May 1997), 106–8.

78   E. Greene, C.J. Cunningham, A. Eustace, N. Kidd, A.W. Clare and B.A. Lawlor, 'Recurrent falls are associated with increased length of stay in elderly psychiatric inpatients', *International Journal of Geriatric Psychiatry*, 16, 10 (October 2001), 965–8.

79   C. Farren, D. McLoughlin and A. Clare, 'Procedures for involuntary admission to public and private psychiatric facilities', *Irish Journal of Psychological Medicine*, 9, 2 (November 1992), 96–100.

80   Clare, *Psychiatry in Dissent*, pp. 325–69.

81   M.F. Bristow and A.W. Clare, 'Prevalence and characteristics of at-risk drinkers among elderly acute medical in-patients', *British Journal of Addiction*, 87, 2 (February 1992), 291–4.

82   G.R.J. Swanwick, H. Lee, A.W. Clare and B.A. Lawlor, 'Consultation-liaison psychiatry: a comparison of two service models for geriatric patients', *International Journal of Geriatric Psychiatry*, 9, 6 (June 1994), 495–9; G. Swanwick and A Clare, 'Inpatient liaison psychiatry: the experience of two Irish general hospitals without psychiatric units', *Irish Journal of Psychological Medicine*, 11, 3 (September 1994), 123–5.

83   G.R.J. Swanwick and A.W. Clare, 'The management of insomnia', *Journal of the Irish Colleges of Physicians and Surgeons*, 20, 4 (October 1991), 249–50.

84   Personal communication: G. Swanwick, email to BK (12 August 2018).

85   J.V. Lucey, G. Butcher, A.W. Clare and T.G. Dinan, 'The clinical characteristics of patients with obsessive compulsive disorder: a descriptive study of an Irish sample', *Irish Journal of Psychological Medicine*, 11, 1 (March 1994), 11–14.

86   A.W. Clare, 'Aggiornamento sull'ansia clinica: Una rassegna della letteratura attuale sulla definizione e classificazione dell'ansia e il dibattito sulle modalità di trattamento' ('Update on clinical anxiety: A review of the current literature on the definition and classification of anxiety and the debate on treatment methods'), *Rivista di Psichiatria*, 24, 2 (April–June 1989), 89–94.

87   J.M. Cooney, C.K. Farren and A.W. Clare, 'Personality disorder among first ever admissions to an Irish public and private hospital', *Irish Journal of Psychological Medicine*, 13, 1 (March 1996), 6–8.

88   M. Cheasty, A.W. Clare and C. Collins, 'Child sexual abuse – predictor of persistent depression in adult rape and sexual assault victims', *Journal of Mental Health*, 11, 1 (2002), 79–84; M. Cheasty, A.W. Clare and C. Collins, 'Relation between sexual abuse in childhood and adult depression: case-control study', *British Medical Journal*, 316, 7126 (17 January 1998), 198–201. See also: A. Clare, 'The courage to be boring', *The Listener*, 26 June 1986.

89   K. Davidson and A.W. Clare, 'Psychotic illness following termination of pregnancy', *British Journal of Psychiatry*, 154, 4 (1 April 1989), 559–60.

90   A.W. Clare and J. Tyrrell, 'Psychiatric aspects of abortion', *Irish Journal of Psychological Medicine*, 11, 2 (June 1994), 92–8. See also: A. Clare, 'A woman's right to choose', *The Listener*, 12 March 1987.

91   A. Clare, 'Proving that life isn't fair', *Literary Review*, September 1998.

92   A. Clare, 'Depression in schizophrenics (book review)', *Irish Journal of Psychological Medicine*, 7, 2 (September 1990), 180–2; A.W. Clare, 'A guide to psychiatry in primary care (book review)', *Irish Journal of Psychological Medicine*, 8, 1 (March 1991), 86.

93   A.W. Clare, 'Health psychology and public health (book review)', *Social Policy and Administration*, 25, 2 (June 1991), 164–6.

94   A.W. Clare, 'Scenes of madness: a psychiatrist at the theatre (book review)', *American Journal of Psychiatry*, 150, 12 (December 1993), 1888.

95   A.W. Clare, 'The two Mr. Gladstones: a study in psychology and history (book review)', *American Journal of Psychiatry*, 155, 12 (December 1998), 1789–90.

96   A.W. Clare, 'Understanding and treating violent psychiatric patients (book review)', *American Journal of Psychiatry*, 158, 10 (October 2001), 1757.

97   A.W. Clare, *Violence, Mental Illness and Society: The Stevens Lectures for the Laity 1994*. London: The Royal Society of Medicine, 1994.

98   A.W. Clare, 'Psychological medicine', in P.J. Kumar and M.L. Clark (eds), *Clinical Medicine: A Textbook for Medical Students and Doctors* (London: Ballière Tindall, 1987), 868–900.

99   A.W. Clare, 'Psychological medicine', in P.J. Kumar and M.L. Clark (eds), *Clinical Medicine: A Textbook for Medical Students and Doctors (Second Edition)* (London: Ballière Tindall, 1990), 965–99.

100 A.W. Clare, 'Psychological medicine', in P. Kumar and M. Clark (eds), *Clinical Medicine: A Textbook for Medical Students and Doctors (Third Edition)* (London: Ballière Tindall, 1994), 957–91.

101 A.W. Clare, 'Psychological medicine', in P. Kumar and M. Clark (eds), *Kumar and Clark: Clinical Medicine: A Textbook for Medical Students and Doctors (Fourth Edition)* (Edinburgh: W.B. Saunders, 1998), 1105–47.

102 P. White and A.W. Clare, 'Psychological medicine', in P. Kumar and M. Clark (eds), *Kumar & Clark: Clinical Medicine (Fifth Edition)* (Edinburgh: W.B. Saunders, 2002), 1225–70.

103 P. White and A.W. Clare, 'Psychological medicine', in P. Kumar and M. Clark (eds), *Kumar & Clark: Clinical Medicine (Sixth Edition)* (Edinburgh: Elsevier Saunders, 2005), 1273–314.

104 P.D. White and A.W. Clare, 'Psychological medicine', in P. Kumar and M. Clark (eds), *Kumar & Clark's Clinical Medicine (Seventh Edition)* (Edinburgh: Saunders Elsevier, 2009), 1185–223.

105 A.W. Clare, 'Commentary on: "Training in psychodynamic psychotherapy: the psychiatric trainee's perspective"', *Irish Journal of Psychological Medicine*, 12, 2 (June 1995), 59–60.

106 A.W. Clare, 'The alcohol problem in universities and the professions', *Alcohol and Alcoholism*, 25, 2–3 (1 January 1990), 277–85.

107 A. Clare, 'The future of postgraduate training in psychiatry in Ireland', *Irish Journal of Psychological Medicine*, 24, 4 (December 2007), 129–31.

108 A.W. Clare, 'Democratic definitely, parochial possibly, challenged certainly: the College at the century's end', *Psychiatric Bulletin*, 23, 1 (1 January 1999), 1–2.

109 A. Clare, R.J. Daly, T.G. Dinan, D. King, B.E. Leonard, C. O'Boyle, J. O'Connor, J. Waddington, N. Walsh and M. Webb, 'Advancement of psychiatric research in Ireland: proposal for a national body', *Irish Journal of Psychological Medicine*, 7, 2 (September 1990), 93. See also: Personal communication: A.W. Clare, correspondence (8 June 1989).

110 D. Newby, 'Review: Safety in Psychiatry: The Mind's Eye', *Psychiatric Bulletin*, 26, 11 (November 2002), 439–40.

111 Personal communication: A.W. Clare, correspondence (4 July 1994).

112 See also: A. Clare, 'Endpiece', *The Listener*, 7 July 1983.

113 A. Clare, 'The concept of care in mental illness', in K. O'Sullivan (ed.), *All in the Mind: Approaches to Mental Health* (Dublin: Gill and Macmillan Ltd., 1986), 16–23.

114 Personal communication: A.W. Clare, correspondence (8 September 1993).

115 Personal communication: A.W. Clare, correspondence to R. Murray (13 December 1989).

116 E. Malcolm, *Swift's Hospital: A History of St Patrick's Hospital, Dublin, 1746–1989.*

117 Personal communication: A.W. Clare, correspondence (2 May 1995).

118 K.R. Jamison, *Touched with Fire: Manic Depressive Illness and the Artistic Temperament* (New York, NY: Free Press, 1993).

119 A.W. Clare, 'Touched with fire: manic depressive illness and the artistic temperament (book review)', *British Journal of Psychiatry*, 171, 4 (1 October 1997), 395.

120 See also: A.W. Clare, 'Psychiatry: beyond analysis (book review)', *Nature*, 314, 6013 (25 April 1985), 696–7.

121 Personal communication: A.W. Clare, correspondence (22 March 1996).

122 Personal communication: P.D. Sutherland, correspondence to A.W. Clare (24 May 1999).

123 J. Walsh, *The Globalist: Peter Sutherland – His Life and Legacy* (London: William Collins, 2019), pp. 7–9, 121.

124 Personal communication: A.W. Clare, correspondence (19 October 1999).

125 Personal communication: A.W. Clare, correspondence to D. Allen (15 April 1992).

126 Personal communication: A.W. Clare, correspondence (25 September 1991).

127 *Swift Times*, Issue 1, Christmas 1991, p. 1.

128 Personal communication: A.W. Clare, correspondence (16 February 1994).

129 A.W. Clare, 'Professor Norman Moore', *Swift Times*, 16 (1996), 1–2.

130 A.W. Clare, 'John Norman Parker Moore (obituary)', *Psychiatric Bulletin*, 20, 12 (1 December 1996), 771–3.

131 A. Clare, 'Norman Moore', *Irish Times*, 29 July 1996.

132 A.W. Clare, *Funeral Address: J.N.P. Moore, MD FRCPI FRCPsych* (Dublin: St Patrick's Cathedral, 1996).

133 Personal communication: D. and C. Moore, correspondence to A. Clare (26 August 1996).

134 Personal communication: A.W. Clare, correspondence (16 June 1999).

135 Personal communication: A.W. Clare, correspondence (22 September 1999).

136 A. Clare, R.J. Daly, T.G. Dinan, D. King, B.E. Leonard, C. O'Boyle, J. O'Connor, J. Waddington, N. Walsh and M. Webb, 'Advancement of psychiatric research in Ireland: proposal for a national body', *Irish Journal of Psychological Medicine*, 7, 2 (September 1990), 93. See also: Personal communication: A.W. Clare, correspondence (8 June 1989).

137 Personal communication: A.W. Clare, correspondence (25 November 1999).

138 Personal communication: A.W. Clare, correspondence (11 April 2000).

139 Anonymous, 'Who is the …', *Daily Mail*, 1 November 1990; J. Hind, 'I ask the questions (such as: how do you FEEL?)', *Mail on Sunday*, 8 October 1995.

140 Personal communication: A.W. Clare, correspondence to the editor of the *Irish Medical News* (16 November 1997). Clare was an early supporter of McAleese.

141 Personal communication: A.W. Clare, correspondence (12 July 1991).

142 Personal communication: A.W. Clare, correspondence (30 March 1995).

143 Personal communication: A.W. Clare, correspondence (29 January 1991).

144 C. Richmond, 'Obituary: Anthony Clare', *Guardian*, 31 October 2007.

145 Personal communication: A.W. Clare, correspondence (24 January 1999).

146 Personal communication: A.W. Clare, correspondence (5 February 1999).

147 Anonymous, 'Mixed up', *Financial Times*, 30 April 1991.

148 Personal communication: M. Browne, email to BK (25 March 2019).

149 J. Hind, 'I ask the questions (such as: how do you FEEL?)', *Mail on Sunday*, 8 October 1995.

150 Personal communication: A.W. Clare, correspondence (8 February 1995).

151 Personal communication: A.W. Clare, correspondence (6 February 1997).

152 Personal communication: A.W. Clare, correspondence (18 October 1993).

153 Personal communication: J. Lucey, interview with BK (30 August 2018).

154 Personal communication: A.W. Clare, correspondence (11 May 1998).

155 Personal communication: A.W. Clare, correspondence (29 October 1993).

156 Personal communication: A.W. Clare, correspondence (11 September 1998).

157 Personal communication: A.W. Clare, correspondence (25 July 2000).

158 Personal communication: T. McMonagle, correspondence (26 August 1999).

159 Personal communication: A.W. Clare, correspondence (8 September 1999).

160 Personal communication: T. McMonagle, email to BK (3 September 2018).

161 Personal communication: A.W. Clare, correspondence to C. Haughey (3 October 1989).

162 Personal communication: A.W. Clare, correspondence to B. Desmond (10 May 1993). For Clare's earlier comments on Desmond, see: A. Clare, 'Eat, drink and be ill', *The Listener*, 12 September 1985.

163 Personal communication: A.W. Clare, correspondence to V. Browne (26 November 1993).

164 Personal communication: A.W. Clare, correspondence to J. Bruton (29 May 1994).

165 Personal communication: A.W. Clare, correspondence to R. O'Hanlon (14 November 1991).

166 Personal communication: A.W. Clare, correspondence to M. O'Rourke (14 November 1991).

167 Personal communication: A.W. Clare, correspondence (25 August 1994).

168 T. Hegarty, 'Private patients may go to public sector if Noonan signs regulations', *Irish Times*, 30 June 1995.

169 P. O'Morain, 'Psychiatrist warns patients face insurance cuts', *Irish Times*, 25 July 1995.

170 *Irish Times*, 'Psychiatric care', *Irish Times*, 25 July 1995.

171 B.D. Kelly, 'Dr Dermot Walsh, 1931–2017', *Irish Journal of Psychological Medicine*, 34, 3 (September 2017), 217–20.

172 D. Walsh, 'Private health insurance', *Irish Times*, 2 August 1995.

173 Personal communication: A.W. Clare, correspondence to D. Walsh (24 August 1995).

174 See, for example: personal communication: A.W. Clare, correspondence (19 September 1995).

175 M. Cummins, 'FF fails to get regulations on mentally ill amended', *Irish Times* (2 May 1996).

176 Anonymous, 'Minister defends regulations on mental illness insurance', *Irish Times*, 29 May 1996.

177 Personal communication: A.W. Clare, correspondence to M. Noonan (29 April 1996).

178 Personal communication: A.W. Clare, correspondence (21 May 1996).

179 Personal communication: A.W. Clare, correspondence to all TDs (29 April 1996).

180 Personal communication: A.W. Clare, correspondence to M. Noonan (30 December 1996).

181 A. Clare, 'Competition is healthy, but not if it discriminates', *Sunday Independent*, 12 January 1997.

182 Personal communication: A.W. Clare, correspondence (7 July 1998).

183 Personal communications: A.W. Clare, correspondence to J. O'Connell (18 June 1992; also: 2 July and 11 August 1992) and correspondence (18 May 1999).

184 Personal communications: A.W. Clare, correspondence to J. O'Connell (27 April 1992) and correspondence (26 April 1993).

185 Personal communication: A.W. Clare, correspondence (16 December 1993).

186 Clare, *Psychiatry in Dissent*, pp. 325–69.

187 A. Clare, 'Tribunal review not the only answer', *Forum*, 9 (September 1992), 16–17.

188 Personal communication: A.W. Clare, correspondence (24 January 1995).

189 Personal communication: A.W. Clare, correspondence (24 March 2000).

190 Personal communications: A.W. Clare, correspondence (24 September 1991 and 19 October 1993).

191 A. Beckett, 'Turn on, check in, dry out', *Guardian*, 5 July 1999.

192 Personal communication: A.W. Clare, correspondence (12 July 1999).

193 Morrissey, *Autobiography* (London: Penguin, 2013), pp. 277–9. See also: S. Maguire, 'Morrissey: TV shrink was no charming man', *Sunday Times*, 20 October 2013.

194 Personal communications: A.W. Clare, correspondence to M. Shepherd (26 September 1994 and 4 May 1995).

7. WORK, LIFE AND THE CRISIS IN MASCULINITY (1989-2007)

1 *Irish Times*, 1 April 2000.

2 Produced and directed by Jim Sherwin of Sherwin Media Group.

3 Personal communication: A.W. Clare, correspondence (19 August 1996).

4 I. Browne, *Music and Madness* (Cork: Atrium/Cork University Press, 2008), pp. 277–83.

5 F. O'Toole, 'Medical body censured Browne but ruled he acted for patient', *Irish Times*, 11 January 1997. See also: F. O'Toole, 'Public has right to know how

doctors are regulated', *Irish Times*, 24 January 1997.

6 Medical Council Fitness to Practise Committee, *Re: Professor Ivor Browne. Inquiry Held at Portobello Court, Lower Rathmines Road, Dublin 6 on 16th–18th October, 1996* (Dublin: Medical Council, 1996). F. O'Toole, 'How Medical Council decided to admonish Ivor Browne', *Irish Times*, 11 January 1997.

7 Personal communication: I. Browne, interview with BK (7 July 2018).

8 Personal communication: J. Lucey, interview with BK (30 August 2018).

9 A.W. Clare, 'Ethical issues in psychiatry', *Practitioner*, 223, 1333 (July 1979), 89–96.

10 G. Brandreth, *Something Sensational to Read in the Train: The Diary of a Lifetime* (London: John Murray, 2009), pp. 666–8; G. Brandreth, 'How to be happy', *Sunday Telegraph*, 30 January 2000.

11 G. Brandreth, *The 7 Secrets of Happiness: An Optimist's Journey* (London: Short Books, 2013).

12 R. Ingle, 'Clare to step down from hot seat at St Patrick's', *Irish Times*, 24 August 1999.

13 P. Casey, 'Farewell to a dear friend and kind mentor', *Irish Independent*, 31 October 2007.

14 Personal communication: A.W. Clare, correspondence (20 November 2000).

15 Personal communication: A.W. Clare, correspondence to M. McAleese (8 November 1999).

16 R. Ingle, 'Clare to step down from hot seat at St Patrick's', *Irish Times*, 24 August 1999.

17 A. Clare, *On Men: Masculinity in Crisis* (London: Chatto & Windus, 2000).

18 A. Clare, 'Men must change', *The Listener*, 13 February 1986; A. Clare, 'The popular front', *The Listener*, 26 January 1989.

19 R. McKie, 'The chair man', *Observer*, 13 May 2001.

20 A. Rissik, 'Men in the psychiatrist's chair', *Guardian*, 12 August 2000. Courtesy of Guardian News & Media Ltd. For more of Clare's thoughts on genetics, see: A. Clare, 'Sturdy offspring', *The Listener*, 30 October 1980.

21 Clare, *On Men: Masculinity in Crisis*, p. 1.

22 Ibid., p. 9.

23 H.J. Friedman, 'Let's talk about male sex drive', *New York Times*, 3 December 2017.

24 G. Younge, 'Nearly every mass killer is a man. We should all be talking more about that', *The Guardian*, 26 April 2018. See also: G. Bowditch, 'Why our fathers need us to stand up for their rights', *Sunday Times*, 15 September 2002.

25 W. Hutton, 'So men are dying because they don't have women's brains. Show me the evidence', *The Observer*, 4 February 2018.

26 D. Ferriter, 'Men struggling to come to terms with post-feminist world', *Irish Times*, 18 November 2017.

27 P. Mishra, 'Not enough man: masculinity in crisis', *The Guardian*, 17 March 2018. Courtesy of Guardian News & Media Ltd.

28 Clare, *On Men: Masculinity in Crisis*, p. 36.

29 Ibid., p. 37.

30 Ibid., p. 56.

31 Ibid., p. 66.

32 J. Bressan, 'A mountain or a mole ill?', *Medicine Weekly*, 6 September 2000. See also: B.D. Kelly, 'Men are so like gorillas', *Medicine Weekly*, 20 September 2000.

33 D. Quinn, 'Men may be in a mess but women suffer too', *Sunday Times*, 23 July 2000.

34 K. Holmquist, 'Men in crisis – or is it just me?', *Irish Times*, 27 July 2000. See also: A. Levin, 'Swapping chairs with Clare', *You Magazine*, 27 September 1992; J. Burns, 'Beckham "a better father than Blair"', *Sunday Times*, 16 July 2000.

35 Clare, *On Men: Masculinity in Crisis*, p. 88

36 Ibid. See also: A. Clare, 'The trouble with men', *Sunday Times*, 16 July 2000.

37 Clare, *On Men: Masculinity in Crisis*, p. 100.

38 Ibid., p. 129.

39 Ibid., p. 135.

40 Ibid., p. 159.

41 Ibid., p. 189.

42 Ibid., p. 193.

43 Ibid., p. 194.

44 Ibid., p. 205.

45 Ibid., pp. 217, 221.

46 L. Fay, 'How the victim culture sparked man trouble', *Sunday Times*, 6 August 2000.

47 H. Ferguson, 'Why can't a man be more like a woman?', *Irish Times*, 12 August 2000.

48 See also: F. Weldon, 'In search of a new role', *Sunday Times*, 30 July 2000; D. Burke, 'Male impotence', *Sunday Times*, 30 July 2000.

49   B.D. Kelly 'Homosexuality and Irish psychiatry: medicine, law and the changing face of Ireland', *Irish Journal of Psychological Medicine*, 34, 3 (September 2017), 209–15.

50   A.W. Clare, 'Homosexuality', *Irish Times*, 9 February 1990.

51   M. Bunting, 'Masculinity in question', *The Guardian*, 2 October 2000. Courtesy of Guardian News & Media Ltd.

52   H. Lynch, 'Men', *Sunday Times*, 6 August 2000; N. Rennison, 'On Men', *Sunday Times*, 10 June 2001.

53   K. Courtney, 'Crisis, what crisis?', *Irish Times*, 4 November 2000.

54   R. Godwin, 'Men after #MeToo: "There's a narrative that masculinity is fundamentally toxic"', *The Guardian*, 10 March 2018. Courtesy of Guardian News & Media Ltd.

55   A. Billen, 'Fame gives you pleasure, like drink or gambling or sex. It doesn't make you happy', *Evening Standard*, 26 July 2000.

56   K. Holmquist, 'Men in crisis – or is it just me?', *Irish Times*, 27 July 2000. See also: A. Clare, 'Langham Diary', *The Listener*, 16 February 1984.

57   Personal communication: J. Clare, interview with BK (23 June 2018).

58   Personal communication: A. Buckley, interview with BK (16 January 2019).

59   T. Real, *How Can I Get Through to You? Closing the Intimacy Gap Between Men and Women* (New York: Fireside, 2002), p. 43.

60   Personal communication: P. Clare, interview with BK (9 February 2019).

61   Personal communication: A.W. Clare, correspondence to BK (7 September 2005).

62   Personal communication: A.W. Clare, correspondence (2 January 1996). See also: Anonymous, 'Don't let parents divorce says radio shrink', *Daily Mail*, 18 April 1994.

63   A. Clare, 'A nation divorced from itself', *Sunday Independent*, 26 November 1995.

64   J. Clare, 'Truth is the first casualty', *Sunday Independent*, 26 November 1995.

65   Personal communication: J. Clare, interview with BK (23 June 2018).

66   J. Clare and M. Keane, *What Will I Be?* (Dublin: Marino Books, 1995). See also: K. MacDermot, 'A mother's counsel for a harsh world', *Irish Independent*, 16

September 1995; J. Clare, 'Parents must fight for choice', *Farmers Journal*, 25 November 2000.

67   Maume, *Dictionary of Irish Biography From the Earliest Times to 2002*; P. Casey, 'Farewell to a dear friend and kind mentor', *Irish Independent*, 31 October 2007.

68   *Constitution of Ireland*, Article 41(1).

69   A. Clare, *Programme: Long Day's Journey into Night* (Dublin: Peri-Talking Theatre Company, 1997).

70   Personal communication: A. Buckley, interview with BK (16 January 2019).

71   Personal communication: M. DelMonte, interview with BK (7 May 2019).

72   Personal communication: F. O'Donoghue, interview with BK (24 January 2019).

73   Personal communication: N. Kennedy, email to BK (22 August 2018).

74   Personal communication: A. Buckley, interview with BK (16 January 2019).

75   Personal communication: F. O'Donoghue, interview with BK (24 January 2019).

76   Personal communication: N. Kennedy, email to BK (22 August 2018).

77   *Medicine Weekly*, 19 March 2008. See also: J. Clare, 'Out of Ireland and into Africa', *Lucan Gazette*, 24 July 2004.

78   C. Richmond, 'Obituary: Anthony Clare', *Guardian*, 31 October 2007.

79   *Irish Times*, 3 November 2007.

80   Personal communication: R. Clare, interview with BK (7 March 2019).

81   Personal communication: A. Buckley, interview with BK (16 January 2019).

82   Personal communication: I. Browne, interview with BK (7 July 2018). See also: A. Billen, 'Fame gives you pleasure, like drink or gambling or sex. It doesn't make you happy', *Evening Standard*, 26 July 2000.

83   Personal communication: J. Clare, interview with BK (23 June 2018).

84   Personal communication: R.M. Murray, interview with BK (25 February 2018).

85   Personal communication: R. Dudley Edwards, interview with BK (14 June 2019). See also: R. Dudley Edwards, 'It is the mischief and laughter that I'll miss most about Tony', *Sunday Independent*, 4 November 2007.

86   Personal communication: J. Lucey, interview with BK (30 August 2018).

87   Personal communication: P. Clare, interview with BK (9 February 2019).

88   R. Dudley Edwards, 'Obituary: Liam Hourican', *Independent*, 16 August 1993.

89 Personal communication: Colm de Barra, email to BK (17 June 2019).

90 E. Oliver, 'Mercy sisters to take action against TV3 over programme alleging abuse', *Irish Times*, 6 November 2000; K. Donaghy, 'Six nuns sue TV3 over rape claims', *Irish Independent*, 24 November 2000.

91 Personal communication: J. Lucey, interview with BK (30 August 2018).

92 Personal communication: A. Buckley, interview with BK (16 January 2019).

93 N. Taylor, 'Why I have lost faith in God', *The Times*, 1 August 2000.

94 R. Gledhill, 'Pope resists moves to soften encyclical', *The Times*, 18 September 1993; Anonymous, 'Priests "turn blind eye to drink"', *Telegraph*, 18 September 1993.

95 P. Casey, 'Farewell to a dear friend and kind mentor', *Irish Independent*, 31 October 2007.

8. THE PSYCHIATRIST IN THE CHAIR

1 Personal communication: correspondence to A.W. Clare (14 September 1989).

2 Personal communication: A.W. Clare correspondence (25 September 1989).

3 Personal communication: Email to BK (26 October 2018).

4 Personal communication: J. Clare, interview with BK (23 June 2018).

5 Personal communication: P. Clare, interview with BK (9 February 2019).

6 Personal communication: R. Clare, interview with BK (7 March 2019).

7 Personal communication: A. Buckley, interview with BK (16 January 2019).

8 C. Byrne, 'Warm tributes to man who changed face of psychiatry', *Irish Independent*, 31 October 2007; S. Cody, 'Anthony Clare', *Guardian*, 31 October 2007; J. McEnroe, 'Tributes for doctor who "demystified psychiatry"', *Irish Examiner*, 31 October 2007.

9 C. Richmond, 'Obituary: Anthony Clare', *Guardian*, 31 October 2007. Courtesy of *Guardian* News & Media Ltd.

10 P. Casey, 'Anthony Clare', *Guardian*, 31 October 2007; P. Casey, 'Farewell to a dear friend and kind mentor', *Irish Independent*, 31 October 2007; M. Houston, 'Prof Anthony Clare dies unexpectedly in Paris', *Irish Times*, 30 October 2007; J. Lucey, 'Dr Anthony Clare remembered', *Irish Medical Times*, 16 November 2007; C. Walsh, 'Remembering a great doctor

and colleague', *Medicine Weekly*, 21 November 2007; M. Fitzgerald, 'Professor Anthony Clare', *Irish Journal of Psychological Medicine*, 24, 4 (1 December 2007), 161; P. Nolan, 'Anthony Clare: a man of compassion', *Mental Health Practice*, 11, 5 (February 2008), 11; R.M. Murray, 'Obituary: Professor Anthony Clare', *Psychiatric Bulletin*, 32, 3 (1 March 2008), 118–19. See also: *Medicine Weekly*, 7 November 2007. For a particular example of Clare's collegial supportiveness and sense of justice, see: Browne, *Music and Madness*, pp. 277–83.

11 Anonymous, 'Obituaries: Professor Anthony Clare', *The Times*, 31 October 2007; A. Cane, 'Obituary: radio psychiatrist who quizzed the famous', *Financial Times*, 31 October 2007.

12 M. Houston, 'Obituary: Anthony Ward Clare', *BMJ*, 335, 7628 (17 November 2007), 1050.

13 BAL, MGTW and TD, 'Professor Anthony Clare: an appreciation of his contribution to psychiatry', *Irish Journal of Psychological Medicine*, 24, 4 (1 December 2007), 127–8.

14 C. Walsh, 'Loss of a vibrant voice', *Irish Times*, 3 November 2007; see also, for example: A.W. Clare, 'More bark than bite', *Irish Times*, 14 July 1990; A. Clare, 'The great university we might have had', *Irish Times*, 18 December 1999.

15 A. Clare, 'Seven types of incongruity', *Irish Times*, 25 February 1995; O. Sacks, *An Anthropologist on Mars: Seven Paradoxical Tales* (New York: Alfred A. Knopf, 1995). See also: A. Clare, 'Disorderly drama', *The Listener*, 5 December 1985; A. Clare, 'Romantic on the loose', *Literary Review*, November 1996.

16 M. Houston, 'Obituaries: Prof Anthony Clare: prolific psychiatrist and incisive interviewer', *Irish Times*, 3 November 2007.

17 R. Dudley Edwards, 'It is the mischief and laughter that I'll miss most about Tony', *Sunday Independent*, 4 November 2007.

18 Personal communication: A. Buckley, interview with BK (16 January 2019).

19 Act 5, Scene 2.

20 Personal communication: R.M. Murray, interview with BK (25 February 2018).

21 Personal communication: R. Jenkins, email to BK (2 August 2018).

22 Personal communication: J. Lucey, interview with BK (30 August 2018).

23   Ibid.

24   Personal communication: R.M. Murray, interview with BK (25 February 2018).

25   Personal communication: J. Shannon, email to MH (28 September 2018).

26   Personal communication: J. Lucey, interview with BK (30 August 2018).

27   Personal communications: A.W. Clare, correspondence to K. Ganter (12 December 1994) and correspondence (6 January 1995).

28   Personal communication: A.W. Clare, correspondence (20 April 1995).

29   Personal communications: A.W. Clare, correspondence (5 December 1994 and 11 August 1995).

30   Personal communication: A.W. Clare, correspondence (24 January 1997).

31   A. Clare, 'Nobody but ourselves to blame for hospital ills', *Sunday Independent*, 21 May 2000.

32   Personal communication: A.W. Clare, correspondence (2 December 1996).

33   Personal communication: A.W. Clare, correspondence (16 December 1999).

34   R. Dudley Edwards, 'It is the mischief and laughter that I'll miss most about Tony', *Sunday Independent*, 4 November 2007.

35   Personal communication: G. Meagan, email to BK (24 August 2018).

36   Personal communication: M. Browne, email to BK (25 March 2019).

37   A. Clare, 'Me and my shadow', *The Listener*, 7 July 1988

38   K.R. Jamison, *Touched with Fire: Manic Depressive Illness and the Artistic Temperament* (New York, NY: Free Press, 1993).

39   Clare, *In the Psychiatrist's Chair III*, pp. 194–5.

40   Ibid., p. 209.

41   Ibid., p. 220.

42   A.W. Clare, 'Touched with fire: manic depressive illness and the artistic temperament (book review)', *British Journal of Psychiatry*, 171, 4 (1 October 1997), 395.

43   K.R. Jamison, *Robert Lowell: Setting the River on Fire: A Study of Genius, Mania and Character* (New York: Alfred A. Knopf, 2017).

44   J. Banville, 'Recovering the poet's reputation', *Irish Times*, 15 April 2017. See also: P. Bosworth, 'Pathologies of a poet', *New York Times (International Edition)*, 8 March 2017; J. Cookson, 'Robert Lowell: setting the river on fire: a study of genius, mania and character

      (book review)', *British Journal of Psychiatry*, 212, 3 (1 March 2018), 185.

45   Jamison, *Robert Lowell: Setting the River on Fire: A Study of Genius, Mania and Character*, pp. 179–80.

46   Milligan and Clare, *Depression and How to Survive It*, p. 121.

47   Ibid., p. 140. See also: S. Brompton, 'Spike: my part in his upturn', *The Times*, 7 January 1993; J. Le Fanu, 'The black dogs of melancholia', *The Times*, 21 January 1993.

48   Personal communication: K.R. Jamison, email to BK (4 May 2018).

49   BBC Radio 4 Extra website: www.bbc. co.uk/programmes/b039dks7 (Accessed 8 December 2019).

50   Personal communication: A.W. Clare, correspondence (4 September 1995).

51   Personal communication: A.W. Clare, correspondence (27 February 1997).

52   Personal communication: A.W. Clare, correspondence (27 August 1990).

53   Clare, *In the Psychiatrist's Chair* (1992).

54   M. Gaffney, 'The view from the chair', *Irish Times*, 26 September 1992.

55   Personal communication: M. Gaffney, email to BK (4 June 2018).

56   Personal communication: A. Mann, interview with BK (2 July 2018).

57   Personal communication: R. Jenkins, email to BK (2 August 2018).

58   Personal communication: I. Browne, interview with BK (7 July 2018).

59   Personal communication: R.M. Murray, interview with BK (25 February 2018).

60   *Medicine Weekly*, 19 March 2008. See also: A. Clare, 'Plan for our children's future', *Medicine Weekly*, 20 June 2007.

61   St Patrick's University Hospital, *Annual Report and Financial Statements 2009* (Dublin: St Patrick's University Hospital, 2010).

62   D. Conroy, 'Marriage of memories behind brace of artistic, cultural carnivals', *Sunday Independent*, 13 May 2018.

63   Amergin Solstice Poetry Gathering, *Unde Scribitur* (An Daingean: Ponc Press, 2018).

64   P. Coleman and A. Clare, 'Me and my family', *Daily Telegraph*, 8 January 1993. See also: A. Clare, 'The nest of love and vipers', *The Listener*, 10 October 1985.

65   See, for example: C. Stott, 'Relative values: shrink resistant', *Sunday Times*, 12 April 1992; P. Deevy, 'In the psychiatrist's lair', *Sunday Independent*, 10 September

1995; M. Lavery, 'Keeper of the Clares', *Farmers Journal*, 25 November 2000.

66 Personal communication: I. Browne, interview with BK (7 July 2018).

67 Personal communication: R. Clare, interview with BK (7 March 2019). See also: J. Clare, 'Family ties', *Sunday Tribune*, 17 September 1995; A. Billen, 'Fame gives you pleasure, like drink or gambling or sex. It doesn't make you happy', *Evening Standard*, 26 July 2000; S. Durrant, 'Clare in the chair', *Guardian*, 31 July 2000.

68 Personal communication: P. Clare, interview with BK (9 February 2019).

69 Personal communication: J. Lucey, interview with BK (30 August 2018).

70 Ibid.

71 Kelly, *Hearing Voices: The History of Psychiatry in Ireland*, pp. 305–6.

72 M. Maher, 'Clare comes a long way from there to here', *Irish Times*, 12 December 1988.

73 Personal communication: correspondence to A. Clare (24 January 1986); World Health Organization, *ICD-10 Classification of Mental and Behavioural Disorders* (Geneva: World Health Organization, 1992), pp. 312, 322.

74 Personal communication: A.W. Clare, correspondence (11 September 1998).

75 B. Levin, 'Society's safety catch', *The Times*, 7 September 1987; B. Levin, 'You analyse; I'd rather just listen', *The Times*, 3 April 1997.

76 N. Browne, 'Laing's theories', *Irish Times*, 28 September 1989. See also: *Irish Times* Reporter, 'Stigma of mental illness persists here, says Clare', *Irish Times*, 15 September 1989; L. Craven, 'Mental illness', *Irish Times*, 26 September 1989.

77 Personal communication: J. Clare, interview with BK (7 June 2018).

78 Personal communication: R. Clare, interview with BK (7 March 2019).

79 Personal communication: J. Clare, interview with BK (23 June 2018).

80 Personal communication: P. Clare, interview with BK (9 February 2019).

81 M. Epstein, *Advice Not Given: A Guide to Getting Over Yourself* (Carlsbad, CA: Hay House, 2018), p. 17.

82 C. Rovelli, *The Order of Time* (London: Allen Lane/Penguin, 2018), p. 21.

83 Personal communication: K.R. Jamison, email to BK (4 May 2018).

84 Personal communication: J. Lucey, interview with BK (30 August 2018).

Anthony Clare: Chronology

Year	Developments in Psychiatry	Anthony Clare's Life and Work
1942	Ireland's mental health service is exclusively asylum-based; Ireland has the highest number of mental hospital beds per head of population of any country in the world.	Anthony Ward Clare is born in Dublin (24 December), the son of Bernard Clare, a solicitor, and Agnes Dunne.
1950s	• Jean Delay and Pierre Deniker in Paris publish data indicating the usefulness of chlorpromazine for the treatment of psychosis, making it the first effective medication for schizophrenia. • The American Psychiatric Association's *Diagnostic and Statistical Manual of Mental Disorders (DSM)* is published (1952).	Clare attends Gonzaga College, a Jesuit second-level school in Ranelagh, Dublin, where he excels academically and helps edit the school newspaper.
1960s	In 1961, three key books appear, challenging the very basis of contemporary psychiatry: Erving Goffman's *Asylums: Essays on the Social Situation of Mental Patients and Other Inmates* (Anchor Books, Doubleday & Co.), Michel Foucault's *Folie et Déraison: Histoire de la Folie à l'Âge Classique* (Plon) and Thomas Szasz's *The Myth of Mental Illness: Foundations of a Theory of Personal Conduct* (Harper & Row).	• Clare studies medicine at University College Dublin (UCD). • Clare is deeply involved in debating with the UCD Literary and Historical Society and wins the *Observer* Mace Trophy with debating colleague, Patrick Cosgrave (1964). • Clare and Cosgrave both write for UCD magazine, *St Stephen's*.

Year	Developments in Psychiatry	Anthony Clare's Life and Work
1966	*The Report of the Commission of Inquiry on Mental Illness* ('the 1966 Report') is written and published (1967), advocating a move away from mental hospitals and towards community-based mental health care in Ireland.	• Clare graduates as a medical doctor from UCD (June). • Clare commences a family practice rotating internship at St Joseph's Hospital, Syracuse, New York (July). • Clare marries Jane Hogan in Dublin (4 October).
1967		Clare commences postgraduate training in psychiatry at St Patrick's Hospital, Dublin, under Professor Norman Moore (July).
1968	The American Psychiatric Association's *Diagnostic and Statistical Manual of Mental Disorders (Second Edition) (DSM-II)* is published, re-classifying mental disorders.	Clare writes in *The Irish Times* about the dilemma that *Humanae Vitae*, a 1968 papal encyclical, presents to doctors who prescribe oral contraceptives (7 August), beginning a long association with national media outlets in Ireland and the United Kingdom.
1970s	Psychiatry goes through a period of radical challenge and change at global and local levels, including the delisting of homosexuality as a mental illness by the American Psychiatric Association (1973).	• Clare commences postgraduate training in psychiatry as a registrar and then senior registrar at the renowned Maudsley Hospital, London (1970). • Clare's first peer-reviewed scientific paper, 'Diazepam, alcohol, and barbiturate abuse', is published in the prestigious *British Medical Journal* (6 November 1971). • Clare authors and co-authors multiple peer-reviewed papers on topics including psychiatric training, alcoholism and mental illness in Irish migrants, clinical responsibility, ethical issues, electro-convulsive therapy (ECT), and 'fringe medicine'. • Clare graduates with an MPhil (*Magister Philosophiae*) in psychiatry for *A Study of Psychiatric Illness in an Immigrant Irish Population* (London University, 1972); he later publishes peer-reviewed papers on this topic (1974).
1976	Miloš Forman's film of Ken Kesey's novel (1962) *One Flew Over the Cuckoo's Nest* is released in the United Kingdom to sustained acclaim; it quickly becomes a classic.	• Clare reviews the film *One Flew Over the Cuckoo's Nest* for the *Lancet* (17 April). • Clare's *Psychiatry in Dissent: Controversial Issues in Thought and Practice* is published by Tavistock.

Year	Developments in Psychiatry	Anthony Clare's Life and Work
		Publications Limited and becomes a classic of the psychiatric literature. A second edition is published by Routledge in 1980. • Clare commences a six-year period in the General Practice Research Unit at the Institute of Psychiatry, London with Professor Michael Shepherd.
1979	The Irish Medical Association, in conjunction with the Health Education Bureau of Ireland, holds an 'International Symposium' on 'Alternatives to Drugs' in Dublin; it is addressed by Mr C.J. Haughey, Minister for Health and Social Welfare, and later Taoiseach (prime minister); Clare speaks about social methods of treatment for neurotic disorders and self-help approaches to mental illness.	Clare co-edits, with Paul Williams, *Psychosocial Disorders in General Practice* (Academic Press and Grune and Stratton) reflecting a key research interest of Clare's: mental disorder in general practice; Clare publishes voluminously on this topic over the course of his career.
1980	The American Psychiatric Association's *Diagnostic and Statistical Manual of Mental Disorders (Third Edition) (DSM-III)* is published, reflecting yet more changes in diagnostic systems in psychiatry.	Clare graduates with an MD (*Doctor of Medicine*, a higher degree) for his thesis titled *Psychiatric and Social Aspects of Premenstrual Complaint* (UCD), and publishes extensively on this topic, most notably a *Psychological Medicine Monograph Supplement*, 'Psychiatric and social aspects of premenstrual complaint' (1983).
1980s	In both the United Kingdom and Ireland, mental healthcare increasingly moves towards the provision of care in the community at large psychiatric hospitals continue to be dismantled and closed.	• Clare authors and co-authors multiple peer-reviewed papers on topics including community mental health, premenstrual syndrome, consent to treatment, psychiatry in general practice, social work, women and mental illness, the death penalty, mood disorders and clinical anxiety. • Clare co-writes, with Sally Thompson, *Let's Talk About Me: A Critical Examination of the New Psychotherapies* (BBC, 1981). • Clare has extensive media involvements including *Stop the Week* on BBC Radio 4.

Year	Developments in Psychiatry	Anthony Clare's Life and Work
1982	The *Irish Journal of Psychological Medicine* is founded by Dr Mark Hartman; Clare contributes extensively (1990, 1991, 1992, 1994, 1995, 1996, 1998, 2002, 2004, 2007).	• Clare co-edits, with Malcolm Lader, *Psychiatry and General Practice* (Academic Press); the book is very well received. • Clare is appointed Vice-Dean of the Institute of Psychiatry, London.
1982–2001	The nature and depth of broadcast interviewing changes substantially, largely in response to Clare's *In the Psychiatrist's Chair*.	Clare presents *In the Psychiatrist's Chair*, the BBC radio series that demystifies psychiatry, combining astute, robust psychological enquiry with unfailing inter-personal empathy; it is widely acclaimed.
1983	The United Kingdom's new Mental Health Act 1983 comes into effect (30 September), bringing significant changes to mental health practices there, especially involuntary care (a long-term interest of Clare's).	Clare is appointed Professor and Head of Psychological Medicine at St Bartholomew's Hospital, London ('Bart's').
1984	A new mental health policy is published in Ireland, *The Psychiatric Services – Planning for the Future*, consolidating the move towards community care.	Clare's *In the Psychiatrist's Chair* (Chatto & Windus/The Hogarth Press) is published, featuring interviews with actor Glenda Jackson, comedian Spike Milligan and others.
1986	Professor Karl O'Sullivan, medical director of St Patrick's Hospital in Dublin, edits *All in the Mind: Approaches to Mental Health* (Gill and Macmillan Ltd), a groundbreaking book on mental health in Ireland; Clare contributes a chapter on 'The concept of care in mental illness'.	Clare's book *Lovelaw: Love, Sex and Marriage Around the World* (BBC Publications) is published.
1987	The American Psychiatric Association's *Diagnostic and Statistical Manual of Mental Disorders (Third Edition, Revised) (DSM-III-R)* is published.	Clare contributes a chapter on 'Psychological medicine' to *Clinical Medicine: A Textbook for Medical Students and Doctors* (Ballière Tindall), edited by P.J. Kumar and M.L. Clark, and later contributes to the second (1990), third (1994), fourth (1998), fifth (2002, with P. White), sixth (2005, with P. White) and seventh editions (2009, with P.D. White); this book becomes a standard text.

Year	Developments in Psychiatry	Anthony Clare's Life and Work
1989	Controversial psychiatrist R.D. Laing, a complex but significant influence on Clare, dies (23 August); Clare writes a generous 'appreciation' (*Psychiatric Bulletin*, February 1990).	Clare returns to Dublin as medical director of St Patrick's Hospital (until 2000) and Clinical Professor of Psychiatry at Trinity College Dublin.
1990s	• The transition to community-based mental health care continues in both the United Kingdom and Ireland. • Christopher Clunis, a person with schizophrenia, kills Jonathan Zito, a bystander, in London (1992); the case commands considerable public attention and Clare comments on it in his 1994 lecture on 'Violence, mental illness and society', the twenty-third in the series of the Stevens Lectures for the Laity at The Royal	• Clare authors and co-authors multiple peer-reviewed papers on topics including depression, psychotherapy, chronic fatigue syndrome, hormones and mental illness, communication and the media, psychiatric classification, anti-depressants, psychiatric aspects of abortion, obsessive-compulsive and personality disorders, suicide and psychiatric history. • As medical director, Clare introduces many changes at St Patrick's Hospital in Dublin: new facilities, funding for research posts, strengthening postgraduate training and attracting world leaders to speak at the annual 'Founder's Day' meeting.
1990	Society of Medicine in London, in which Clare robustly highlights deficits in community mental healthcare.	Clare leads a group of colleagues and collaborators in an editorial in the *Irish Journal of Psychological Medicine* focused on the 'Advancement of psychiatric research in Ireland: proposal for a national body' (September).
1991		Clare contributes a chapter on 'The mad Irish?' to *Mental Health in Ireland* (Gill and Macmillan and Radio Telefís Éireann), edited by Colm Keane.
1991–7		Clare chairs the Prince of Wales's Advisory Group on Disability.
1992	The World Health Organisation's *ICD-10 Classification of Mental and Behavioural Disorders* is published (1992) and receives considerable public attention; Clare is involved in its preparation.	Clare's *In the Psychiatrist's Chair* (William Heinemann Ltd) is published, featuring interviews with Anthony Hopkins, Eartha Kitt and R.D. Laing, among others.
1993		Clare co-writes, with comedian Spike Milligan, *Depression and How to Survive It* (Ebury Press/Random House Group); it becomes an enduring feature of the popular literature on depression.

Year	Developments in Psychiatry	Anthony Clare's Life and Work
1994	The American Psychiatric Association's *Diagnostic and Statistical Manual of Mental Disorders (Fourth Edition) (DSM-IV)* is published, once again re-classifying mental disorders.	Clare co-writes a series of papers relating to obsessive compulsive disorder, discontinuation of anti-depressants, consultation-liaison psychiatry, abortion, and violence, mental illness and society.
1995	The sixth series of Linacre Lectures (1995/6), a high-profile public lecture series focused on issues of environment and cross-disciplinary research, takes place at Linacre College, a graduate college of the University of Oxford; Clare contributes with a lecture titled 'Meeting of minds: the import of family and society'.	Clare's *In the Psychiatrist's Chair II* (Mandarin/William Heinemann Ltd) is published, featuring interviews with Ruth Rendell, Joanna Lumley and Cecil Parkinson, among others.
1996		Clare writes a moving obituary of Professor Norman Moore, a huge influence on Clare's career and on Irish psychiatry (*Psychiatric Bulletin*, December).
1998	Leading figures in world psychiatry accept Clare's invitations to speak at 'Founder's Day' in St Patrick's Hospital throughout the 1990s, including Professor Kenneth Kendler from Virginia Commonwealth University (1998).	Clare's *In the Psychiatrist's Chair III* (Chatto & Windus/Random House) is published, featuring interviews with Stephen Fry, Nigel Kennedy, Uri Geller and Paul Theroux, among others.
2000	The American Psychiatric Association's *Diagnostic and Statistical Manual of Mental Disorders (Fourth Edition, Text Revision)* (DSM-IV-TR) is published, with added information.	Clare's *On Men: Masculinity in Crisis* (Chatto & Windus) is published and widely discussed in the media.
2000s	New mental health legislation is developed and introduced in Ireland, the Mental Health Act 2001 (fully implemented in 2006).	Clare authors and co-authors multiple peer-reviewed papers on topics including psychiatry of later life, depression following child sexual abuse, immigration and mental health, suicide attempts and the future of psychiatric training.

Year	Developments in Psychiatry	Anthony Clare's Life and Work
2003	Ian Falloon's paper on 'Family interventions for mental disorders: efficacy and effectiveness' is published in *World Psychiatry* (February 2003); like Clare, Falloon worked at the Institute of Psychiatry in London and Clare is a strong supporter of Falloon's emphasis on family involvement in mental health care.	• Clare co-writes, with Caroline Smyth and Malcolm MacLachlan, *Cultivating Suicide? Destruction of Self in a Changing Ireland* (The Liffey Press). • Clare becomes a director of Plan Ireland, a development and humanitarian organisation that advances children's rights and equality for girls (www.plan.ie).
2006	A new mental health policy is published in Ireland, *A Vision for Change*; it re-affirms a commitment to community-based mental healthcare and urges renewed focus on developing and sustaining mental health services.	Clare writes: 'There is a book to be written about the current controversies in psychiatry … There is still an enormous conceptual problem regarding psychiatric illness … That is why the stigma concerning psychiatric illness exhibits such robustness. That is why there is such fear and denial and rejection … Perhaps I will write something on these issues but at the present time I have other things preoccupying me and this will have to wait' (1 September).
2007	The Royal College of Psychiatrists awards honorary fellowship to Clare; it is psychiatry's highest honour.	Clare dies suddenly in Paris (28 October); he is widely and deeply mourned.

Acknowledgements

· ·

We are very grateful to everyone who spoke with us, wrote to us, and emailed us during the preparation of this book. Your insights and comments have added immeasurably to our work and we thank you for your generosity and assistance. We are especially grateful to Jane Clare, Rachel Clare, Peter Clare and all of the Clare family who were incredibly helpful, supportive and generous from the outset; without them, this book could not have been written.

We greatly appreciate the support and guidance of our agent, Ms Vanessa O'Loughlin of the Inkwell Group (www.inkwellwriters.ie), Professor Lesley Rees, Mr Gareth Rees, Mr Sebastian Cody, Ms Laura Cook, Dr Mary Canning, Professor Ivor Browne, Dr Mary O'Hanlon, Ms Caroline Sherlock (St Patrick's Mental Health Services), Ms Harriet Wheelock (Heritage Centre, Royal College of Physicians of Ireland), Ms Geraldine Meagan (MedMedia Group, Dún Laoghaire, County Dublin), Ms June Shannon, Brenda Fitzsimons (picture editor, *The Irish Times*), Eoin McVey (managing editor, *The Irish Times*), Ms Liz Kearney (*Irish Independent* and *The Herald*) and Mr Michael Bevan (Gonzaga College SJ).

Brendan Kelly would like to thank, first and foremost, Regina, Eoin and Isabel. I am also very grateful to my parents (Mary and Desmond), sisters (Sinéad and Niamh) and nieces (Aoife and Aisling). Mention must also be made of Trixie, Terry and, of course, Sheldon. I appreciate the ongoing advice and guidance of Dr Larkin Feeney, Dr John Bruzzi and Dr Aidan Collins. I am also very grateful to Professor Veronica O'Keane, Ms Alison Collie and all my colleagues at Trinity College Dublin and Tallaght University Hospital, Professor Sharlene Walbaum (Quinnipiac University), Dr Cathy Smith (University of Northampton), Professor Jon Stobart (Manchester Metropolitan University) and my teachers at Scoil Chaitríona, Renmore, Galway; St Joseph's Patrician College, Nun's Island, Galway (especially my history teacher, Mr Ciaran Doyle); and the School of Medicine at NUI Galway.

Muiris Houston would like to thank, firstly, Marion, Críosa, Fionán, Dearbhaile and Aoibheann. I appreciate the guidance and advice of Dr

257

Damian Mohan, Prof Tom O'Dowd, Prof Bill Shannon, Prof Davis Coakley, Dr Gerry Cummins and Dr Michael Boland. I am grateful to the editors of *The Irish Times*, from Conor Brady to Paul O'Neill, who have supported my work as a medical journalist. I wish to thank the former editor of the IT health page, Sheila Wayman, and the editors of the *Health and Family* supplement from Kevin O'Sullivan to Damian Cullen for their encouragement and collegiality. Willy Clingan, my first news editor, deserves a medal for his patience in helping me develop as a rookie news correspondent. And I would like to acknowledge the influence of the late Kathryn Holmquist and Sylvia Thompson, *Irish Times* journalists of the highest quality. I wrote my first 'second opinion' column for *Medicine Weekly* with the encouragement of editor Robert Love; I am also grateful to Dara Gantly, editor of *The Irish Medical Times*, and Paul Mulholland, editor of the *Medical Independent*. In Trinity College Dublin, I wish to thank Dr Aileen Patterson, Professor of Medical Education, for facilitating the development of my narrative medicine module for medical students. I would like to thank Prof Orla Hardiman in the Department of Academic Neurology and her colleagues Miriam Galvin and Deirdre Murray for encouraging my research into the stories of people with motor neurone disease. In NUI Galway, I wish to acknowledge the support of Dr Ger Flaherty, Professor of Medical Education, and Prof Declan Devane, Cochrane and Evidence Synthesis enthusiast *par excellence*.

Permissions

We are very grateful to *The Irish Times* for permission to quote from that newspaper. All extracts from the *Guardian* and *Observer* are courtesy of Guardian News & Media Ltd. Material adapted from B.D. Kelly and L. Feeney, 'Psychiatry: no longer in dissent?', *Psychiatric Bulletin*, 30, 9 (1 September 2006), 344–5, is reprinted with permission of Cambridge University Press. Quotations from A.W. Clare, *Violence, Mental Illness and Society: The Stevens Lectures for the Laity 1994* (London: The Royal Society of Medicine, 1994) are reproduced by kind permission of the Royal Society of Medicine. Material from *Studies: An Irish Quarterly Review* is reproduced by kind permission of the editor.

We are very grateful to the editors, publishers, authors and copyright holders who permitted reuse of material in this book. All reasonable efforts have been made to contact the copyright holders for all material used. If any have been omitted, please contact the publisher.

Bibliography

● ●

Works by Anthony W. Clare

Books (Anthony W. Clare) (Chronological Order)

Clare, A., *Psychiatry in Dissent: Controversial Issues in Thought and Practice* (London: Tavistock Publications Ltd, 1976).

Clare, A., *Psychiatry in Dissent: Controversial Issues in Thought and Practice (Second Edition)* (London and New York: Routledge, 1980).

Clare, A.W. and S. Thompson, *Let's Talk About Me: A Critical Examination of the New Psychotherapies* (London: British Broadcasting Corporation, 1981).

Clare, A., *In the Psychiatrist's Chair* (London: Chatto & Windus/The Hogarth Press, 1984).

Clare, A., *Lovelaw: Love, Sex and Marriage Around the World* (London: BBC Publications, 1986).

Clare, A., *In the Psychiatrist's Chair* (London: William Heinemann Ltd, 1992).

Milligan, S. and A. Clare, *Depression and How to Survive It* (London: Ebury Press/Random House Group, 1993).

Clare, A.W., *Violence, Mental Illness and Society: The Stevens Lectures for the Laity 1994.* London: The Royal Society of Medicine, 1994.

Clare, A., *In the Psychiatrist's Chair II* (London: Mandarin/William Heinemann Ltd, 1995).

Clare, A., *In the Psychiatrist's Chair III* (London: Chatto & Windus/Random House, 1998).

Clare, A., *On Men: Masculinity in Crisis* (London: Chatto & Windus, 2000).

Smyth, C., M. MacLachlan and A. Clare, *Cultivating Suicide? Destruction of Self in a Changing Ireland* (Dublin: The Liffey Press, 2003).

Books Co-edited (Anthony W. Clare) (Chronological Order)

Williams, P. and A. Clare (eds), *Psychosocial Disorders in General Practice* (London and New York: Academic Press and Grune and Stratton, 1979).

Clare, A.W. and M. Lader (eds), *Psychiatry and General Practice* (London: Academic Press, 1982).

Book Chapters and Book Contributions (Anthony W. Clare) (Chronological Order)

Williams, P. and A.W. Clare, 'Preface', in P. Williams and A. Clare (eds), *Psychosocial Disorders in General Practice* (London and New York: Academic Press and Grune and Stratton, 1979), xi–xii.

Williams, P. and A.W. Clare, 'Introduction', in P. Williams and A. Clare (eds), *Psychosocial Disorders in General Practice* (London and New York: Academic Press and Grune and Stratton, 1979), 3–7.

Clare, A.W. and V.E. Cairns, 'A standardized interview to assess social maladjustment and dysfunction', in P. Williams and A. Clare (eds), *Psychosocial Disorders in General Practice* (London and New York: Academic Press and Grune and Stratton, 1979), 29–43.

A.W. Clare and P. Williams, 'Future trends in research into primary care psychiatry: a personal view', in P. Williams and A. Clare (eds), *Psychosocial Disorders in General Practice* (London and New York: Academic Press and Grune and Stratton, 1979), 325–32.

Shepherd, M. and A. Clare, 'Addendum: developments since 1966', in M. Shepherd, B. Cooper, A.C. Brown and G. Kalton, *Psychiatric Illness in General Practice*

(Second Edition) (Oxford: Oxford University Press, 1981), 208–27.

Clare, A.W. and M. Lader, 'Preface', in A.W. Clare and M. Lader (eds), *Psychiatry and General Practice* (London: Academic Press, 1982), xi–xiv.

Clare, A.W., 'Problems of psychiatric classification in general practice', in A.W. Clare and M. Lader (eds), *Psychiatry and General Practice* (London: Academic Press, 1982), 15–25.

Clare, A.W. and K. Sabbagh, 'Appendix: general practice consultation video exercise', in A.W. Clare and M. Lader (eds), *Psychiatry and General Practice* (London: Academic Press, 1982), 26–32.

Clare, A., 'The concept of care in mental illness', in K. O'Sullivan (ed.), *All in the Mind: Approaches to Mental Health* (Dublin: Gill and Macmillan Ltd, 1986), 16–23.

Clare, A.W., 'Psychological medicine', in P.J. Kumar and M.L. Clark (eds), *Clinical Medicine: A Textbook for Medical Students and Doctors* (London: Ballière Tindall, 1987), 868–900.

Clare, A.W., 'Psychological medicine', in P.J. Kumar and M.L. Clark (eds), *Clinical Medicine: A Textbook for Medical Students and Doctors (Second Edition)* (London: Ballière Tindall, 1990), 965–99.

Clare, A., 'Foreword', in N. Kfir and M. Slevin, *Challenging Cancer: From Chaos to Control* (London and New York: Tavistock/Routledge, 1991), xi.

Clare, A., 'The mad Irish?', in C. Keane (ed.), *Mental Health in Ireland* (Dublin: Gill and Macmillan and Radio Telefís Éireann, 1991), 4–17.

Clare, A.W., 'Foreword', in P.J. Taylor (ed.), *Violence in Society* (London: Royal College of Physicians of London, 1993), iii–iv.

Clare, A.W., 'Psychological medicine', in P. Kumar and M. Clark (eds), *Clinical Medicine: A Textbook for Medical Students and Doctors (Third Edition)* (London: Ballière Tindall, 1994), 957–91.

Clare, A., 'Nervous breakdown', in C. Keane (ed.), *Nervous Breakdown* (Cork and Dublin: Mercier Press and Radio Telefís Éireann, 1994), 17–26.

Clare, A., 'Foreword', in E. Lee, *Mental Health Care: A Workbook for Care Workers* (London: Palgrave Macmillan, 1997), v.

Clare, A.W., 'Meeting of minds: the import of family and society', in B. Cartledge (ed.), *Mind, Brain and the Environment: The Linacre Lectures 1995–6* (Oxford: Oxford University Press, 1998), 144–57.

Clare, A.W., 'Psychological medicine' in P. Kumar and M. Clark (eds), *Kumar and Clark: Clinical Medicine: A Textbook for Medical Students and Doctors (Fourth Edition)* (Edinburgh: W.B. Saunders, 1998), 1105–47.

White, P. and A.W. Clare, 'Psychological medicine', in P. Kumar and M. Clark (eds), *Kumar & Clark: Clinical Medicine (Fifth Edition)* (Edinburgh: W.B. Saunders, 2002), 1225–70.

Clare, A.W., 'Foreword to the first edition', in M. Slevin and N. Kfir, *Challenging Cancer: Fighting Back, Taking Control, Finding Options (Second Edition)* (London: Class Publishing, 2002), xiii.

Clare, A.W., 'Foreword', in R.S. Kirby, C.C. Carson, M.G. Kirby and R.N. Farah (eds), *Men's Health (Second Edition)* (London: Taylor & Francis, 2004), xiii.

White, P. and A.W. Clare, 'Psychological medicine', in P. Kumar and M. Clark (eds), *Kumar & Clark: Clinical Medicine (Sixth Edition)* (Edinburgh: Elsevier Saunders, 2005), 1273–314.

White, P.D. and A.W. Clare, 'Psychological medicine', in P. Kumar and M. Clark (eds), *Kumar & Clark's Clinical Medicine (Seventh Edition)* (Edinburgh: Saunders Elsevier, 2009), 1185–223.

University Theses (Anthony W. Clare) (Chronological Order)

Clare, A.W., 'A Study of Psychiatric Illness in an Immigrant Irish Population' (MPhil (Psychiatry) Thesis, London University, 1972).

Clare, A.W., 'Psychiatric and Social Aspects of Premenstrual Complaint' (MD Thesis, University College Dublin, 1980).

Papers in Peer-Reviewed Journals (Anthony W. Clare) (Chronological Order)

Bird, J., P. Campbell, A. Clare, J. Hamilton, A. Maiden, W. Marsh, A. McDowall, P. O'Farrell, E. Owens, D. Storer, R. Symonds, and E. Worrall, 'Association of Psychiatrists in Training', *Lancet*, 298, 7724 (11 September 1971), 597.

Adams, R.C., and over 300 others including A.W. Clare, 'Examination for the MRCPsych', *Lancet*, 298, 7724 (11 September 1971), 598–9.

Clare, A.W., 'Diazepam, alcohol, and barbiturate abuse', *British Medical Journal*, 4, 5783 (6 November 1971), 340.

Clare, A.W., 'Training of psychiatrists', *Lancet*, 300, 7780 (7 October 1972), 753–6.

Clare, A.W. and J.G. Cooney, 'Alcoholism and road accidents', *Journal of the Irish Medical Association*, 66, 11 (9 June 1973), 281–6.

Bowden, P. and A.W. Clare, 'Redeployment of registrar and senior-registrar posts', *Lancet*, 302, 7833 (13 October 1973), 856–7.

Clare, A.W., 'Mental illness in the Irish emigrant', *Journal of the Irish Medical Association*, 67, 1 (12 January 1974), 20–4.

Clare, A.W., 'Alcoholism and schizophrenia in Irishmen in London – a reassessment', *British Journal of Addiction to Alcohol and Other Drugs*, 69, 3 (September 1974), 207–12.

Clare, A.W., 'The mind of the kidnapper', *Nursing Mirror and Midwives Journal*, 142, 15 (8 April 1976), 47–8.

Clare, A.W., 'One Flew Over the Cuckoo's Nest (film review)', *Lancet*, 307, 7964 (17 April 1976), 851.

Clare, A.W., 'Psychiatry in dissent', *Nursing Mirror and Midwives Journal*, 143, 15 (7 October 1976), 61–2.

Clare, A.W., 'Psychological profiles of women complaining of premenstrual symptoms', *Current Medical Research and Opinion*, 4, suppl. 4 (1977), 23–8.

Clare, A.W., 'Handbook for inceptors and trainees in psychiatry (book review)', *Psychiatric Bulletin*, 1, 2 (1 August 1977), 15.

Clare, A.W., 'Clinical responsibility: II. Where does the patient stand? When did you last see your psychiatrist?', *British Medical Journal*, 2, 6103 (24–31 December 1977), 1637–42.

Clare, A.W., 'Therapeutic and ethical aspects of electro-convulsive therapy: a British perspective', *International Journal of Law and Psychiatry*, 1, 3 (1978), 237–5.

Clare, A.W., 'In defence of compulsory psychiatric intervention', *Lancet*, 311, 8075 (3 June 1978), 1197–8.

Clare, A.W., 'Treatment or torture', *Midwife, Health Visitor and Community Nurse*, 14, 7 (July 1978), 205–6.

Clare, A.W. and V.E. Cairns, 'Design, development and use of a standardised interview to assess social maladjustment and dysfunction in community studies', *Psychological Medicine*, 8, 4 (November 1978), 589–604.

Cutting, J.C., A.W. Clare and A.H. Mann, 'Cycloid psychosis: an investigation of the diagnostic concept', *Psychological Medicine*, 8, 4 (November 1978), 637–48.

Clare, A.W., 'Fringe medicine and beyond', *Journal of the Irish Medical Association*, 72, 12 (suppl) (1979), 30–4.

Toone, B.K., R. Murray, A. Clare, F. Creed and A. Smith, 'Psychiatrists' models of mental illness and their personal backgrounds', *Psychological Medicine*, 9, 1 (February 1979), 165–78.

Clare, A.W., 'The causes of alcoholism', *British Journal of Hospital Medicine*, 21, 4 (April 1979), 403–11.

Clare, A.W., 'Ethical issues in psychiatry', *Practitioner*, 223, 1333 (July 1979), 89–96.

Clare, A.W., 'The treatment of premenstrual symptoms', *British Journal of Psychiatry*, 135, 6 (December 1979), 576–9.

Clare, A.W., 'Community mental health centres', *Journal of the Royal Society of Medicine*, 73, 1 (January 1980), 75–6.

Bebbington, P., J.L.T. Birley, A.W. Clare, J. Cutting, R. Kumar, A. Mann, P. Mullen, P. Williams and D.H. Bennett, 'Unmodified ECT', *Lancet*, 315, 8168 (Pt 1) (15 March 1980), 599.

Williams, P., A. Tarnopolsky and A.W. Clare, 'Recent advances in the epidemiological study of minor psychiatric disorder', *Journal of the Royal Society of Medicine*, 73, 9 (September 1980), 679–80.

Clare, A.W., 'Progesterone, fluid, and electrolytes in premenstrual syndrome', *British Medical Journal*, 281, 6234 (20 September 1980), 810–11.

Clare, A.W., 'Premenstrual syndrome', *British Journal of Psychiatry*, 138, 1 (1 January 1981), 82–3.

Clare, A.W., 'Consent to treatment', *Journal of the Royal Society of Medicine*, 74, 11 (November 1981), 787–9.

Murray, J., P. Williams and A. Clare, 'Health and social characteristics of long-term psychotropic drug-takers', *Social Science and Medicine*, 16, 18 (1982), 1595–8.

Williams, P., J. Murray and A. Clare, 'A longitudinal study of psychotropic drug prescription', *Psychological Medicine*, 12, 1 (February 1982), 201–6.

Briscoe, M.E. and A.W. Clare, 'The health visitor and prevention', *British Medical Journal (Clinical Research Edition)*, 285, 6343 (11 September 1982), 740.

Corney, R.H., A. W. Clare and J. Fry, 'The development of a self-report questionnaire to identify social problems: a pilot study',

Psychological Medicine, 12, 4 (November 1982), 903–9.

Clare, A.W., 'The dying don't need analytic psychotherapy', *Journal of Medical Ethics*, 8, 4 (December 1982), 213.

Clare, A.W., 'Psychiatric and social aspects of premenstrual complaint', *Psychological Medicine Monograph Supplement*, 4 (1983), 1–58.

Clare, A.W, 'Psycho-social morbidity in general practice', *Practitioner*, 227, 1375 (January 1983), 35–44.

Corney, R.H. and A.W. Clare, 'The effectiveness of attached social workers in the management of depressed women in general practice', *British Journal of Social Work*, 13, 1 (1 January 1983), 57–74.

Clare, A.W., 'Psychiatry in general practice', *Journal of the Royal College of General Practitioners*, 33, 249 (April 1983), 195–8.

Clare, A.W., 'Premenstrual tension: psychological aspects', *Irish Journal of Medical Science*, 152 (suppl. 2) (June 1983), 33–43.

Clare, A.W., 'The relationship between psychopathology and the menstrual cycle', *Women and Health*, 8, 2–3 (Summer–Fall 1983), 125–36.

O'Sullivan, K., P. Whillans, M. Daly, B. Carroll, A. Clare and J. Cooney, 'A comparison of alcoholics with and without co-existing affective disorder', *British Journal of Psychiatry*, 143, 2 (August 1983), 133–8.

Clare, A.W., 'Behavior and the menstrual cycle (sexual behavior series, vol. 1) (book review)', *Journal of Psychosomatic Research*, 28, 4 (1984), 349.

Clare, A.W., R.H. Corney and V.E. Cairns, 'Social adjustment: the design and use of an instrument for social work and social work research', *British Journal of Social Work*, 14, 1 (1 January 1984), 323–36.

Clare, A.W., 'Alcohol education and the medical student', *Alcohol and Alcoholism*, 19, 4 (1 January 1984), 291–6.

Corney, R.H., A. Cooper and A.W. Clare, 'Seeking help for marital problems: the role of the general practitioner', *Journal of the Royal College of General Practitioners*, 34, 265 (August 1984), 431–3.

Clare, A.W., 'Sex and mood', *Health and Hygiene: Journal of the Royal Institute of Public Health and Hygiene*, 6 (1985), 43–60.

Clare, A.W., 'Hormones, behaviour and the menstrual cycle', *Journal of Psychosomatic Research*, 29, 3 (1985), 225–33.

Clare, A.W., '"The other half of medicine" and St Bartholomew's Hospital', *British Journal of Psychiatry*, 146, 2 (1 February 1985), 120–6.

Clare, A., K. Rawnsley and M. Roth, 'Dr Anatoly Koryagin', *Psychiatric Bulletin*, 9, 4 (1 April 1985), 80.

Clare, A.W., 'Psychiatry: beyond analysis (book review)', *Nature*, 314, 6013 (25 April 1985), 696–7.

Corney, R.H. and A.W. Clare, 'The construction, development and testing of a self-report questionnaire to identify social problems', *Psychological Medicine*, 15, 3 (August 1985), 637–49.

Clare, A. W., 'Myth, magic and the common solution (book review)', *Nature*, 316, 6029 (15 August 1985), 584.

Clare, A.W., 'Premenstrual syndrome: single or multiple causes?', *Canadian Journal of Psychiatry*, 30, 7 (November 1985), 474–82.

Clare, A.W., 'Where lies the science? (book review)', *Nature*, 318, 6042 (14 November 1985), 112–13.

Jenkins, R. and A.W. Clare, 'Women and mental illness', *British Medical Journal (Clinical Research Edition)*, 291, 6508 (30 November 1985), 1521–2.

Blacker, C.V. and A.W. Clare, 'Depression in general practice', *British Journal of Psychiatry*, 148, 3 (1 March 1986), 333–5.

Besser, G.M., A.W. Clare, C.J. Dickinson, N. Joels, O.J. Lewis, D.F.J. Mason, G.M. Rees, M.R. Salkind, E.D.R. Stone and R.F.M. Wood, 'Future of Bart's preclinical school', *Lancet*, 327, 8483 (29 March 1986), 741.

Friedman, D.E., A.W. Clare, L.H. Rees and A. Grossman, 'Should impotent males who have no clinical evidence of hypogonadism have routine endocrine screening?', *Lancet*, 327, 8488 (3 May 1986), 1041.

Clare, A.W., 'Going into a trance (book review)', *Nature*, 324, 6098 (18 December 1986), 624.

Adshead, F. and A.W. Clare, 'Doctors' double standards on alcohol', *British Medical Journal (Clinical Research Edition)*, 293, 6562 (20–27 December 1986), 1590–1.

Clare, A.W., 'Developing a policy for a district alcohol service', *Practitioner*, 231, 1425 (8 March 1987), 318–21.

Clare, A.W., 'Doctors and the death penalty: an international issue', *British Medical Journal (Clinical Research Edition)*, 294, 6581 (9 May 1987), 1180–1.

Blacker, C.V. and A.W. Clare, 'Depressive disorder in primary care', *British Journal of Psychiatry*, 150, 6 (1 June 1987), 737–51.

Clare, A.W., 'The clinical process in psychiatry (book review)', *Journal of Neurology, Neurosurgery and Psychiatry*, 50, 8 (August 1987), 1089–90.

Clare, A. and M. Bristow, 'Drinking drivers: the needs for research and rehabilitation', *British Medical Journal (Clinical Research Edition)*, 295, 6611 (5 December 1987), 1432–3.

Blacker, C.V. and A.W. Clare, 'The prevalence and treatment of depression in general practice', *Psychopharmacology*, 95, 1 (suppl.) (March 1988), S14–17.

O'Sullivan, K., C. Rynne, J. Miller, S. O'Sullivan, V. Fitzpatrick, M. Hux, J. Cooney and A. Clare, 'A follow-up study on alcoholics with and without co-existing affective disorder', *British Journal of Psychiatry*, 152, 6 (1 June 1988), 813–9.

Corney, R.H. and A.W. Clare, 'The treatment of premenstrual syndrome', *Practitioner*, 233, 1463 (22 February 1989), 233–6.

Davidson, K. and Clare, A.W., 'Psychotic illness following termination of pregnancy', *British Journal of Psychiatry*, 154, 4 (1 April 1989), 559–60.

Clare, A.W., 'Aggiornamento sull'ansia clinica: Una rassegna della letteratura attuale sulla definizione e classificazione dell'ansia e il dibattito sulle modalità di trattamento' ('Update on clinical anxiety: A review of the current literature on the definition and classification of anxiety and the debate on treatment methods'), *Rivista di Psichiatria*, 24, 2 (April–June 1989), 89–94.

Corney, R.H., R. Stanton, R. Newell and A.W. Clare, 'Comparison of progesterone, placebo and behavioural psychotherapy in the treatment of premenstrual syndrome', *Journal of Psychosomatic Obstetrics and Gynecology*, 11, 3 (1990), 211–20.

Clare, A.W., 'The alcohol problem in universities and the professions', *Alcohol and Alcoholism*, 25, 2–3 (1 January 1990), 277–85.

Clare, A.W., 'Ronald David Laing 1927–1989: an appreciation', *Psychiatric Bulletin*, 14, 2 (1 February 1990), 87–8.

Ball, R.A. and A.W. Clare, 'Symptoms and social adjustment in Jewish depressives', *British Journal of Psychiatry*, 156, 3 (1 March 1990), 379–83.

Clare, A., R.J. Daly, T.G. Dinan, D. King, B.E. Leonard, C. O'Boyle, J. O'Connor, J. Waddington, N. Walsh and M. Webb, 'Advancement of psychiatric research in Ireland: proposal for a national body', *Irish Journal of Psychological Medicine*, 7, 2 (September 1990), 93.

Clare, A., 'Depression in schizophrenics (book review)', *Irish Journal of Psychological Medicine*, 7, 2 (September 1990), 180–2.

Corney, R.H., R. Stanton, R. Newell, A. Clare and P. Fairclough, 'Behavioural psychotherapy in the treatment of irritable bowel syndrome', *Journal of Psychosomatic Research*, 35, 4–5 (1991), 461–9.

O'Hanlon, M., S. Barry, A.W. Clare and T.G. Dinan, 'Serum thyrotropin responses to thyrotropin-releasing hormone in alcohol-dependent patients with and without depression', *Journal of Affective Disorders*, 21, 2 (February 1991), 109–15.

Sharpe, M.C., L.C. Archard, J.E. Banatvala, L.K. Borysiewicz, A.W. Clare, A. David, R.H.T. Edwards, K.E.H. Hawton, H.P. Lambert, R.J.M. Lane, E.M. McDonald, J.F. Mowbray, D.J. Pearson, T.E.A. Peto, V.R. Preedy, A.P. Smith, D.G. Smith, D.J. Taylor, D.A.J. Tyrrell, S. Wessely, P.D. White, P.O. Behan, F. Clifford Rose, T.J. Peters, P.G. Wallace, D.A. Warrell and D.J.M Wright, 'A report: chronic fatigue syndrome: guidelines for research', *Journal of the Royal Society of Medicine*, 84, 2 (February 1991), 118–21.

Clare, A.W., 'A guide to psychiatry in primary care (book review)', *Irish Journal of Psychological Medicine*, 8, 1 (March 1991), 86.

Clare, A.W., 'Health psychology and public health (book review)', *Social Policy and Administration*, 25, 2 (June 1991), 164–6.

Lucey, J.V., V. O'Keane, K. O'Flynn, A.W. Clare and T.G. Dinan, 'Gender and age differences in the growth hormone response to pyridostigmine', *International Clinical Psychopharmacology*, 6, 2 (Summer 1991), 105–9.

Swanwick, G.R.J. and A.W. Clare, 'The management of insomnia', *Journal of the Irish Colleges of Physicians and Surgeons*, 20, 4 (October 1991), 249–50.

Clare, A.W., 'Mental health and the media', *Journal of Mental Health*, 1, 1 (1992), 1–2.

Bristow, M.F. and A.W. Clare, 'Prevalence and characteristics of at-risk drinkers among elderly acute medical in-patients', *British Journal of Addiction*, 87, 2 (February 1992), 291–4.

Lucey, J.V., G. Butcher, A.W. Clare and T.G. Dinan, 'Buspirone induced prolactin responses in obsessive-compulsive disorder (OCD): is OCD a 5-HT2 receptor disorder?', *International Clinical*

Psychopharmacology, 7, 1 (Spring 1992), 45–9.

Clare, A., W. Gulbinat and N. Sartorius, 'A triaxial classification of health problems presenting in primary health care: a World Health Organization multi-centre study', *Social Psychiatry and Psychiatric Epidemiology*, 27, 3 (May 1992), 108–16.

Ur, E., T.G. Dinan, V. O'Keane, A.W. Clare, L. McLoughlin, L.H. Rees, T.H. Turner, A. Grossman and G.M. Besser, 'Effect of metyrapone on the pituitary-adrenal axis in depression: relation to dexamethasone suppressor status', *Neuroendocrinology*, 56, 4 (October 1992), 533–8.

Lucey, J.V., V. O'Keane, G. Butcher, A.W. Clare and T.G. Dinan, 'Cortisol and prolactin responses to d-fenfluramine in non-depressed patients with obsessive-compulsive disorder: a comparison with depressed and healthy controls', *British Journal of Psychiatry*, 161, 4 (1 October 1992), 517–21.

Farren, C., D. McLoughlin and A. Clare, 'Procedures for involuntary admission to public and private psychiatric facilities', *Irish Journal of Psychological Medicine*, 9, 2 (November 1992), 96–100.

Clare, A., 'The 1992 Jansson Memorial Lecture: communication in medicine', *European Journal of Disorders of Communication*, 28, 1 (1993), 1–12.

Lucey, J.V., G. Butcher, A.W. Clare and T.G. Dinan, 'The anterior pituitary responds normally to protirelin in obsessive-compulsive disorder: evidence to support a neuroendocrine serotonergic deficit', *Acta Psychiatrica Scandinavica*, 87, 6 (June 1993), 384–8.

Lucey, J.V., G. Butcher, A.W. Clare and T.G. Dinan, 'Elevated growth hormone responses to pyridostigmine in obsessive-compulsive disorder: evidence of cholinergic supersensitivity', *American Journal of Psychiatry*, 150, 6 (June 1993), 961–2.

Clare, A.W., 'Scenes of madness: a psychiatrist at the theatre (book review)', *American Journal of Psychiatry*, 150, 12 (December 1993), 1888.

Lucey, J.V., G. Butcher, K. O'Flynn, A.W. Clare and G. Dinan, 'The growth hormone response to baclofen in obsessive compulsive disorder: does the GABA-B receptor mediate obsessive anxiety?', *Pharmacopsychiatry*, 27, 1 (January 1994), 23–6.

Montgomery, S.A., J. Henry, G. McDonald, T. Dinan, M. Lader, I. Hindmarch, A.

Clare and D. Nutt, 'Selective serotonin reuptake inhibitors: meta-analysis of discontinuation rates', *International Clinical Psychopharmacology*, 9, 1 (Spring 1994), 47–53.

Lucey, J.V., G. Butcher, A.W. Clare and T.G. Dinan, 'The clinical characteristics of patients with obsessive compulsive disorder: a descriptive study of an Irish sample', *Irish Journal of Psychological Medicine*, 11, 1 (March 1994), 11–14.

Swanwick, G.R.J., H. Lee, A.W. Clare and B.A. Lawlor, 'Consultation-liaison psychiatry: a comparison of two service models for geriatric patients', *International Journal of Geriatric Psychiatry*, 9, 6 (June 1994), 495–9.

Clare, A.W. and J. Tyrrell, 'Psychiatric aspects of abortion', *Irish Journal of Psychological Medicine*, 11, 2 (June 1994), 92–8.

Bruce-Jones, W.D.A., P.D. White, J.M. Thomas and A.W. Clare, 'The effect of social adversity on the fatigue syndrome, psychiatric disorders and physical recovery, following glandular fever', *Psychological Medicine*, 24, 3 (August 1994), 651–9.

Swanwick, G. and A Clare, 'Inpatient liaison psychiatry: the experience of two Irish general hospitals without psychiatric units', *Irish Journal of Psychological Medicine*, 11, 3 (September 1994), 123–5.

White, P.D., W.D. Bruce-Jones, J.M. Thomas, J. Amess and A.W. Clare, 'Viruses, neurosis and fatigue', *Journal of Psychosomatic Research*, 39, 3 (April 1995), 379.

Farren, C.K., A.W. Clare and T.G. Dinan, 'Basal serum cortisol and dexamethasone-induced growth hormone release in the alcohol dependence syndrome', *Human Psychopharmacology*, 10, 3 (May/June 1995), 207–13.

Clare, A.W., 'Commentary on: "Training in psychodynamic psychotherapy: the psychiatric trainee's perspective"', *Irish Journal of Psychological Medicine*, 12, 2 (June 1995), 59–60.

White, P.D., J.M. Thomas, J. Amess, S.A. Grover, H.O. Kangro and A.W. Clare, 'The existence of a fatigue syndrome after glandular fever', *Psychological Medicine*, 25, 5 (September 1995), 907–16.

White, P.D., S.A. Grover, H.O. Kangro, J.M. Thomas, J. Amess and A.W. Clare, 'The validity and reliability of the fatigue syndrome that follows glandular fever', *Psychological Medicine*, 25, 2 (September 1995), 917–24.

Farren, C.K., A.W. Clare, D. Ziedonis, F.A. Hammeedi and T.G. Dinan, 'Evidence for reduced dopamine D2 receptor sensitivity in postwithdrawal alcoholics', *Alcoholism, Clinical and Experimental Research*, 19, 6 (December 1995), 1520–4.

Farren, C.K., D. Ziedonis, A.W. Clare, F.A. Hammeedi and T.G. Dinan, 'D-fenfluramine-induced prolactin responses in postwithdrawal alcoholics and controls', *Alcoholism, Clinical and Experimental Research*, 19, 6 (December 1995), 1578–82.

Cooney, J.M., C.K. Farren and A.W. Clare, 'Personality disorder among first ever admissions to an Irish public and private hospital', *Irish Journal of Psychological Medicine*, 13, 1 (March 1996), 6–8.

Clare, A.W., 'John Norman Parker Moore (obituary)', *Psychiatric Bulletin*, 20, 12 (1 December 1996), 771–3.

Swanwick, G.R. and A.W. Clare, 'Suicide in Ireland 1945–1992: social correlates', *Irish Medical Journal*, 90, 3 (April–May 1997), 106–8.

Clare, A.W., 'Touched with fire: manic depressive illness and the artistic temperament (book review)', *British Journal of Psychiatry*, 171, 4 (1 October 1997), 395.

Cheasty, M., A.W. Clare and C. Collins, 'Relation between sexual abuse in childhood and adult depression: case-control study', *British Medical Journal*, 316, 7126 (17 January 1998), 198–201.

Farren, C.K., A.W. Clare, K.F. Tipton and T.G Dinan, 'Platelet MAO activity in subtypes of alcoholics and controls in a homogenous population', *Journal of Psychiatric Research*, 32, 1 (January–February 1998), 49–54.

Clare, A.W., 'Swift, mental illness and St Patrick's Hospital', *Irish Journal of Psychological Medicine*, 15, 3 (September 1998), 100–4.

Clare, A.W., 'St. Patrick's Hospital', *American Journal of Psychiatry*, 155, 11 (November 1998), 1599.

White, P.D., J.M. Thomas, J. Amess, D.H. Crawford, S.A. Grover, H.O. Kangro and A.W. Clare, 'Incidence, risk and prognosis of acute and chronic fatigue syndromes and psychiatric disorders after glandular fever', *British Journal of Psychiatry*, 173, 6 (December 1998), 475–81.

Clare, A.W., 'The two Mr. Gladstones: a study in psychology and history (book review)', *American Journal of Psychiatry*, 155, 12 (December 1998), 1789–90.

Clare, A.W., 'Psychiatry's future: psychological medicine or biological psychiatry?', *Journal of Mental Health*, 8, 2 (1999), 109–11.

Clare, A.W., 'Democratic definitely, parochial possibly, challenged certainly: the College at the century's end', *Psychiatric Bulletin*, 23, 1 (1 January 1999), 1–2.

Clare, A.W., 'Understanding and treating violent psychiatric patients (book review)', *American Journal of Psychiatry*, 158, 10 (October 2001), 1757.

Greene, E., C.J. Cunningham, A. Eustace, N. Kidd, A.W. Clare and B.A. Lawlor, 'Recurrent falls are associated with increased length of stay in elderly psychiatric inpatients', *International Journal of Geriatric Psychiatry*, 16, 10 (October 2001), 965–8.

White, P.D., J.M. Thomas, H.O. Kangro, W.D. Bruce-Jones, J. Amess, D.H. Crawford, S.A. Grover and A.W. Clare, 'Predictions and associations of fatigue syndromes and mood disorders that occur after infectious mononucleosis', *Lancet*, 358, 9297 (8 December 2001), 1946–54.

Cheasty, M., A.W. Clare and C. Collins, 'Child sexual abuse – predictor of persistent depression in adult rape and sexual assault victims', *Journal of Mental Health*, 11, 1 (2002), 79–84.

Clare, A.W., 'Immigration: new challenges for psychiatry and mental health services in Ireland', *Irish Journal of Psychological Medicine*, 19, 1 (March 2002), 3.

O'Connell, H. and A. Clare, 'Nearly lethal suicide attempt: implications for research and prevention', *Irish Journal of Psychological Medicine*, 21, 4 (December 2004), 131–3.

Clare, A., 'The future of postgraduate training in psychiatry in Ireland', *Irish Journal of Psychological Medicine*, 24, 4 (December 2007), 129–31.

Medical Press and Popular Press (Non-Peer Reviewed) (Anthony W. Clare) (Chronological Order)

Clare, A.W., 'General Costello and NATO', *Irish Times*, 20 February 1962.

Clare, A.W., 'A question of numbers', *St Stephen's* (Michaelmas, 1963), 9–11.

Clare, A.W., 'Students and intellectual freedom', *Hibernia*, 28, 1 (January 1964), 7–8.

Clare, A.W., 'Doctors and the pill', *Irish Times*, 7 August 1968.

Clare, A.W., 'Is aggression instinctive? Konrad Lorenz's theories re-assessed', *Studies: An Irish Quarterly Review*, 58, 230 (Summer 1969), 153–65.

Clare, A., 'The humanist and abortion', *Irish Times*, 25 May 1970.

Clare, A., 'Explorers of inner space', *Irish Times*, 27 June 1970.

Clare, A.W., 'Ireland's smug medicine', *Irish Times*, 7 January 1971.

Clare, A., 'Does psychoanalysis work?', *Irish Times*, 20 January 1971.

Clare, A., 'Psychoanalysis on the defensive?', *Irish Times*, 17 July 1971.

Clare, A., 'Eysenck and the Irish', *Irish Times*, 5 August 1971.

Clare, A., 'The new neurosis', *Irish Times*, 14 August 1971.

Clare, A., 'How sick is the North?', *Irish Times*, 30 August 1971.

Clare, A., 'The new inquisition', *Irish Times*, 16 March 1972.

Clare, A., 'What are psychiatrists doing?', *The Spectator*, 12 August 1972.

Clare, A.W., 'Laing returns to the fold', *The Spectator*, 3 February 1973.

Clare, A.W., 'Laing's return', *The Spectator*, 17 March 1973.

Clare, A.W., 'Eysenck the controversialist', *The Spectator*, 21 April 1973.

Clare, A.W., 'Controversial Eysenck', *The Spectator*, 19 May 1973.

Clare, A.W., 'Jung confusions', *The Spectator*, 30 June 1973.

Clare, A.W., 'Jensen's reply', *The Spectator*, 18 August 1973.

Clare, A., 'Herrema siege', *The Spectator*, 15 November 1975.

Clare, A., 'Balls up', *The Spectator*, 26 June 1976.

Clare, A., 'Standard works', *New Society*, 21 April 1977.

Clare, A., 'Neurotics anonymous', *The Listener*, 16 June 1977.

Clare, A., 'Obsessed with being reasonable', *Irish Times*, 5 July 1977.

Clare, A., 'Is Nixon nuts?', *Sunday Telegraph*, 31 July 1977.

Clare, A., 'Depth psychology', *The Listener*, 15 December 1977.

Clare, A., 'The drugging of prisoners', *The Spectator*, 17 December 1977.

Clare, A., 'Autistic brilliance', *The Listener*, 23 February 1978.

Clare, A., 'Freud for fun', *New Society*, 6 April 1978.

Clare, A., 'Flagellomania', *The Listener*, 20 July 1978.

Clare, A., '"Let's talk about me" – the other person's need for therapy', *The Listener*, 5 October 1978.

Clare, A., 'The time for grown-up talk – and the time for screaming', *The Listener*, 19 October 1978.

Clare, A., 'Psychotherapy and the search for meaning', *The Listener*, 9 November 1978.

Clare, A., 'The guilty sick', *The Listener*, 22 February 1979.

Clare, A., 'Massification and personhood', *The Listener*, 3 May 1979.

Clare, A., 'Sigmund's stories', *The Listener*, 27 September 1979.

Clare, A., 'Facing up to cancer', *The Listener*, 29 November 1979.

Clare, A. and L. Gostin, 'More than a second opinion needed about Broadmoor', *Guardian*, 2 February 1980.

Clare, A., 'Lucky loonies?', *The Listener*, 26 June 1980.

Clare, A., 'Lucky loonies?', *The Listener*, 3 July 1980.

Clare, A., 'Sturdy offspring', *The Listener*, 30 October 1980.

Clare, A.W., 'Premenstrual problems', *The Times*, 26 November 1981.

Clare, A., 'Mother or someone', *The Listener*, 18 February 1982.

Gostin, L. and A. Clare, 'How health charges will put extra strain on mental patients', *Guardian*, 2 March 1982.

Clare, A.W., 'Letter to the editor', *Guardian*, 24 April 1982.

Clare, A., 'Fears after Freud', *The Listener*, 29 April 1982.

Clare, A., 'The recurrent message is that none of us is free from flaw', *The Listener*, 5 August 1982.

Clare, A., 'Langham Diary', *The Listener*, 4 November 1982.

Clare, A., 'Dickens has much to answer for', *The Listener*, 23 December 1982.

Clare, A., 'Langham Diary', *The Listener*, 12 May 1983.

Clare, A., 'Margaret Thatcher: a psychiatrist's view', *The Listener*, 9 June 1983.

Clare, A., 'Endpiece', *The Listener*, 30 June 1983.

Clare, A.W., 'Implications in N. Ireland of hanging', *The Times*, 6 July 1983.

Clare, A., 'Endpiece', *The Listener*, 7 July 1983.

Clare, A., 'Endpiece', *The Listener*, 14 July 1983.

Clare, A., 'Endpiece', *The Listener*, 21 July 1983.

Clare, A., 'Endpiece', *The Listener*, 28 July 1983.

Clare, A., 'Endpiece', *The Listener*, 4 August 1983.

Clare, A., 'Endpiece', *The Listener*, 11 August 1983.

Clare, A., 'How to be professional moms and dads', *The Listener*, 24 November 1983.

Clare, A., 'Langham Diary', *The Listener*, 16 February 1984.

Clare, A., 'Truth and treachery', *The Listener*, 19 April 1984.

Clare, A., 'Scepticism is the first refuge of the wise', *The Listener*, 26 April 1984.

Clare, A., 'A suitable case for treatment?', *The Listener*, 24 May 1984.

Clare, A., 'Rage for happiness', *The Listener*, 21 June 1984.

Clare, A., 'Off the air, on the couch: a life in the day of Anthony Clare', *Sunday Times*, 8 July 1984.

Clare, A., 'Triumph of the will', *The Listener*, 26 July 1984.

Clare, A., 'Cinderella story', *The Listener*, 30 August 1984.

Clare, A., 'El Vino veritas', *The Listener*, 27 September 1984.

Clare, A., 'A moderate's voice', *The Listener*, 25 October 1984.

Clare, A., 'Animals and man', *The Listener*, 22 November 1984.

Clare, A. *Power and the Public Man (Lecture)* (London: Institute of Contemporary Arts, 1985).

Clare, A., 'What is an acceptable risk?', *The Listener*, 3 January 1985.

Clare, A., 'Answers for everything', *The Listener*, 31 January 1985.

Clare, A., 'Righteous indignation', *The Listener*, 28 February 1985.

Clare, A., 'The phone-in physician', *The Listener*, 28 March 1985.

Clare, A., 'A challenge to honour', *The Listener*, 25 April 1985.

Clare, A., 'Psychoanalysis has been overtaken by knowledge and events', *The Listener*, 2 May 1985.

Clare, A., 'Tomorrow's golden eggs', *The Listener*, 23 May 1985.

Clare, A., 'The price Laing paid', *The Listener*, 6 June 1985.

Clare, A., 'The writing on the wall', *The Listener*, 20 June 1985.

Clare, A., 'At Her Majesty's pleasure ...', *The Listener*, 18 July 1985.

Clare, A., 'Face to face with a TV megastar', *The Listener*, 15 August 1985.

Clare, A., 'Eysenck is a behavioural conquistador with eyes on Freud's territory', *The Listener*, 29 August 1985.

Clare, A., 'Eat, drink and be ill', *The Listener*, 12 September 1985.

Clare, A., 'Is analysis a Freudian slip?', *The Times*, 8 July 1985.

Clare, A., 'Myth or medicine?', *The Times*, 9 July 1985.

Clare, A., 'The nest of love and vipers', *The Listener*, 10 October 1985.

Clare, A., 'Help at the end of the phone', *The Listener*, 7 November 1985.

Clare, A., 'The seductive lady problem', *The Listener*, 5 December 1985.

Clare, A., 'Disorderly drama', *The Listener*, 5 December 1985.

Clare, A., 'Sense and desensitisation', *The Listener*, 9 January 1986.

Clare, A., 'Sport's smokescreen', *The Listener*, 6 February 1986.

Clare, A., 'Men must change', *The Listener*, 13 February 1986.

Clare, A., 'Eskimo Bernard', *The Listener*, 6 March 1986.

Clare, A., 'No sense of proportion', *The Listener*, 3 April 1986.

Clare, A., 'Peer pressure', *The Listener*, 29 May 1986.

Clare, A., 'The courage to be boring', *The Listener*, 26 June 1986.

Clare, A., 'Why success means more than winning', *The Listener*, 31 July 1986.

Clare, A., 'Sex and the confused parent', *The Listener*, 2 October 1986.

Clare, A., 'Sex education: who'll tell the children?', *Time Out*, 29 October 1986.

Clare, A., 'Keeping violence in the family', *The Listener*, 6 November 1986.

Clare, A., 'AIDS and medical hubris', *The Listener*, 1 January 1987.

Clare, A., 'Secrecy in the personal interest', *The Listener*, 5 February 1987.

Clare, A., 'A woman's right to choose', *The Listener*, 12 March 1987.

Clare, A., 'The Royal Touch', *The Listener*, 23 April 1987.

Clare, A., 'How to put spice into politics', *The Listener*, 21 May 1987.

Clare, A., 'Safe in a grip of iron', *The Listener*, 9 July 1987.

Clare, A., 'Looking after number one', *The Listener*, 6 August 1987.

Clare, A., 'Jumping the gun', *The Listener*, 17 September 1987.

Clare, A., 'The despotism of desperate times', *The Listener*, 3 March 1988.

Clare, A., 'Living death', *The Listener*, 31 March 1988.

Clare, A., 'Me and my shadow', *The Listener*, 7 July 1988.

Clare, A., 'Brain scan', *The Listener*, 15 September 1988.

Clare, A., 'My hero: Anthony Clare on John Hume', *Independent*, 7 January 1989.

Clare, A., 'The popular front', *The Listener*, 26 January 1989.

Clare, A., 'Television and the death of literacy', *Irish Times*, 29 June 1998.

Clare, A.W., 'Homosexuality', *Irish Times*, 9 February 1990.

Clare, A., 'The relationship', *Daily Telegraph*, 13 June 1989.

Clare, A.W., 'More bark than bite', *Irish Times*, 14 July 1990.

Clare, A., 'Come to think of it, I must be mad to be a psychiatrist', *Daily Mail*, 17 September 1991.

Clare, A., 'Taking "real" illness to the psychiatrist', *Daily Mail*, 1 October 1991.

Clare, A., 'Just another one for the road', *Daily Mail*, 8 October 1991.

Clare, A., 'Stressed doctors and angry patients can make each other feel better', *Daily Mail*, 15 October 1991.

Clare, A., 'Searching for the truth will never be an easy task', *Daily Mail*, 29 October 1991.

Clare, A., 'Menopause for thought on sexual politics …', *Daily Mail*, 12 November 1991.

Clare, A., 'Tribunal review not the only answer', *Forum*, 9 (September 1992), 16–17.

Clare, A., 'Why closing Bart's is an act of madness', *Evening Standard*, 17 December 1992.

Coleman, P. and A. Clare, 'Me and my family', *Daily Telegraph*, 8 January 1993.

Clare, A., 'Wounded minds that find no peace when the war is over', *Sunday Express*, 17 January 1993.

Clare, A., 'Let's talk, and keep peace hopes alive', *Sunday Times*, 1 August 1993.

Clare, A., 'Relative values that Albert Einstein forgot', *Sunday Express*, 5 September 1993.

Clare, A., 'The prisoner', *Sunday Times*, 3 October 1993.

Clare, A., 'A beneficial treatment hijacked by the affluent', *The Times*, 21 February 1994.

Clare, A., 'Seven types of incongruity', *Irish Times*, 25 February 1995.

Clare, A., 'Pick of the year', *Sunday Times*, 19 November 1995.

Clare, A., 'A nation divorced from itself', *Sunday Independent*, 26 November 1995.

Clare, A., 'Norman Moore', *Irish Times*, 29 July 1996.

Clare, A., 'Romantic on the loose', *Literary Review*, November 1996.

Clare, A.W., 'Professor Norman Moore', *Swift Times*, 16 (1996), 1–2.

Clare, A., 'Competition is healthy, but not if it discriminates', *Sunday Independent*, 12 January 1997.

Kewley, V. and A. Clare, 'My hols', *Sunday Times*, 5 October 1997.

Clare, A., 'Proving that life isn't fair', *Literary Review*, September 1998.

Lynch, F. and A. Clare, 'Chronic fatigue syndrome', *Modern Medicine of Ireland*, 29, 5 (May 1999), 22–4.

Clare, A., 'The great university we might have had', *Irish Times*, 18 December 1999.

Clare, A., 'Nobody but ourselves to blame for hospital ills', *Sunday Independent*, 21 May 2000.

Clare, A., 'The trouble with men', *Sunday Times*, 16 July 2000.

Clare, A., 'Truths my father told me', *Sunday Independent*, 23 July 2000.

Clare, A., 'A rust bowl', *New Statesman*, 18 December 2000.

Clare, A., 'The lust for life', *New Statesman*, 16 April 2001.

Clare, A., 'Plan for our children's future', *Medicine Weekly*, 20 June 2007.

Personal Communications (Anthony W. Clare) (Chronological Order)

Clare, A.W., correspondence to BK (7 September 2005).

Clare, A.W., correspondence to BK (1 September 2006).

(All other correspondence to and from A.W. Clare cited in the text are drawn from Clare's papers at St Patrick's Mental Health Services, Dublin, accessed with permission in 2018.)

Reports and Manuscripts (Anthony W. Clare) (Chronological Order)

Clare, A.W., *St Patrick's Hospital: A Discussion Document Concerning its Current Status and Future Plans in the Light of Trends in Contemporary Psychiatric Theory and Practice* (Dublin: St Patrick's Hospital, 1989).

Clare, A.W., *Funeral Address: J.N.P. Moore, MD FRCPI FRCPsych* (Dublin: St Patrick's Cathedral, 1996).

Clare, A., *Programme: Long Day's Journey into Night* (Dublin: Peri-Talking Theatre Company, 1997).

Primary Sources

Printed (pre-1970)

American Psychiatric Association, *Diagnostic and Statistical Manual of Mental Disorders (First Edition) (DSM-I)* (Washington DC: American Psychiatric Association, 1952).

American Psychiatric Association, *Diagnostic and Statistical Manual of Mental Disorders (Second Edition) (DSM-II)* (Washington DC: American Psychiatric Association, 1968).

Anonymous, 'School curriculum "deplored"', *Irish Times*, 28 November 1960.

Anonymous, 'Sees Ireland as fount of labour for Europe', *Irish Times*, 20 November 1962.

Anonymous, 'Students look at Irish parents', *Irish Times*, 10 December 1962.

Anonymous, '*Irish Times* trophy won by UCD', *Irish Times*, 15 February 1963.

Anonymous, 'The winning team', *Irish Times*, 16 February 1963.

Anonymous, '*Irish Times* debating trophy won by UCD', *Irish Times*, 6 May 1963.

Anonymous, 'UCD "ban" on two churchmen', *Irish Times*, 11 January 1964.

Anonymous, 'Highest semi-final standard so far', *Irish Times*, 25 January 1964.

Anonymous, '*Irish Times* debating trophy winners', *Irish Times*, 2 March 1964.

Anonymous, 'UCD debaters through to final', *Irish Times*, 10 April 1964.

Anonymous, '*Observer* debate won by UCD', *Irish Times*, 29 June 1964.

Commission of Inquiry on Mental Illness, *Report of the Commission of Inquiry on Mental Illness* (Dublin: The Stationery Office, 1967).

Foucault, M., *Folie et Déraison: Histoire de la Folie à l'Âge Classique* (Paris: Plon, 1961).

Frank, R.T., 'The hormonal causes of premenstrual tension', *Archives of Neurology and Psychiatry*, 26, 5 (November 1931), 1053–7.

Goffman, E., *Asylums: Essays on the Social Situation of Mental Patients and Other Inmates* (New York: Anchor Books, Doubleday & Co., 1961).

Greene, R. and K. Dalton, 'The premenstrual syndrome', *British Medical Journal*, 1, 4818 (9 May 1953), 1007–14.

Irish Times Reporter, 'UCD reach final of *Observer* tournament', *Irish Times*, 18 March 1963.

Irish Times Reporter, 'Glasgow students win debating tournament', *Irish Times*, 8 May 1963.

Irish Times Reporter, 'Ireland has high mental illness rate', *Irish Times*, 29 March 1967.

Kesey, K., *One Flew Over the Cuckoo's Nest* (New York: Viking Press, 1962).

Laing, R.D., *The Divided Self* (Harmondsworth, Middlesex: Penguin, 1960).

Lewis, A., 'Health as a social concept', *British Journal of Sociology*, 4, 2 (June 1953), 109–14.

Lewis, A., 'Edward Mapother and the making of the Maudsley Hospital', *British Journal of Psychiatry*, 115, 529 (December 1969), 1349–66.

Lorenz, K., *On Aggression* (London: Methuen, 1966).

Moos, R.H., 'The development of a menstrual distress questionnaire', *Psychosomatic Medicine*, 30, 6 (November–December 1968), 853–67.

Moos, R.H., 'Assessment of psychological concomitants of oral contraceptives', in H.A. Salhanick, D.M. Kipnis and R.L. Vande Wiele (eds), *Metabolic Effects of Gonadal Hormones and Contraceptive Steroids* (New York: Plenum, 1969), 676–705.

Moos, R.H., 'Typology of menstrual cycle symptoms', *American Journal of Obstetrics and Gynecology*, 103, 3 (1 February 1969), 390–402.

Shepherd, M., B. Cooper, A.C. Brown and G.W. Kalton (eds), *Psychiatric Illness in General Practice* (Oxford: Oxford University Press, 1966).

Stafford-Clark, D., *Psychiatry Today* (Harmondsworth, Middlesex: Penguin, 1952).

Szasz, T., *The Myth of Mental Illness: Foundations of a Theory of Personal Conduct* (New York: Harper & Row, 1961).

Taylor, F.K., 'Prokaletic measures derived from psychoanalytic technique', *British Journal of Psychiatry*, 115, 521 (April 1969), 407–19.

Veale, J., 'Men speechless', *Studies: An Irish Quarterly Review*, 46, 183 (Autumn 1957), 322–39.

Personal communications

Ashkenazy, V., interview with BK (15 May 2018).

Bevan, M., emails to BK (24 June and 4 October 2019).

Browne, I., interview with BK (7 July 2018).

Browne, M., email to BK (25 March 2019).

Buckley, A., interview with BK (16 January 2019).

Burns, T., email to BK (26 September 2018).

Butler, B., interview with BK (30 January 2019).

Campbell (nee Clare), J., interview with MH (8 May 2019).

Clare, J., interviews with BK (10 May, 7 and 23 June, 2018).

Clare, J., email to MH and BK (14 January 2019).

Clare, P., interview with BK (9 February 2019).

Clare, R., interview with BK (7 March 2019).

Cody, S., emails to BK and MH (6 and 7 April 2019).

Currie, E., email to BK (11 May 2018).

De Barra, C., email to BK (17 June 2019).

DelMonte, M., interview with BK (7 May 2019).

Dinan, T., email to BK (3 July 2018).

Dudley Edwards, R., interview with BK (14 June 2019).

Fahy, T., email to BK (26 February 2018).

Gaffney, M., email to BK (4 June 2018).

Geller, U., interview with BK (8 May 2018).

Geoghegan, R., *Tony Clare (Private Memoir)* (4 November 2007).

Greenfield, S., interview with BK (1 June 2018).

Horlick, N., email to BK (8 May 2018).

Jamison, K.R., email to BK (4 May 2018).

Jenkins, R., email to BK (2 August 2018).

Kennedy, N., email to BK (22 August 2018).

Kent, B., email to BK (7 May 2018).

Knight, B., correspondence to BK (20 May 2018).

Knowles, D., interview with MH (12 November 2018).

Lawson, N., email to BK (9 May 2018).

Lucey, J., interview with BK (30 August 2018).

Lumley, J., email to BK (21 May 2018).

MacLachlan, M., email to BK (16 August 2018).

Mann, A., interview with BK (2 July 2018).

Meagan, G., email to BK (24 August 2018).

Mohan, D., interview with MH (8 November 2018).

Moriarty, J., email to BK (14 August 2018).

Murray, R.M., interview with BK (25 February 2018).

O'Donoghue, F., interview with BK (24 January 2019).

Philbin Bowman, E., email to BK (1 June 2018).

Rantzen, E., interview with BK (18 May 2018).

Savage, W., email to BK (30 September 2018).

Shannon, J., email to MH (28 September 2018).

Slovo, G., email to BK (15 May 2018).

Swanwick, G., email to BK (12 August 2018).

Wessely, S., interview with BK (2 October 2017).

Widdecombe, A., interview with BK (10 May 2018).

Newspapers and Magazines

Cara
Daily Express
Daily Mail
Daily Mirror
Daily Telegraph
Evening Standard
Financial Times
Gonzaga Observer
Guardian
Hibernia
Hong Kong Sunday Post
Independent
Irish Examiner
Irish Independent
Irish Medical Times
The Irish Times
Listener
Luxembourg Weekly
Mail on Sunday
New Society
New Statesman
New York Times
Observer
Radio Times
Spectator
Sunday Correspondent
Sunday Express
Sunday Independent
Sunday Telegraph
Sunday Times
Sunday Tribune
Swift Times
Telegraph
Time Out
Times
Today
World Medicine
Yorkshire Post

Secondary Sources (1970 onwards)

Ackroyd, P., 'Modest virtues', *The Times*, 2 August 1983.

Adams, J., 'He tried to shrink away but we got him to expand on love', *Today*, 18 August 1990.

Amergin Solstice Poetry Gathering, *Unde Scribitur* (An Daingean: Ponc Press, 2018).

American Psychiatric Association, *Diagnostic and Statistical Manual of Mental Disorders (Third Edition) (DSM-III)* (Washington DC: American Psychiatric Association, 1980).

American Psychiatric Association, *Diagnostic and Statistical Manual of Mental Disorders*

(Third Edition, Revised) (DSM-III-R) (Washington DC: American Psychiatric Association, 1987).

American Psychiatric Association, *Diagnostic and Statistical Manual of Mental Disorders (Fourth Edition) (DSM-IV)* (Washington DC: American Psychiatric Association, 1994).

American Psychiatric Association, *Diagnostic and Statistical Manual of Mental Disorders (Fourth Edition, Text Revision) (DSM-IV-TR)* (Washington DC: American Psychiatric Association, 2000).

American Psychiatric Association, *Diagnostic and Statistical Manual of Mental Disorders (Fifth Edition) (DSM-5)* (Washington DC: American Psychiatric Association, 2013).

Andreasen, N.C., *Brave New Brain: Conquering Mental Illness in the Era of the Genome* (Oxford: Oxford University Press, 2001).

Anonymous, 'Sobering plight of student doctors', *Guardian*, 24 April 1982.

Anonymous, 'How to couch the best questions', *Guardian*, 14 August 1982.

Anonymous, 'Dinners', *The Times*, 20 September 1986.

Anonymous, 'A loner "living in fantasy world of violence"', *The Times*, 20 August 1987.

Anonymous, 'Schizophrenia video launch', *The Times*, 8 September 1987.

Anonymous, 'Dinners', *The Times*, 18 September 1987.

Anonymous, 'The powers that will be', *Sunday Times*, 22 November 1987.

Anonymous, 'Emotional problems', *Evening Standard*, 3 March 1988.

Anonymous, 'Who is the …', *Daily Mail*, 1 November 1990.

Anonymous, 'Mixed up', *Financial Times*, 30 April 1991.

Anonymous, 'Priests "turn blind eye to drink"', *Telegraph*, 18 September 1993.

Anonymous, 'Don't let parents divorce says radio shrink', *Daily Mail*, 18 April 1994.

Anonymous, 'Christie: UK lacks respect', *Sunday Times*, 3 September 1995.

Anonymous, 'Minister defends regulations on mental illness insurance', *Irish Times*, 29 May 1996.

Anonymous, 'Obituaries: Professor Anthony Clare', *The Times*, 31 October 2007.

Anonymous, 'AGM Minutes – 2007 Thirty-Sixth Annual Meeting [of the Royal College of Psychiatrists]', *Psychiatric Bulletin*, 31, 12 (1 December 2007), 470–9.

Anonymous, 'Michael Ember, BBC Radio "talks" producer – obituary', *The Telegraph*, 11 April 2017.

Arnold-Forster, V., 'Sounds of battle', *Guardian*, 7 August 1982.

Arnold-Forster, V., 'All huff and puff', *Guardian*, 17 June 1983.

Arnold-Forster, V., 'Crime on the couch', *Guardian*, 5 July 1985.

Arnold-Forster, V., 'Electric chair', *Guardian*, 30 August 1986.

Bailey, P., 'The gentle persuader', *Sunday Times*, 24 July 1983.

Ballantyne, A., 'Psychiatrist says long hours harm junior doctors' health', *Guardian*, 10 April 1989.

Banks-Smith, N., 'Macho', *Guardian*, 2 August 1983.

Banville, J., 'Recovering the poet's reputation', *Irish Times*, 15 April 2017.

Barnes, J., 'Shrink wrapped', *Sunday Times*, 19 July 1998.

Baruk, H., 'Book review: *Psychiatry in Dissent: Controversial Issues in Thought and Practice*', *International Journal of Social Psychiatry*, 25, 3 (1 September 1979), 227.

Beckett, A., 'Turn on, check in, dry out', *Guardian*, 5 July 1999.

Bell, J.M., 'Responsibilities', *Irish Times*, 3 September 1971.

Berger, J., 'Book review: *Psychiatry in Dissent: Controversial Issues in Thought and Practice*', *Canadian Journal of Psychiatry*, 24, 1 (1 February 1979), 95–7.

Berrington, L., 'Weldon fails to lift curse of therapy', *The Times*, 24 February 1994.

Berry, D., 'All in the mind', *Guardian*, 6 August 1986.

Beveridge, A., 'Ten books', *British Journal of Psychiatry*, 191, 6 (1 November 2007), 567–70.

Bewley, T., *Madness to Mental Illness: A History of the Royal College of Psychiatrists* (London: RCPsych Publications, 2008),

Billen, A., 'Fame gives you pleasure, like drink or gambling or sex. It doesn't make you happy', *Evening Standard*, 26 July 2000.

Billen, A., 'Face to face with an ice maiden', *The Times*, 4 April 2007.

Binchy, M., 'The race that God made mad', *Irish Times*, 7 June 1976.

Binchy, M., 'If you're Irish … come into the media', *Irish Times*, 31 March 1984.

Bloch, S. and P. Reddaway, *Soviet Psychiatric Abuse: The Shadow Over World Psychiatry* (London: Victor Gollancz Ltd., 1984).

Boston, R., 'In the late 1960s confusion of the psychic, the psychotic and the psychedelic, Dr Laing's homage to catatonia went down beautifully', *Guardian*, 3 August 1976.

Bosworth, P., 'Pathologies of a poet', *New York Times (International Edition)*, 8 March 2017.

Bowditch, G., 'Why our fathers need us to stand up for their rights', *Sunday Times*, 15 September 2002.

Bowman, R., 'Does psychoanalysis work?', *Irish Times*, 25 January 1971.

Bradberry, G., 'In the chair and off guard', *The Times*, 20 August 1996.

Brandreth, G., 'How to be happy', *Sunday Telegraph*, 30 January 2000.

Brandreth, G., *Something Sensational to Read in the Train: The Diary of a Lifetime* (London: John Murray, 2009).

Brandreth, G., *The 7 Secrets of Happiness: An Optimist's Journey* (London: Short Books, 2013).

Brankin, M., 'The legacy of Anthony Clare', *Irish Times*, 15 November 2007.

Brennan, D., *Irish Insanity, 1800–2000* (Abingdon, Oxon.: Routledge, 2014).

Bressan, J., 'A mountain or a mole ill?', *Medicine Weekly*, 6 September 2000.

Bridgstock, G. and A. Clare, 'Stress sense', *Evening Standard*, 28 July 1989.

Brompton, S., 'Spike: my part in his upturn', *The Times*, 7 January 1993.

Browne, I., *Music and Madness* (Cork: Atrium/ Cork University Press, 2008).

Browne, N., 'Laing's theories', *Irish Times*, 28 September 1989.

Browne, V., 'Wasted lives', in F. Callanan (ed.), *The Literary and Historical Society, 1955–2005* (Dublin: A&A Farmar, 2005), 117–19.

Bunce, K., 'Life, death, footie – and Phil Collins', *The Observer*, 22 October 2000.

Bunting, M., 'Masculinity in question', *The Guardian*, 2 October 2000.

Burke, D., 'Male impotence', *Sunday Times*, 30 July 2000.

Burns, J., 'Beckham "a better father than Blair"', *Sunday Times*, 16 July 2000.

Burns, T., *Our Necessary Shadow: The Nature and Meaning of Psychiatry* (London: Allen Lane/Penguin Group, 2013).

Burt, P., 'The man who meets the minds of the famous', *Evening Standard*, 25 July 1991.

Byrne, C., 'Warm tributes to man who changed face of psychiatry', *Irish Independent*, 31 October 2007.

C., R.H., 'Obituary: Sir (John) Denis Hill, formerly Professor of Psychiatry, Institute of Psychiatry, London SE5', *Bulletin of the Royal College of Psychiatrists*, 6, 11 (November 1982), 206–7.

Campbell-Johnston, R., 'A life as ordinary', *The Times*, 8 August 1998.

Candy, J., 'Shock wave', *Guardian*, 16 May 1978.

Cane, A., 'Obituary: radio psychiatrist who quizzed the famous', *Financial Times,* 31 October 2007.

Cannon, M., *Carrying the Songs* (Manchester: Carcanet Press Limited, 2007).

Casey, P., 'Anthony Clare', *Guardian*, 31 October 2007.

Casey, P., 'Farewell to a dear friend and kind mentor', *Irish Independent*, 31 October 2007.

City Diary, 'Unshrinking', *The Times*, 26 September 1998.

Cheston, P., 'Flirting, arrogance and me by Edwina', *Evening Standard*, 17 August 1988.

Clare, J., 'Family ties', *Sunday Tribune*, 17 September 1995.

Clare, J., 'Truth is the first casualty', *Sunday Independent*, 26 November 1995.

Clare, J., 'Parents must fight for choice', *Farmers Journal*, 25 November 2000.

Clare, J., 'Out of Ireland and into Africa', *Lucan Gazette*, 24 July 2004.

Clare, J. and M. Keane, *What Will I Be?* (Dublin: Marino Books, 1995).

Cody, S., 'Anthony Clare', *Guardian*, 31 October 2007.

Coleman, P. and A. Clare, 'Me and my family', *Daily Telegraph*, 8 January 1993.

Coles, J., 'BBC pays for Whitehouse slur on Potter's mother', *Guardian*, 4 October 1990.

Conroy, D., 'Marriage of memories behind brace of artistic, cultural carnivals', *Sunday Independent*, 13 May 2018.

Cook, S., 'An arguably interesting session on the couch with Edwina Currie', *Guardian*, 18 August 1988.

Cookson, J., 'Robert Lowell: setting the river on fire: a study of genius, mania and character (book review)', *British Journal of Psychiatry*, 212, 3 (1 March 2018), 185.

Cosgrave, P., 'The ambiguities of attitude', *St Stephen's* (Trinity, 1962), 18–22.

Cosgrave, P., 'The Marxist legacy', *St Stephen's* (Trinity, 1963), 39–45.

Cosgrave, P., *Margaret Thatcher: A Tory and Her Party* (London: Hutchinson, 1978).

Courtney, K., 'Crisis, what crisis?', *Irish Times*, 4 November 2000.

Crammer, J., 'Unmodified ECT', *Lancet*, 315, 8166 (1 March 1980), 486.

Crane, A., 'Radio psychiatrist who quizzed the famous', *Financial Times*, 31 October 2007.

Craven, L., 'Mental illness', *Irish Times*, 26 September 1989.

Crawley, H., 'Applause is a hard drug: 1961–6', in F. Callanan (ed.), *The Literary and Historical Society, 1955–2005* (Dublin: A&A Farmar, 2005), 97–114.

Crowley, J., 'Patrick Cosgrave: immigrant chic', *Irish Times*, 28 January 1978.

Cummins, M., 'FF fails to get regulations on mentally ill amended', *Irish Times* (2 May 1996).

Cunningham, J., 'Mental health plans', *Guardian*, 3 March 1973.

Cunningham Owens, D., 'Ten books', *British Journal of Psychiatry*, 199, 2 (1 August 2011), 160–3.

Curran, E., 'Ripe for expansion: 1998–2002', in F. Callanan (ed.), *The Literary and Historical Society, 1955–2005* (Dublin: A&A Farmar, 2005), 326–37.

Dalton, K., 'Progesterone, fluid, and electrolytes in premenstrual syndrome', *British Medical Journal*, 281, 6232 (5 July 1980), 61.

Dalton, K., 'Premenstrual syndrome', *British Journal of Psychiatry*, 137, 2 (1 August 1980), 199.

Dalton, K., 'Progesterone, fluid, and electrolytes in premenstrual syndrome', *British Medical Journal*, 281, 6246 (11 October 1980), 1008–9.

Davies, M.M., 'Reasons why', *Radio Times*, 23 June 1983.

Deevy, P., 'In the psychiatrist's lair', *Sunday Independent*, 10 September 1995.

Deitch, R., 'Commentary from Westminster', *Lancet*, 315, 8165 (23 February 1980), 433–4.

Deitch, R., 'Commentary from Westminster', *Lancet*, 315, 8169 (22 March 1980), 663–4.

Delaney, E., 'Where politics and culture collide', *Irish Times*, 30 March 2004.

Dickson, E.J., 'Hometown: Anthony Clare, Dublin', *The Times*, 14 October 1995.

Diski, J., 'Who's been sitting in my chair?', *Observer*, 9 August 1998.

Donaghy, K., 'Six nuns sue TV3 over rape claims', *Irish Independent*, 24 November 2000.

Donovan, P., 'Parkinson's sadness over daughter he has never seen', *Sunday Times*, 25 July 1993.

Double, D.B., 'Twenty years of the Critical Psychiatry Network', *British Journal of Psychiatry*, 214, 2 (1 February 2019), 61–2.

Dowling, B., 'An exercise in comedy: 1966–8', in F. Callanan (ed.), *The Literary and Historical Society, 1955–2005* (Dublin: A&A Farmar, 2005), 120–31.

Dudley Edwards, R., 'Obituary: Liam Hourican', *Independent*, 16 August 1993.

Dudley Edwards, R., 'Patrick Cosgrave – Tory rebel', in F. Callanan (ed.), *The Literary and Historical Society, 1955–2005* (Dublin: A&A Farmar, 2005), 87–9.

Dudley Edwards, R., 'It is the mischief and laughter that I'll miss most about Tony', *Sunday Independent*, 4 November 2007.

Duggan, J., 'The humanist and abortion', *Irish Times*, 30 May 1970.

Dunn, P., 'Putting Dr Clare in the chair', *Sunday Times*, 12 September 1982.

Durrant, S., 'Clare in the chair', *Guardian*, 31 July 2000.

Earley, W., 'A natural resting place: 1968–70', in F. Callanan (ed.), *The Literary and Historical Society, 1955–2005* (Dublin: A&A Farmar, 2005), 137–47.

Ellis, A.T., 'Speaking their minds', *The Times*, 14 October 1995.

Epstein, M., *Advice Not Given: A Guide to Getting Over Yourself* (Carlsbad, CA: Hay House, 2018).

Erlichman, J., '"IQ" vitamin claims prompt inquiry', *Guardian*, 15 June 1988.

Expert Group on Mental Health Policy, *A Vision for Change* (Dublin: The Stationery Office, 2006).

Eysenck, H.J., 'Controversial Eysenck', *The Spectator*, 5 May 1973.

Falloon, I.R., 'Family interventions for mental disorders: efficacy and effectiveness', *World Psychiatry*, 2, 1 (February 2003), 20–8.

Faulks, S., 'It's my chair and I'll ask what I like', *The Independent*, 19 September 1992.

Fay, L., 'How the victim culture sparked man trouble', *Sunday Times*, 6 August 2000.

Ferguson, H., 'Why can't a man be more like a woman?', *Irish Times*, 12 August 2000.

Ferriman, A., '"Threat" of institutional psychiatry described at mental health meeting', *The Times*, 9 December 1977.

Ferriman, A., 'Aspirin "could prevent strokes"', *Observer*, 3 July 1988.

Ferriter, D., 'Men struggling to come to terms with post-feminist world', *Irish Times*, 18 November 2017.

Fitzgerald, M., 'Professor Anthony Clare', *Irish Journal of Psychological Medicine*, 24, 4 (1 December 2007), 161.

Foster, P., 'High-profile victims mourn their quiet but unyielding interrogator', *The Times*, 31 October 2007.

Foucault, M., *History of Madness* (London and New York: Routledge, 2006).

France, L., 'I was never good enough for my mother', *Daily Mail*, 22 July 1995.

Friedman, D., 'Myth or medicine?', *The Times*, 15 July 1985.

Friedman, H.J., 'Let's talk about male sex drive', *New York Times*, 3 December 2017.

Gaffney, M., 'The view from the chair', *Irish Times*, 26 September 1992.

Geoghegan, R., 'Joseph Veale, SJ', *Irish Times*, 4 November 2002.

Geoghegan, R., 'Remembering Joseph Veale', *Interfuse*, 114 (Christmas 2002), 4–9.

Geoghegan, R., 'John Charles McQuaid and the L&H', in F. Callanan (ed.), *The Literary and Historical Society, 1955–2005* (Dublin: A&A Farmar, 2005), 95–6.

Gibb, F., 'Society takes the Mickey', *The Times*, 26 October 1999.

Gledhill, R., 'Pope resists moves to soften encyclical', *The Times*, 18 September 1993.

Godwin, R., 'Men after #MeToo: "There's a narrative that masculinity is fundamentally toxic"', *The Guardian*, 10 March 2018.

Goldberg, D., *The Detection of Psychiatric Illness by Questionnaire (Maudsley Monograph No. 21)* (London: Oxford University Press, 1972).

Goldberg, D.P. and B. Blackwell, 'Psychiatric illness in general practice: a detailed study using a new method of case identification', *British Medical Journal*, 1, 5707 (23 May 1970), 439–43.

Goldie, L., 'The ethics of telling the patient', *Journal of Medical Ethics*, 8, 3 (September 1982), 128–33.

Goodwin, S., 'The health visitor and prevention', *British Medical Journal (Clinical Research Edition)*, 285, 6336 (17 July 1982), 182–3.

Goudsmit, E., 'Chronic fatigue syndrome', *Modern Medicine of Ireland*, 29, 7/8 (July/August 1999), 67–9.

Gray, D. and P. Watt, *Giving Victims a Voice: Joint Report into Sexual Allegations Made Against Jimmy Savile* (London: National Society for the Prevention of Cruelty to Children and the Metropolitan Police, 2013).

Griffey, H., 'Falling from a great Hite', *Guardian*, 23 September 1996.

Grove, V., 'Behind the psychiatrist's mask', *Sunday Times*, 14 August 1988.

Grove, V., 'Wedding bells ring again for Bayley at 74', *The Times*, 12 January 2000.

Guardian, 'Battles beyond the mind', *Guardian*, 22 April 1982.

Hackett, D., 'A model of self-possession', *The Times*, 26 July 1983.

Hanks, R., 'In the psychiatrist's easy chair', *The Independent*, 3 August 1992.

Hardcastle, E., 'Authoress Gitta Sereny ...', *Daily Mail*, 2 June 1998.

Hartston, W., 'The armchair confessions of an agony uncle', *The Independent*, 19 October 1992.

Haughey, C.J., 'Opening address', *Journal of the Irish Medical Association*, 72, 12 (suppl) (1979), 7–8.

Healy, D. and D. Cattell, 'Interface between authorship, industry and science in the domain of therapeutics', *British Journal of Psychiatry*, 183, 1 (1 July 2003), 22–7.

Heaney, S., *Field Work* (London: Faber & Faber, 1979).

Hebert, H., 'The end of the affair', *Guardian*, 10 November 1986.

Hegarty, T., 'Private patients may go to public sector if Noonan signs regulations', *Irish Times*, 30 June 1995.

Hendy, D., *Life On Air: A History of Radio Four* (Oxford: Oxford University Press, 2007).

Hepburn, J., 'Heard the one about radio's new comics?', *The Times*, 21 August 1993.

Hickling, M., 'Clare thoughts', *Yorkshire Post*, 22 October 1982.

Hildrew, 'Old hands on new body', *Guardian*, 28 February 1987.

Hind, J., 'I ask the questions (such as: how do you FEEL?)', *Mail on Sunday*, 8 October 1995.

Hislop, A., 'If at first you don't succeed', *The Times*, 20 October 1986.

Hogan, S., *History of Irish Steel* (Dublin: Gill and Macmillan Ltd., 1980).

Holmes, J., 'Ten books', *British Journal of Psychiatry*, 179, 5 (1 November 2001), 468–71.

Holmquist, K., 'Men in crisis – or is it just me?', *Irish Times*, 27 July 2000.

Holmquist, K., 'Where the sharpest pit their wits', *Irish Times*, 19 February 2010.

Hourican, L., 'Louis Courtney and Flann O'Connor take America by storm', in F. Callanan (ed.), *The Literary and Historical Society, 1955–2005* (Dublin: A&A Farmar, 2005), 90–2.

Hourican, P., 'The audience howled for blood', in F. Callanan (ed.), *The Literary and Historical Society, 1955–2005* (Dublin: A&A Farmar, 2005), 93–4.

Houston, M., 'Prof Anthony Clare dies unexpectedly in Paris', *Irish Times*, 30 October 2007.

Houston, M., 'Obituaries: Prof Anthony Clare: prolific psychiatrist and incisive interviewer', *Irish Times*, 3 November 2007.

Houston, M., 'Obituary: Anthony Ward Clare', *BMJ*, 335, 7628 (17 November 2007), 1050.

Hoyle, M., 'Curious character', *The Times*, 9 August 1983.

Hsieh, D.K. and S.A. Kirk, 'The effect of social context on psychiatrists' judgements of adolescent antisocial behaviour', *Journal of Child Psychology and Psychiatry*, 44, 6 (September 2003), 877–87.

Hussey, G., *At the Cutting Edge: Cabinet Diaries 1982–1987* (Dublin: Gill and Macmillan Ltd., 1990).

Hutton, W., 'So men are dying because they don't have women's brains. Show me the evidence', *The Observer*, 4 February 2018.

Ingle, R., 'Clare to step down from hot seat at St Patrick's', *Irish Times*, 24 August 1999.

Irish Times, 'Psychiatric care', *Irish Times*, 25 July 1995.

Irish Times Reporter, 'Stigma of mental illness persists here, says Clare', *Irish Times*, 15 September 1989.

Jamison, K.R., *Touched with Fire: Manic Depressive Illness and the Artistic Temperament* (New York, NY: Free Press, 1993).

Jamison, K.R., *Robert Lowell: Setting the River on Fire: A Study of Genius, Mania and Character* (New York: Alfred A. Knopf, 2017).

Jenner, F.A., 'Compulsory psychiatry', *Lancet*, 311, 8074 (27 May 1978), 1150.

Johnson, R., 'Somehow it's less frightening in full colour', *The Times*, 29 April 1995.

Johnston, M., 'Pioneer psychiatrist brought families in', *New Zealand Herald*, 21 July 2006.

Keane, C., 'Introduction', in C. Keane (ed.), *Mental Health in Ireland* (Dublin: Gill and Macmillan and Radio Telefís Éireann, 1991), 1–3.

Kelly, B.D., 'Men are so like gorillas', *Medicine Weekly*, 20 September 2000.

Kelly, B.D., *Hearing Voices: The History of Psychiatry in Ireland* (Dublin: Irish Academic Press, 2016).

Kelly, B.D., 'Homosexuality and Irish psychiatry: medicine, law and the changing face of Ireland', *Irish Journal of Psychological Medicine*, 34, 3 (September 2017), 209–15.

Kelly, B.D., 'Dr Dermot Walsh, 1931–2017', *Irish Journal of Psychological Medicine*, 34, 3 (September 2017), 217–20.

Kelly, B.D., 'Mental health services: where does Ireland stand internationally?', *Medical Independent*, 15 March 2018.

Kelly, B.D., P. Bracken, H. Cavendish, N. Crumlish, S. MacSuibhne, T. Szasz and T. Thornton, '*The Myth of Mental Illness* 50 years after publication: what does it mean today?', *Irish Journal of Psychological Medicine*, 27, 1 (March 2010), 35–43.

Kelly, B.D. and L. Feeney, 'Psychiatry: no longer in dissent?', *Psychiatric Bulletin*, 30, 9 (1 September 2006), 344–5.

Kelly, H., 'Move over McGonagall', in F. Callanan (ed.), *The Literary and Historical Society, 1955–2005* (Dublin: A&A Farmar, 2005), 132–6.

Kennedy, P., 'In the chair with Doctor Clare', *Daily Express*, 29 August 1988.

King, A., 'Agony in the office', *The Times*, 7 September 1988.

Kinlay, H., 'Sessions with the shrink', *Irish Times*, 21 August 1984.

Knott, B., 'Julie's returns', *Financial Times*, 19 October 2019.

Lancet, 'College capers', *Lancet*, 298, 7724 (11 September 1971), 587–8.

Lancet, 'ECT at Broadmoor', *Lancet*, 315, 8164 (16 February 1980), 348–9.

L., B.A., M.G.T.W. & T.D., 'Professor Anthony Clare: an appreciation of his contribution to psychiatry', *Irish Journal of Psychological Medicine*, 24, 4 (1 December 2007), 127–8.

Lavery, M., 'Keeper of the Clares', *Farmers Journal*, 25 November 2000.

Lawson, N., 'Great shrink show', *The Spectator*, 29 April 1995.

Le Fanu, J., 'The black dogs of melancholia', *The Times*, 21 January 1993.

Leahy, P., 'A good time for debating: 1990–2', in F. Callanan (ed.), *The Literary and Historical Society, 1955–2005* (Dublin: A&A Farmar, 2005), 279–87.

Levin, A., 'Swapping chairs with Clare', *You Magazine*, 27 September 1992.

Levin, B., 'Society's safety catch', *The Times*, 7 September 1987.

Levin, B., 'You analyse; I'd rather just listen', *The Times*, 3 April 1997.

Lewis, A., 'Foreword', in M. Shepherd, B. Cooper, A.C. Brown and G. Kalton (eds), *Psychiatric Illness in General Practice (Second Edition)* (Oxford: Oxford University Press, 1981), v–vi.

Lewis, P., 'What drives people to the top?', *Daily Mail*, 19 September 1995.

Lucey, J., 'Dr Anthony Clare remembered', *Irish Medical Times*, 16 November 2007.

Lynch, H., 'Men', *Sunday Times*, 6 August 2000.

Lysaght, C., 'First stirring of dissent, 1958–62', in F. Callanan (ed.), *The Literary and*

Historical Society, 1955–2005 (Dublin: A&A Farmar, 2005), 50–63.

Lysaght, C., 'Memories of the 1950s', in M. Bevan (ed.), *Gonzaga At Sixty: A Work in Progress* (Dublin: Messenger Publications, 2010), 46–55.

MacDermot, K., 'A mother's counsel for a harsh world', *Irish Independent*, 16 September 1995.

MacÉinrí, P., *Immigration into Ireland* (Cork: Irish Centre For Migration Studies, 2001).

MacNicholas, M., 'Seedy glamour: 1992–6', in F. Callanan (ed.), *The Literary and Historical Society, 1955–2005* (Dublin: A&A Farmar, 2005), 288–304.

Maguire, 'Morrissey: TV shrink was no charming man', *Sunday Times*, 20 October 2013.

Maher, M., 'Clare comes a long way from there to here', *Irish Times*, 12 December 1988.

Malcolm, E., *Swift's Hospital: A History of St Patrick's Hospital, Dublin, 1746–1989* (Dublin: Gill and Macmillan, 1989).

Maume, P., 'Clare, Anthony Ward', in J. McGuire and J. Quinn (eds), *Dictionary of Irish Biography From the Earliest Times to 2002* (Dublin and Cambridge: Royal Irish Academy and Cambridge University Press, 2014).

McCartney, D., 'The L&H – windbag factory for Ireland's gilded youth?', *Irish Independent*, 24 July 2005.

McDowell, M., 'Braving the cockpit of controversy', *Irish Times*, 12 March 2005.

McEnroe, J., 'Tributes for doctor who "demystified psychiatry"', *Irish Examiner*, 31 October 2007.

McGarry, P., 'Schizophrenia Ireland's "Lucia Day" highlights Joyce family's tragedy to heighten awareness of mental illness', *Irish Times*, 27 July 1998.

McGrath, P.G., 'ECT at Broadmoor', *Lancet*, 315, 8167 (8 March 1980), 550.

McKie, R., 'The chair man', *Observer*, 13 May 2001.

McPhail, T., 'Dr Clare praises wife's bravery', *Evening Standard*, 28 April 1993.

McTeirnan, A., 'Momentous occasion for future president', *Irish Times*, 31 January 1992.

Medical College of Saint Bartholomew's Hospital in the City of London, *Annual Report 1986* (London: University of London, 1986).

Medical Council Fitness to Practise Committee, *Re: Professor Ivor Browne. Inquiry Held at Portobello Court, Lower Rathmines Road, Dublin 6, on 16th–18th October, 1996* (Dublin: Medical Council, 1996).

Midgley, C., 'Questionmaster in the hot seat', *The Times*, 21 May 1997.

Miller, G., 'David Stafford-Clark (1916–1999): seeing through a celebrity psychiatrist', *Wellcome Open Research*, 2 (2017), 30.

Mishra, P., 'Not enough man: masculinity in crisis', *The Guardian*, 17 March 2018.

Monick, S. and O.E.F. Baker, 'Mega, February 1941: The role of the 1st South African Irish Regiment', *Scientia Militaria: South African Journal of Military Studies*, 20, 4 (1990), 27–53.

Morrell, D., 'Foreword', in P. Williams and A. Clare (eds), *Psychosocial Disorders in General Practice* (London and New York: Academic Press and Grune and Stratton, 1979), ix.

Morrissey, *Autobiography* (London: Penguin, 2013).

Munro, R., 'Judicial psychiatry in China and its political abuses', *Columbia Journal of Asian Law*, 14, 1 (Spring 2000), 1–125.

Murray, R.M., 'Obituary: Professor Anthony Clare', *Psychiatric Bulletin*, 32, 3 (1 March 2008), 118–19.

Neeleman, J. and A.H. Mann, 'Treatment of hysterical aphonia with hypnosis and prokaletic therapy', *British Journal of Psychiatry*, 163, 6 (December 1993), 816–19.

Neustatter, A., 'Mental disorder', *Guardian*, 5 May 1976.

Newby, D., 'Review: *Safety in Psychiatry: The Mind's Eye*', *Psychiatric Bulletin*, 26, 11 (November 2002), 439–40.

Nicholson, B., 'Revealing languages of love', *The Times*, 27 September 1986.

Nolan, P., 'Anthony Clare: A man of compassion', *Mental Health Practice*, 11, 5 (February 2008), 11.

Norell, J.S., 'Book review: *Psychiatry in Dissent: Controversial Issues in Thought and Practice (Second Edition)*', *Journal of the Royal College of General Practitioners*, 30, 220 (November 1980), 702.

Oliver, E., 'Mercy sisters to take action against TV3 over programme alleging abuse', *Irish Times*, 6 November 2000.

O'Brien, A., 'Did the mirth move for you? How it was for me', in F. Callanan (ed.), *The Literary and Historical Society, 1955–2005* (Dublin: A&A Farmar, 2005), 84–6.

O'Donoghue, D., 'Shrink rap', *RTÉ Guide*, 1 May 1999.

O'Morain, P., 'Psychiatrist warns patients face insurance cuts', *Irish Times*, 25 July 1995.

O'Toole, F., 'Medical body censured Browne but ruled he acted for patient', *Irish Times*, 11 January 1997.

O'Toole, F., 'How Medical Council decided to admonish Ivor Browne', *Irish Times*, 11 January 1997.

O'Toole, F., 'Public has right to know how doctors are regulated', *Irish Times*, 24 January 1997.

Ottaway, R., 'Highlights this week', *Radio Times*, 31 July – 6 August 1982.

Our Medical Reporter, 'GMC wants details of psychiatry training', *The Times*, 13 November 1971.

Pearce, E., 'Patrick Cosgrave: English-loving Irish journalist who blasted Edward Heath', *Guardian*, 17 September 2001.

Perera, S., 'Currie claims success for anti-drug campaign', *Guardian*, 30 October 1987.

Pereira Gray, D., 'Psychiatry and general practice (book review)', *Psychological Medicine*, 14, 1 (February 1984), 233–6.

Philbin Bowman, E., 'Clare's chair', *Irish Times*, 2 June 1984.

Phillips, L.D., 'Myth or medicine?', *The Times*, 15 July 1985.

Picard, A., 'Shrink wrapped in an enigma', *Sunday Telegraph*, 5 September 1999.

Picardie, J. and D. Wade, 'Closure call for women's jail wing', *Sunday Times*, 28 July 1985.

Pond, D.A., 'ECT at Broadmoor', *Lancet*, 315, 8165 (23 February 1980), 430.

Prentice, T., 'Doctors back lower drink-drive limit and random testing', *The Times*, 5 December 1987.

Prentice, T., 'Daily spending on mentally ill "only cost of a cup of tea"', *The Times*, 31 August 1991.

Proops, M., 'What's your problem with agony aunts like me?', *Daily Mirror*, 24 April 1995.

Purcell, D., 'Clare headed', *Sunday Tribune*, 11 January 1987.

Quinn, D., 'Men may be in a mess but women suffer too', *Sunday Times*, 23 July 2000.

Rayment, T. and K. Symon, 'Adams tells of his Protestant loves', *Sunday Times*, 6 August 1995.

Rayner, C., 'Foreword to this edition', in M. Slevin and N. Kfir, *Challenging Cancer: Fighting Back, Taking Control, Finding Options (Second Edition)* (London: Class Publishing, 2002), xi–xii.

Real, T., *How Can I Get Through to You? Closing the Intimacy Gap Between Men and Women* (New York: Fireside, 2002).

Rennison, N., 'On Men', *Sunday Times*, 10 June 2001.

Richmond, C. 'Obituary: Anthony Clare', *Guardian*, 31 October 2007.

Riddell, M., 'A grumpy psychiatrist in the chair', *The Times*, 5 August 1996.

Rissik, A., 'Men in the psychiatrist's chair', *Guardian*, 12 August 2000.

Rook, J., 'A shrink who cuts everyone down to size', *Daily Express*, 7 August 1991.

Roth, M., 'Obituary: Kenneth Rawnsley, CBE, formerly Professor of Psychiatry in the Welsh National School of Medicine and President of the Royal College of Psychiatrists', *Psychiatric Bulletin*, 16, 9 (September 1992), 587–9.

Rovelli, C., *The Order of Time* (London: Allen Lane/Penguin, 2018).

Rowan, I., 'Dr Clare gets a grilling', *Sunday Telegraph*, 14 August 1983.

Russell, G., 'Michael Shepherd (obituary)', *Psychiatric Bulletin*, 20, 10 (October 1996), 632–7.

Russell, G., 'Obituary: Mr Leslie Paine MA (Oxon), OBE, formerly House Governor of the Bethlem Royal and Maudsley Hospital (1963–1985)', *Psychiatric Bulletin*, 38, 5 (October 2013), 253–4.

S., M., 'Obituary: Frederick Kräupl Taylor', *Psychiatric Bulletin*, 13, 7 (July 1989), 394–5.

Sackett, D.L., W.M.C. Rosenberg, J.A. Gray, R.B. Haynes and W.S. Richardson, 'Evidence based medicine: what it is and what it isn't', *BMJ*, 312, 7023 (13 January 1996), 71–2.

Sacks, O., *An Anthropologist on Mars: Seven Paradoxical Tales* (New York: Alfred A. Knopf, 1995).

Sampson, G.A., 'Premenstrual syndrome: a double-blind controlled trial of progesterone and placebo', *British Journal of Psychiatry*, 135, 3 (1 September 1979), 209–15.

Sang, R., 'Letter to the editor', *Guardian*, 24 April 1982.

Sedgwick, P., 'Shrinking world', *Guardian*, 27 May 1976.

Sedgwick, P., *PsychoPolitics* (London: Pluto Press, 1982).

Shakespeare, N., 'Naughty but nicely done', *The Times*, 10 November 1986.

Shepherd, M., 'Aubrey Lewis 1900–1975', *American Journal of Psychiatry*, 132, 8 (August 1975), 872.

Shepherd, M., 'Foreword', in P. Williams and A. Clare (eds), *Psychosocial Disorders in General Practice* (London and New York: Academic Press and Grune and Stratton, 1979), vii–viii.

Shepherd, M., B. Cooper, A.C. Brown and G. Kalton (eds), *Psychiatric Illness in General*

Practice (Second Edition) (Oxford: Oxford University Press, 1981).

Shorter, E., *A History of Psychiatry: From the Era of the Asylum to the Age of Prozac* (New York: John Wiley & Sons, Inc., 1997).

Sibley, B., 'Compelling illusion', *The Times*, 2 July 1983.

Simpson, R., 'On a Clare day you can see for ever', *Daily Express*, 28 July 1992.

Sinnott, G., 'Hip hiatuses and a return to history: 1996–8', in F. Callanan (ed.), *The Literary and Historical Society, 1955–2005* (Dublin: A&A Farmar, 2005), 314–23.

Smyth, P., 'Drama and Life', in F. Callanan (ed.), *The Literary and Historical Society, 1955–2005* (Dublin: A&A Farmar, 2005), 342–3.

Snaith, R.P., 'The health visitor and prevention', *British Medical Journal (Clinical Research Edition)*, 285, 6340 (14 August 1982), 512.

Sontag, S., *Illness as Metaphor* (London: Allen Lane, 1979).

St Patrick's University Hospital, *Annual Report and Financial Statements 2009* (Dublin: St Patrick's University Hospital, 2010).

Stott, C., 'Relative values: shrink resistant', *Sunday Times*, 12 April 1992.

Study Group on the Development of the Psychiatric Services, *The Psychiatric Services – Planning for the Future* (Dublin: Stationery Office, 1984).

Syal, R., 'Absolutely furious: Lumley's sister demands apology for sanity slur', *Sunday Times*, 9 July 1995.

Szasz, T., 'The case against compulsory psychiatric interventions', *Lancet*, 311, 8072 (13 May 1978), 1035–6.

Szasz, T.S., *The Manufacture of Madness* (London: Routledge and Kegan Paul, 1972).

Tattler, 'Out to lunch', *Sunday Express*, 19 July 1992.

Taylor, J., 'Putting Anthony Clare in a psychiatrist's chair', *Daily Express*, 29 September 1995.

Taylor, L., 'Are you sitting uncomfortably? Then I'll begin …', *Mail on Sunday*, 5 June 1983.

Taylor, L., 'Curiouser and curiouser', *The Times*, 13 April 1984.

Taylor, L., 'New tunes from Joanna', *The Times*, 16 July 1994.

Taylor, N., 'Why I have lost faith in God', *The Times*, 1 August 2000.

Taylor, R.W., 'Book review: Psychiatric and social aspects of premenstrual complaint',

Psychological Medicine, 14, 3 (August 1984), 706–7.

Thomas, P. and P. Bracken, 'Critical psychiatry in practice', *Advances in Psychiatric Treatment*, 10, 5 (1 August 2004), 361–70.

Timmins, N., 'Depression in women "caused by poor life"', *The Times*, 29 November 1985.

Tirbutt, S., 'Bedtime is something our brains have dreamed up', *Guardian*, 28 January 1983.

Toynbee, P., 'The unequal partnership', *Guardian*, 22 September 1986.

Treneman, A., 'Ran's hand is twice its normal size. It is the hand of a witch', *The Times*, 14 March 2000.

Trethowan, W.H., 'Book review: *Psychiatry in Dissent*', *British Medical Journal*, 2, 6041 (16 October 1976), 948.

Turner, T., 'Henry Maudsley – psychiatrist, philosopher and entrepreneur', *Psychological Medicine*, 18, 3 (August 1988), 551–74.

Turner, T., 'Ten books', *British Journal of Psychiatry*, 209, 2 (1 August 2016), 175–7.

Twisk, R., 'Doctor, what's wrong here?', *Observer*, 5 August 1990.

Tyrer, P., 'From the Editor's Desk', *British Journal of Psychiatry*, 192, 1 (1 January 2008), 82.

Veitch, A., 'MIND adviser quits over law change', *Guardian*, 24 April 1982.

Verdoux, H. and J. van Os, 'Psychotic symptoms in non-clinical populations and the continuum of psychosis', *Schizophrenia Research*, 54, 1–2 (1 March 2002), 59–65.

Vincent, S., 'The elusive self', *Guardian*, 23 September 1995.

Wade, D., 'The public face of privacy', *The Times*, 14 August 1982.

Wade, D., 'Minds matter', *The Times*, 21 November 1988.

Wainwright, M., 'Touch of Venus beyond our Ken', *Guardian*, 26 September 1986.

Wallace, A., 'Ireland's greatest rugby legislator', *Irish Times*, 2 March 2018.

Wallace, M., R. Bluglass, F. Caldicott, A. Clare, M. Lader, C. Thompson, A. Tylee and M. Weller, 'Mental health propaganda', *Independent*, 13 June 1995.

Walsh, C., 'Loss of a vibrant voice', *Irish Times*, 3 November 2007.

Walsh, C., 'Remembering a great doctor and colleague', *Medicine Weekly*, 21 November 2007.

Walsh, D., 'Private health insurance', *Irish Times*, 2 August 1995.

Walsh, J., *The Globalist: Peter Sutherland – His Life and Legacy* (London: William Collins, 2019).

Webb, M., *Trinity's Psychiatrists: From Serenity of the Soul to Neuroscience* (Dublin: Trinity College, 2011).

Weekes, T., 'Sitting and waiting', in F. Callanan (ed.), *The Literary and Historical Society, 1955–2005* (Dublin: A&A Farmar, 2005), 46–7.

Weldon, F., 'In search of a new role', *Sunday Times*, 30 July 2000.

Wessely, S., 'Ten books', *British Journal of Psychiatry*, 181, 1 (1 July 2002), 81–4.

Wheatley, J., 'The face: A lonely road', *The Times*, 13 January 2006.

White, A., 'Compulsory psychiatry', *Lancet*, 311, 8074 (27 May 1978), 1150.

White, S.M., 'Preventive detention must be resisted by the medical profession', *Journal of Medical Ethics*, 28, 2 (April 2002), 95–8.

Whyms, P., 'Gentle speakers conquered: 1979–83', in F. Callanan (ed.), *The Literary and Historical Society, 1955–2005* (Dublin: A&A Farmar, 2005), 236–45.

Wilkinson, D.G., 'Compulsory psychiatry', *Lancet*, 311, 8074 (27 May 1978), 1150.

Wilkinson, G., 'Medicine and the media', *British Medical Journal*, 287, 6393 (3 September 1983), 683.

Williams, M., 'Laing's return?', *The Spectator*, 24 February 1973.

Wilson, T., 'Shall we swap livers?', *The Guardian*, 21 October 2000.

Wood, N., 'Parkinson dispute revived', *The Times*, 23 August 1986.

World Health Organization, *The ICD-9 Classification of Mental and Behavioral Disorders: Clinical Descriptions and Diagnostic Guidelines* (Geneva: World Health Organization, 1978).

World Health Organization, *ICD-10 Classification of Mental and Behavioural Disorders* (Geneva: World Health Organization, 1992).

Yorke, C., 'Analytical slips on Freudian analysis', *The Times*, 13 July 1985.

Young, D., 'Writer's mother libelled by BBC', *The Times*, 4 October 1990.

Young, G., 'Foreword', in A.W. Clare and M. Lader (eds), *Psychiatry and General Practice* (London: Academic Press, 1982), vii–x.

Young, R., 'Baby's kidnapper was convinced she gave birth to twins', *The Times*, 14 September 1993.

Younge, G., 'Nearly every mass killer is a man. We should all be talking more about that', *The Guardian*, 26 April 2018.

Index